Mathematical Modeling of Atherosclerosis, Cancer, and Diabetes

Diabetes, atherosclerosis, and cancer are the three diseases that contribute to most morbidity and mortality in the world. ***Mathematical Modeling of Atherosclerosis, Cancer, and Diabetes: Analysis and Simulation*** provides state-of-art mathematical models describing the dynamical behavior of these three diseases, focusing not only on numerical simulations but also on the mathematical analysis of the models themselves. Mathematical analysis in this context means rigorously studying some theoretical issues such as the 'well-posedness' of the models, steady solutions and their stability, and asymptotical behavior of the solutions.

The book is aimed at professional mathematical analysts, applied mathematicians, biophysicists, and biomedical engineers. The book can be used to teach graduate students, while it should be valuable reference for researchers in mathematical biology, dynamical systems, PDEs, and stochastic differential equations.

Features

- Collects the most recent research on both mathematical analysis and numerical simulation of mathematical models for diabetes, atherosclerosis, and cancer
- Includes both analysis and simulation of stochastic models for the diseases
- Provides a self-contained review of dynamical systems, partial differential equations, and stochastic differential equations
- Software code for readers who wish to practice data on any one of the existing models. The code is available in the programming languages of MATLAB® and/or Python.

Xuming Xie is Professor of Mathematics at Morgan State University in the U.S.A. He earned his BS and MS in Applied Mathematics at Huazhong (Central China) University of Science and Technology and his PhD in Mathematics at The Ohio State University. His research interests are in mathematical biology and free boundary problems arising from fluid mechanics and material sciences.

Chapman & Hall/CRC Mathematical Biology Series
Series Editors
Ruth Baker, Mark Broom, Adam Kleczkowski, Doron Levy, Sergei Petrovskiy

About the Series
This series aims to capture new developments in mathematical biology, as well as high quality work summarizing or contributing to more established topics. Publishing a broad range of textbooks, reference works, and handbooks, the series is designed to appeal to students, researchers, and professionals in mathematical biology.

We will consider proposals on all topics and applications within the field, including but not limited to stochastic modelling, differential equation modelling, dynamical systems, game theory, machine learning, data science, evolutionary biology, cell biology, oncology, epidemiology, ecology, and more.

An Introduction to Physical Oncology
How Mechanistic Mathematical Modeling Can Improve Cancer Therapy Outcomes
Vittorio Cristini, Eugene Koay, Zhihui Wang

Introduction to Mathematical Oncology
Yang Kuang, John D. Nagy, Steffen E. Eikenberry

Stochastic Dynamics for Systems Biology
Christian Mazza, Michel Benaim

Systems Biology
Mathematical Modeling and Model Analysis
Andreas Kremling

Cellular Potts Models
Multiscale Extensions and Biological Applications
Marco Scianna, Luigi Preziosi

Quantitative Biology
From Molecular to Cellular Systems
Edited By Michael E. Wall

Game-Theoretical Models in Biology, Second Edition
Mark Broom, Jan Rychtář

Mathematical Modeling in Biology
A Research Methods Approach
Shandelle M. Henson, James L. Hayward

Complex Population Dynamics
Theory and Data
Shandelle M. Henson, Robert A. Desharnais, J. M. Cushing, Brian Dennis, R. F. Costantino

Mathematical Modeling of Atherosclerosis, Cancer, and Diabetes
Analysis and Simulation
Xuming Xie

For more information about the series, visit: https://www.routledge.com/Chapman--HallCRC-Mathematical-Biology-Series/book-series/CRCMBS

Mathematical Modeling of Atherosclerosis, Cancer, and Diabetes

Analysis and Simulation

Xuming Xie

CRC Press
Taylor & Francis Group
Boca Raton London New York

CRC Press is an imprint of the
Taylor & Francis Group, an **informa** business
A CHAPMAN & HALL BOOK

Designed cover image: Janice Xie

First edition published 2026
by CRC Press
2385 NW Executive Center Drive, Suite 320, Boca Raton FL 33431

and by CRC Press
4 Park Square, Milton Park, Abingdon, Oxon, OX14 4RN

CRC Press is an imprint of Taylor & Francis Group, LLC

ISBN: 978-1-032-45320-0 (hbk)
ISBN: 978-1-032-45377-4 (pbk)
ISBN: 978-1-003-37667-5 (ebk)

DOI: 10.1201/9781003376675

Typeset in Latin Modern font
by KnowledgeWorks Global Ltd.

*Publisher's note:*This book has been prepared from camera-ready copy provided by the authors.

To my family
and in memory of my parents: Shuiying Li and
Shurong Xie

Contents

Preface

Atherosclerosis and cancer are two leading causes of death in many parts of the world, while nearly 463 million people worldwide have diabetes. Studies aimed at understanding these diseases need to be broad in scope and integrative in nature. As these diseases are medical conditions that affect critical organs and circulatory systems, studying human subjects poses logistical and ethical problems, as access to live tissue is limited and disturbances risk human lives. As a result, it is compelling to study these diseases by mathematical models which are biologically relevant and can be used to simulate pathway dynamics of the diseases. A mathematical modeling approach can provide many profits. Principally, it yields a platform for therapeutic hypothesis generation and for in silico drug target identification. The past five decades have seen huge growth in research on these diseases based on mathematical modeling in the literature. There are usually two types of research articles in the literature: the first type articles, which usually appear in medical journals and biomedical engineering journals, focus on mathematical modeling and numerical simulation; second type of articles, which appear in mathematical journals, focus on mathematical analysis. One of the aims in this book is to collect up-to-date mathematical models of these three diseases and perform both mathematical analysis and numerical simulation of these models. *Mathematical analysis* in this book means rigorously studying theoretical issues such as the well-posedness of the models, steady solutions and their stability, and asymptotical behavior of the solutions. Tools and techniques from the theories of dynamical systems, functional analysis, partial differential equations (PDE), and stochastic differential equations (SDE) will be employed. It is hoped that this book will be beneficial to both pure mathematicians and researchers in the fields of bioengineering, applied mathematics, and medicine.

Chapter One will cover mathematical models for diabetes, a disease where patients' cells cannot efficiently take in dietary sugar, causing it to build up in the blood. When insulin secretion by the pancreas is insufficient or absent, due to (autoimmune) destruction of β-cells, the clinical picture of Type 1 Diabetes Mellitus (T1DM) results; when insulin is secreted in normal or supernormal amounts but it is ineffective in lowering glycemia to normal levels, Type 2 Diabetes Mellitus (T2DM) is said to be present. As the first approximation, we model the glucose-insulin homeostasis in different scales. In a subcellular/cellular/organ, we will model insulin secretion and glucose-insulin oscillations. In an organ level, the modeling concerns the glucose-insulin dynamics after an external perturbation such as a glucose bolus injection (intravenous glucose tolerance test, IVGTT), an oral glucose consumption (oral glucose tolerance test, OGTT), or continuous glucose and insulin infusions like the Euglycemic Hyperinsulinemic Clamp (EHC), within a relatively short period of a few hours. Diabetes is a chronic condition that is the culmination of a series of gradual changes. There are several pathways to diabetes: insulin resistance and β-cell disfunction contribute to diabetes pathogenesis. Section 1.3 includes several long-term models that account for dynamics of β-cell mass, insulin, and glucose. We will cover mathematical analysis of the models in the form of delay differential equations and integro-differential equations. The last section of Chapter One will cover stochastic models for IVGTT and β-cell, insulin, and glucose kinetics using stochastic differential equations (SDE).

Chapter 2 will cover mathematical models for atherosclerosis. We will mostly focus on models that consist of partial differential equations (PDE) with a free boundary. Atherosclerosis is a condition where plaque builds up in the artery. It emerges because of multiple dynamical cell processes including hemodynamic, endothelial damage, innate immunity, and sterol biochemistry. One recognizes the critical role of low-density lipoprotein (LDL) and high-density lipoprotein (HDL) in determining whether a plaque, once formed, will grow or shrink. The simplified model in section 2.1 has only variables LDL, HDL, macrophage, and foam cells, and is tractable for rigorous analysis. A comprehensive model of more variables, representing different proteins and cells, is then given in section 2.2. Diabetes causes endothelial cell dysfunction due to inflammation and oxidative stress. In hyperglycemia, chronic inflammation increases vascular permeability, promotes the generation of adhesion molecules and chemokines, and stimulates accumulation of monocytes in the artery wall. Diabetic patients have an increased risk of cardiovascular disease (CVD) and have a more than twofold increase in the risk of dying from CVD. Very recent results in diabetic atherosclerosis are discussed in section 2.3. A compartment model is established in section 2.4, describing blood flow dynamics, hypertension risk, and LDL penetration from lumen to intima. A stochastic free boundary model in terms of partial differential equations (SPDE) is discussed in 2.5. To account for the uncertainty of parameters and free boundaries, the stochastic free boundary problem is proposed by incorporating the white noises into the PDEs for cells and the condition on the free boundary.

Chapter 3 discusses mathematical modeling of cancer and therapy. Cancer is a disease of tissue growth failure, and it is the result of normal cells transforming into cancer cells because of mutations in genes that regulate cell growth and differentiation. Cancer therapy is a broad area of research which may have three subfields: immunotherapy, gene therapy, and oncolytic virotherapy. Immunotherapy relies on the concept of stimulating the body's immune system to recognize and destroy cancer cells. Oncolytic viral therapy involves the use of oncolytic viruses, namely genetically modified viruses to selectively infect cancer cells and induce cell death through lysis and further propagation of the virus. In terms of modeling the tumor growth, we will focus on PDE free boundary models that involve tumor-immune interactions. Section 3.1 will include three models. Model One consists of only cancer cells, and Model Two consists of two cells. These two models are tractable for mathematical analysis. A more comprehensive model, containing more variables for different cells and cytokines, is also discussed. Section 3.2 covers cancer therapy that includes virotherapy and immunotherapy. Section 3.3 discusses stochastic models for virotherapy and immunotherapy. The stochastic models are established by incorporating environmental noise and stochastic effects into some basic deterministic model.

There are three appendices in the book. Appendix 1 reviews the theory of ordinary differential equations and dynamical systems. Appendix 2 reviews the theory of PDEs, and Appendix 3 reviews the theory of stochastic differential equations (SDEs and SPDEs).

Some existing books on mathematical biology have discussed cancer and atherosclerosis in terms of both analysis and simulation. What makes this book unique is that it includes both analysis and simulation of stochastic models for these diseases. Given the large number of inputs to the models, several sources of uncertainty exist. For example, uncertainty may come from clinical measurements, estimation of parameters, image-based geometries, biological properties, boundary conditions, choice of models, etc. Rigorously assessing the impact of uncertainty on simulation predictions must be considered a priority. Stochastic modeling and analysis now offer means to rigorously quantify confidence in the outputs from the models.

The book is aimed at graduate students, mathematical analysts, applied mathematicians, computational biologists, biomedical physicists, and engineers.

The author acknowledges the support from the Department of Mathematics at Morgan State University that granted the author a sabbatical leave. Several sections were written while the author was visiting the Department of Mathematics at Southern University of Science and Technology (SUSTech) in Shenzhen, China. Thanks go to Professor Qing Xiang of SUSTech for his invitation and hospitality. Some results in this book were presented in the School of Mathematics at Guangdong University of Education in Guangzhou, China. I thank Professor Yangming Li of Guangdong University of Education for his hospitality. Thanks go to Janice Xie for help with several figures in the book and Changhui Yang for help with LaTex typing.

Xuming Xie

CHAPTER 1

Mathematical Modeling of Diabetes

The glucose-insulin system is one of the clearest and simplest examples of homeostatic control in the organism. The level of glucose in the blood needs to be kept within a narrow range. Since it represents the main metabolic substrate, or energy source, for brain tissue, abnormally low glucose concentrations give rise to anxiety, tremors, aggressiveness, obfuscation, coma and eventually death. On the other hand, excessive plasma glucose concentrations produce microvascular damages (notably in the retina and kidney) and neural damages, leading among others to blindness and chronic renal insufficiency. Essentially, a single hormone (insulin) is secreted by the β-cells of the pancreas in response to rising glucose concentrations (hyperglycemia). Insulin effects include increasing peripheral tissue glucose uptake (mainly by the muscle and fat tissues) and decreasing spontaneous glucose output by the liver. When insulin secretion by the pancreas is insufficient or absent, due to (autoimmune) destruction of β-cells, the clinical picture of type 1 diabetes mellitus (T1DM) results; when insulin is secreted in normal amount, but it is ineffective in lowering glycemia to normal levels, type 2 diabetes mellitus (T2DM) is said to be present. A number of hormones contribute to rescuing the organism from hypoglycemia (adrenalin, glucagon, growth hormone, cortisol); however, since in clinical practice the situation of interest is normally inappropriately high glycemia, concentrating attention on the response to hyperglycemia by insulin seems justified, at least as a first modeling approach. We may therefore consider, as a first approximation, a simplified system in which a single metabolite (glucose) is controlled by a single hormone (insulin). This system will have to maintain glycemia in the absence of food intake, and will have to suppress hyperglycemia rapidly after meals, without incurring in dangerous hypoglycemias. We see therefore that the glucose insulin system could be viewed, at least approximately, as a feedback control with a controller (the

DOI: 10.1201/9781003376675-1

pancreas) and multiple effectors (muscle, liver, fat tissue), but where the only state variables of interest are glycemia and insulinemia.

Mathematical models of diabetes [35, 93, 211] aim to (i) describe physiological glucose–insulin–counterregulatory dynamics, (ii) quantify disease progression (particularly type 2 diabetes, T2D), (iii) support glucose control systems (insulin pumps, closed-loop/artificial pancreas), and (iv) enable personalised decision support (digital twins, prediction and optimization). Models range from simple compartmental "minimal" models to detailed multi-compartment mechanistic simulators, stochastic/process models [225–227, 303], insulin therapy models [274, 275], and fully data-driven machine-learning models [271, 303]. Foundational minimal and meal models laid the groundwork for much later simulator and control design. Early modeling efforts focused on glucose–insulin feedback regulation at the systemic level, such as the classic Bergman minimal model [21, 22, 264], while later studies expanded toward β-cell electrophysiology, intracellular calcium oscillations, pulsatile insulin release, and whole-body dynamics across multiple organs. Recent advances—ranging from multiscale modeling, stochastic control, and machine learning (ML) to digital twins—aim to enable precision medicine and fully automated diabetes management [129, 143, 173].

1.1 MINIMAL MODELS

The early linear models of the glucose–insulin homeostasis, which have been validated by means of an IVGTT, date back to Bolie [33] and the Ackerman's research group [2, 3, 130] in the sixties. However, the most famous and still greatly widespread model used in clinical assessments, such as the estimate of the insulin sensitivity index, is the so-called Minimal Model (MM), proposed by Bergman and collaborators in the late seventies [21,22,264]. For a historical review see [20, 23, 24].

1.1.1 Minimal Model for IVGTT

The IVGTT (Intra-Venous Glucose Tolerance Test) is a clinical experiment where a glucose bolus is rapidly injected intra-venously into a subject. Glucose and insulin samples are acquired in the following 3 h during which glycemia and insulinemia return to their basal values. The glucose injection is modeled as an instantaneous change in the plasma glucose concentration. In healthy subjects the glucose-induced pancreatic response of insulin release consists of two contributions: a first phase release, which is a quick response to a sudden change in glycemia, and a second phase release, which occurs some ten minutes after the bolus injection. The first phase is usually modeled as an instantaneous change in the plasma insulin concentration. The second phase is described by the model equations, and the difference among the many existing mathematical models are evaluated by their ability to capture the observed dynamics correctly. The models being studied are the minimal model and dynamical model, and models with time delays (DDE models). The minimal model follows early papers [21,22,264]. The minimal model (MM) is composed of two separate parts: one describing the dynamics of the glucose uptake after the external stimulus, regarding the insulin concentration as a known forcing function; the other describing the dynamics of the pancreatic insulin release in response to the glucose stimulus, with the glucose concentration regarded as a known forcing function. The second part of the MM concerns the insulin kinetics and consists of a single compartment model. The equations can be expressed in [92] as follows:

$$\frac{dG(t)}{dt} = -[p_1 + X(t)]G(t) + p_1 G_b, \quad G(0) = p_0 \tag{1.1}$$

$$\frac{dX(t)}{dt} = -p_2 X(t) + p_3[I(t) - I_b], \quad X(0) = 0 \tag{1.2}$$

$$\frac{dI(t)}{dt} = p_4[G(t) - p_5]^+ t - p_6[I(t) - I_b], \quad I(0) = p_7 + I_b, \tag{1.3}$$

where the parameters are as follows:
$G(t)$ [mg/dl] is the blood glucose concentration at time t [min];
$I(t)$ [μ UI/ml] is the blood insulin concentration;
$X(t)$ [min^{-1}] is an auxiliary function representing insulin-excitable tissue glucose uptake activity, proportional to insulin concentration in a "distant" compartment;
G_b [mg/dl] is the subject's baseline glycemia;
I_b [μ UI/ml] is the subject's baseline insulinemia;
p_0 [mg/dl] is the theoretical glycemia at time 0 after the instantaneous glucose bolus;
p_1 [min^{-1}] is the glucose "mass action" rate constant, i.e. the insulin-independent rate constant of tissue glucose uptake, "glucose effectiveness";
p_2 [min^{-1}] is the rate constant expressing the spontaneous decrease of tissue glucose uptake ability;
p_3 [min^{-2}] (μ UI/ml)$^{-1}$] is the insulin-dependent increase in tissue glucose uptake ability, per unit of insulin concentration excess over baseline insulin;
p_4 [(μ UI/ml) (mg/dl)$^{-1}$ min^{-1}] is the rate of pancreatic release of insulin after the bolus, per minute and per mg/dl of glucose concentration above the "target" glycemia;
p_5 [mg/dl] is the pancreatic "target glycemia";
p_6 [min^{-1}] is the first order decay rate constant for insulin in plasma;
p_7 [μUI/ml] is the theoretical plasma insulin concentration at time 0, above basal insulinemia, immediately after the glucose bolus.

1.1.2 Mathematical Analysis and Simulation of IVGTT Minimal Models

In this section we wish to provide a mathematical analysis of the minimal model stated in section 1.1.1. Some proofs were given in [92, 202].

Lemma 1.1 *If $(G(t), X(t), I(t)) \in C^1[0,\infty)$ is a solution of system (1.1) (1.2) and (1.3), $I(0) > I_b$, then $I(t) > I_b, X(t) \geq 0, 0 \leq G(t) \leq G_b + [G(0) - G_b]e^{-p_1 t}$, for all $t \geq 0$. In particular, if $G(T) \leq G_b$ for some $T \geq 0$, then $G(t) \leq G_b$ for all $t \geq T$.*

Proof. Rewrite equation (1.3) as

$$\frac{d}{dt}(I - I_b) + p_6[I(t) - I_b] \quad = \quad p_4[G(t) - p_5]^+ t.$$

Using integrating factor, we obtain

$$I(t) = I_b + p_7 e^{-p_6 t} + \int_0^t e^{p_6(s-t)}[p_4(G(s) - p_5)^+ s]ds, \tag{1.4}$$

which leads to $I(t) \geq I_b$. Solving for $X(t)$ from (1.2), we obtain

$$X(t) = p_3 \int_0^t e^{p_2(s-t)}(I(s) - I_b)ds, \tag{1.5}$$

which leads to $X(t) \geq 0$. Solving for $G(t)$ from (1.1) on $[T, t]$, we obtain

$$G(t) = G(T)e^{-\int_T^t [p_1 + X(s)]ds} + p_1 G_b \int_T^t e^{-\int_s^t [p_1 + X(\tau)]d\tau} ds, \tag{1.6}$$

which leads to the lemma using $X(t) \geq 0$. ■

Theorem 1.2 *If $I(0) \geq I_b$, then there exists a unique solution $(G(t), X(t), I(t)) \in C^1[0,\infty)$ to the system of (1.1), (1.2) and (1.3).*

Proof. From the classical local existence theorem, there exists a solution $(G(t), X(t), I(t)) \in C^1[0, T]$ for some $T > 0$, the solution interval $[0, T]$ can be extended indefinitely as long as $G(t), I(t)$ and $X(t)$ are bounded at any finite time. which we are going to show by deriving some estimates.
From (1.6) we can see

$$G(t) \leq G_b + G(0), \text{ for all } t > 0. \tag{1.7}$$

(1.7) and (1.4) imply that

$$I(t) \leq I_b + p_7 + \frac{[G_b + G(0) - p_5]^+ t}{p_6} \text{ for all } t > 0. \tag{1.8}$$

Using (1.8) and (1.5), we have

$$X(t) \leq p_3 p_7 + \frac{p_3[G_b + G(0) - p_5]^+ t^2}{p_6} \text{ for all } t > 0. \tag{1.9}$$

(1.7), (1.8) and (1.9) show that the solution does not blow up in finite time. so the global solution exists. ■

Lemma 1.3 *Suppose* $G_b > p_5, \limsup_{t\to\infty} G(t) > p_5$. *Then* $\limsup_{t\to\infty} X(t) = \infty$.

Proof. The idea to prove this statement will be to use the solution of $I(t)$ and substitute that into the $\frac{dX}{dt}$ equation to show $\limsup_{t\to\infty} X(t) = \infty$. So substituting (1.4) into the $X(t)$ equation from lemma, we have

$$\begin{aligned}
X(t) &= p_3 \int_0^t e^{-p_2(t-u)} \left[p_7 e^{-p_6 t} + \int_0^u e^{-p_6(u-s)} [p_4(G(s)-p_5)^+ s] ds \right] du \\
&= p_3 p_7 e^{-p_6 t} \left(\frac{1}{p_2} - e^{-p_2 t} \right) \\
&\quad + p_3 p_4 \int_0^t \left[e^{-p_2(t-u)} \int_0^u e^{-p_6(u-s)} [(G(s)-p_5)^+ s] ds \right] du \\
&= p_3 p_7 e^{-p_6 t} \left(\frac{1}{p_2} - e^{-p_2 t} \right) \\
&\quad + p_3 p_4 \int_0^t \left[\int_s^t e^{-p_2(t-u)} e^{-p_6(u-s)} [(G(s)-p_5)^+ s] du \right] ds \\
&= p_3 p_7 e^{-p_6 t} \left(\frac{1}{p_2} - e^{-p_2 t} \right) \\
&\quad + p_3 p_4 \int_0^t e^{(-p_2 t + p_6 s)} [(G(s)-p_5)^+ s] \left[\int_s^t e^{(p_2-p_6)u} du \right] ds.
\end{aligned}$$

From here we can look at two cases for $X(t)$. Case 1 being $p_2 = p_6$ and the other $p_2 \neq p_6$. Suppose Case 1 is true. Then we have

$$X(t) = p_3 p_7 e^{-p_6 t} \left(\frac{1}{p_2} - e^{-p_2 t} \right) + p_3 p_4 \int_0^t e^{(-p_2 t + p_6 s)} [(G(s)-p_5)^+ s](t-s) ds.$$

From here we can see that the integral will approach infinity due to the t variable multiple introduced after completing the first integration, and also the fact that each term within the integral is positive as well. Thus for case 1 $\limsup_{t\to\infty} X(t) = \infty$. Now suppose case 2 where $p_2 \neq p_6$. Then we have

$$X(t) = p_3 p_7 e^{-p_6 t} \left(\frac{1}{p_2} - e^{-p_2 t} \right) + p_3 p_4 \int_0^t \frac{e^{-p_6(t-s)} - e^{-p_2(t-s)}}{p_2 - p_6} [(G(s)-p_5)^+ s] ds.$$

Now by assumption we know $G_b > p_5$ and $\limsup_{t\to\infty} G(t) > p_5$. Thus we know $\exists t_n \in \mathbb{R}$ such that as $t_n \to \infty, \exists h > 0$ and $T > 0$ where $\forall n \in \mathbb{N}, G(s) \geq p_5 + h$ for $t_n \leq s \leq t_n + T$. So for $t_n \leq s \leq t_n + T$, we have

$$X(t_n + T) \geq X(t_n + T) - X(t_n) \geq p_3 p_4 h t_n \int_0^t \frac{e^{-p_6(t-s)} - e^{-p_2(t-s)}}{p_2 - p_6} ds.$$

Lastly we know $X(t_n) \to \infty$ as $t_n \to \infty$. Therefore $\limsup_{t\to\infty} X(t) = \infty$. ∎

Lemma 1.4 *If* $\limsup_{t\to\infty} G(t) < p_5$, *then* $G_b \le p_5$.

Proof. Suppose $G(t) < p_5$ and $G_b > p_5$. Then we have $\frac{dI}{dt} = -p_6[I(t) - I_b]$ since $(G(t) - p_5)^+ = 0$. Solving for $I(t)$ we get $I(t) = p_7 e^{-p_6 t} + I_b$. Thus as $t \to \infty, I \to I_b$. Since $I \to I_b$ that implies $\frac{dX}{dt} = -p_2 X(t) \Rightarrow X(t) = 0$ by (1.2). If $X(t) = 0$, then $\frac{dG}{dt} = -p_1 G(t) + p_1 G_b \Rightarrow G(t) = (G_b - p_0)e^{-p_1 t} + G_b \Rightarrow G(t) \to G_b$ as $t \to \infty$ which is a contradiction. ■

Lemma 1.5 *If* $p_5 < G_b$, *then the system does not permit an equilibrium.*

Proof. Suppose the system has an equilibrium. Let $\frac{dX}{dt} = \frac{dI}{dt} = \frac{dG}{dt} = 0$. The only possible equilibrium point solving such system would be $(G_b, 0, I_b)$. If this is the case then by equation (1.1), $\frac{dI(t)}{dt} = p_4[G(t) - p_5]^+ t - p_6[I(t) - I_b]$. Thus when $p_5 < G_b$, and the equilibrium point $(G_b, 0, I_b)$ is substituted, we have $\frac{dI(t)}{dt} = p_4[G_b - p_5]^+ t > 0$ which is a contradiction since $\frac{dI}{dt} = 0$. ■

Lemma 1.6 *If* $G_b \le p_5$, *then the equilibrium point provided by the system will be asymptotically stable.*

Proof. Suppose $G_b < p_5$. From (1.1) to (1.3) we see that a equilibrium point is $(G_b, 0, I_b)$. From this then we have the following using equation (1.3) and lemma 1.1.

$$\frac{dI}{dt} \ge -p_6(I(t) - I_b) \Rightarrow \liminf_{t\to\infty} I(t) \ge I_b \Rightarrow \liminf_{t\to\infty} X(t) \ge 0.$$

We also have the following from equation (1.1) and lemma 1.3 for $\epsilon > 0$ sufficiently small

$$\frac{dG}{dt} \le -(p_1 - \epsilon)G(t) + p_1 G_b; t \ge T \Rightarrow \limsup_{t\to\infty} G(t) \le G_b.$$

Therefore we know

$$\exists T \text{ such that } t \ge T \Rightarrow G(t) \le G_b + \epsilon < p_5 \Rightarrow \frac{dI}{dt} = -p_6(I(t) - I_b)$$

which implies that $I(t) \to I_b, X(t) \to 0, G(t) \to G_b$. ■

We give numerical simulation of the IVGTT minimal model in Figures 1.1 and 1.2. We used values stated in [22] for parameters p_1, p_2, p_3, I_b and G_b values specified in [92], and parameters stated in [264] for p_4, p_5, p_6. Parameters p_0 and p_7 are theoretical; therefore, we chose values ourselves to illustrate the aforementioned results.

1.1.3 OGTT Model

In the OGTT (Oral Glucose Tolerance Test), plasma glucose and insulin concentrations are measured at time 0, 30, 60, 90, and 120 min, following an oral

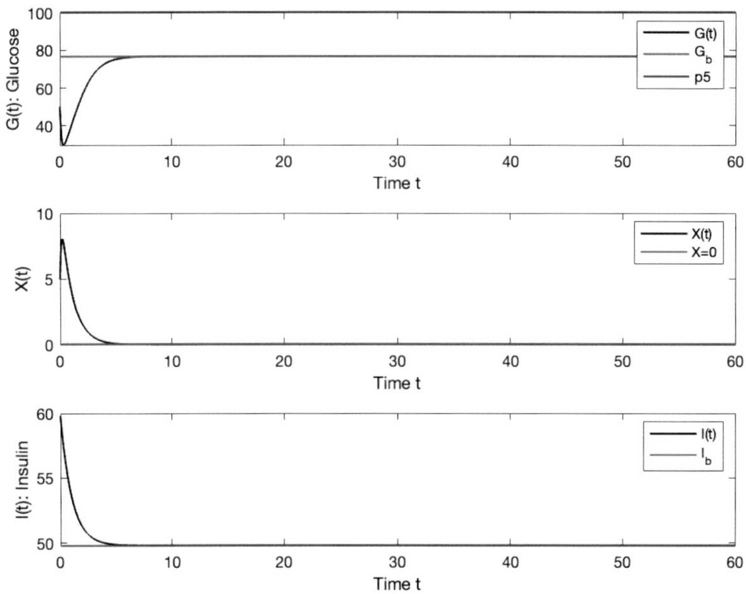

Figure 1.1 Here we have solution curve for $G(t)$, $X(t)$, and $I(t)$. These graphs were produced numerically by MATLAB with parameters $p_0 = 140, p_1 = 4.9, p_2 = 9.1, p_3 = 8.96, p_4 = .038, p_5 = 100, p_6 = .99, p_7 = 10, G_b = 50, I_b = 49.8$. These graphs here show us how the system does reach equilibrium $(G_b, 0, I_b)$ in the case where $G_b < p_5$.

glucose load of 75 g. C-peptide must also be measured to compute indexes of the insulin secretion. The OGTT is a simple clinical test currently used to aid diagnosis of glucose intolerance and T2DM.

Mathematical models for the Oral Glucose Tolerance Test (OGTT) play a crucial role in understanding glucose metabolism dynamics, predicting outcomes, and optimizing diagnostic and therapeutic strategies. Various mathematical models have been used in the context of OGTT. The OGTT minimal model [54, 88, 197] extends to the oral test the basic model proposed for the IVGTT, with the modification that glucose administration does no longer appear as a bolus dose in the initial condition of the equation for glucose kinetics, but as an input function that specifies the rate of appearance of oral glucose in plasma. The OGTT minimal model has also been used in conjunction with models of C-peptide secretion [14, 37, 69, 70, 198, 206, 207, 222] and models that include the effect of incretins [38].

The OGTT mimics the physiological conditions of the glucose-insulin system more closely than the IVGTT. However, the analysis of the OGTT data

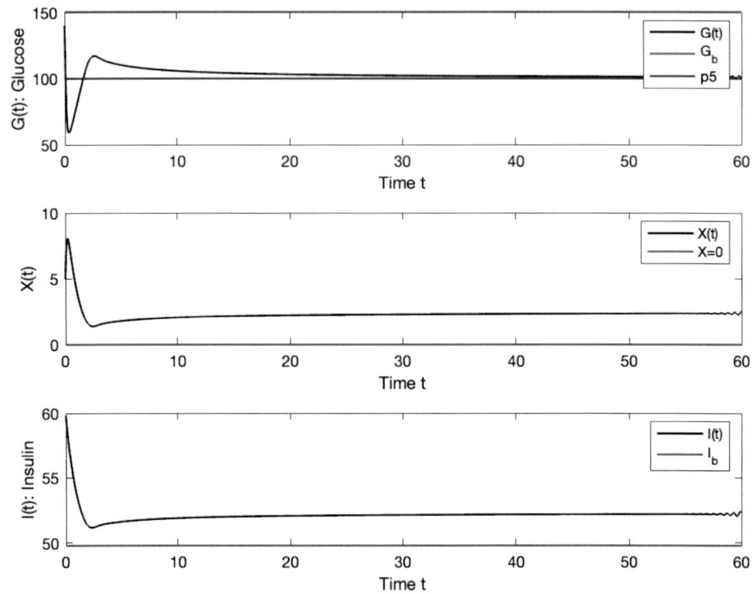

Figure 1.2 Here we have solution curves for $G(t), X(t)$, and $I(t)$. These graphs were produced numerically by MATLAB with parameters $p_0 = 140, p_1 = 4.9, p_2 = 9.1, p_3 = 8.96, p_4 = .038, p_5 = 100, p_6 = .99, p_7 = 10, G_b = 150, I_b = 49.8$. These graphs here show us how the system does not reach equilibrium in the case where $G_b > p_5$.

by a mathematical model is affected by the complication that the time course of the delivery to plasma of exogenous glucose and even the total amount of glucose delivered are unknown. In fact, the rate of appearance, Ra, of exogenous glucose in plasma is influenced by several factors: the rate of gastric emptying of ingested glucose, the extent of absorption during the intestinal transit, glucose amount used by the gut as an energy substrate, and hepatic uptake. Moreover, gut-derived hormones, secreted in response to glucose delivery to the small intestine, markedly increase the insulin secretion with respect to that observed after an intravenous glucose infusion that produces the same elevation of plasma glucose (incretin effect).

More recent models [140–142] retains a glucose-insulin feedback loop of the minimal model, but also include insulin secretion by β cells, the effect of ATP-sensitive K (KATP) channel density to shift the glucose dependence of secretion and insulin granule exocytosis. Here we present the model proposed in [141]. The variables of the model are shown in Table 1.1.

TABLE 1.1 Variables and units

Variables	Units	Description
G	mg/dl	plasma glucose concentration
I	$\mu U/ml$	plasma insulin concentration
γ	$(unitless)$	dose-response curve shift
σ	$\mu U/\mu g \cdot d$	β-cell function
β	mg	β cell mass
S_I	$ml/\mu U \cdot d$	insulin sensitivity
t	d	time

The core element is a glucose-insulin feedback loop, represented by two differential equations adapted from the minimal model:

$$\frac{dG(t)}{dt} = OGTT(t) - (E_{G0} + S_I I(t))G(t) \tag{1.10}$$

$$\frac{dI(t)}{dt} = \left(\frac{\beta}{V} ISR(\sigma, G) - kI(t)\right) \tag{1.11}$$

The glucose (G) equation (Eq. 1.10) says that G increases on a timescale of hours as a result of meal influx and hepatic glucose production (HGP) decreases as a result of uptake, which has both insulin-independent (E_{G0}) and insulin-dependent components. The factor S_I in the insulin-dependent term is closely related to the well-known sensitivity to insulin reported by the minimal model. The insulin (I) equation (Eq. 1.11) says that I decreases because of removal, mainly in the liver, with rate constant k, and increases because of secretion by beta-cells, where β is the beta-cell mass, ISR is the insulin secretion rate per unit mass, and V is the volume of distribution. ISR depended only on G, through the rate of beta-cell metabolism M:

$$ISR = \sigma \frac{(M + \gamma)^{kISR}}{\alpha_{ISR}^{kISR} + (M + \gamma)^{kISR}} \tag{1.12}$$

where M was assumed to be a sigmoidally increasing function of G:

$$M = \frac{G^{kM}}{\alpha_M^{kM} + G^{kM}} \tag{1.13}$$

The parameter γ in Eq. 1.12 represents the effect of ATP-sensitive K (KATP) channel density to shift the glucose dependence of secretion; when the channel density is low, γ is high and shifts the dependence to the left, increasing secretion for the same level of M because Ca^{2+} is higher. This can be viewed as the first line of defense through enhanced beta-cell function against insulin resistance over a timescale of days (e.g., holiday overeating).

The value of depends on glucose, which is taken into account by adding a third differential equation to the system:

$$\frac{d\gamma(t)}{dt} = \frac{\gamma_\infty(G) - \gamma}{\tau_\gamma} \tag{1.14}$$

where γ_∞ is an increasing sigmoidal function of G and τ_γ is the time constant.

Insulin resistance that persists over longer periods (months in humans) despite reduced KATP channel density is assumed to trigger a further level of compensatory increased beta-cell function via, the maximal insulin secretion capacity (Eq. 1.12). This corresponds to the amplifying effects of metabolism and/or modulators such as glucagon-like peptide 1 (GLP-1) and ACh (Acetylcholine) on the efficacy of Ca^{2+} to drive insulin granule exocytosis. This second aspect of beta-cell functional compensation entails a fourth differential equation:

$$\frac{d\sigma(t)}{dt} = \frac{\sigma_\infty(ISR, M) - \sigma}{\tau_\sigma} \tag{1.15}$$

We assume that increased ISR leads to an increase in σ whereas increased M leads to a decrease in γ.

The slowest and final form of compensation for insulin resistance is increased beta-cell mass, β, which develops over years in humans. We assume that β is increased by proliferation, P, and decreased by apoptosis, A. We assume that P increases when ISR increases. We further assume that apoptosis is largely driven by metabolic stress (e.g., through increased production of reactive oxygen species) when glucose is high, so we make A an increasing function of M:

$$\frac{d\beta(t)}{dt} = \frac{(P(ISR) - A(M))\beta}{\tau_\beta} \tag{1.16}$$

The parameters defining P and A are chosen such that modest increases in G result in a net increase in β but large increases in G result in a net decrease in β. This leads to a shift from compensation (negative feedback) to decompensation (positive feedback). It can be shown that this can account for the threshold behavior observed in both rodents and humans, that is, nearly steady G followed by a sharp, essentially irreversible increase. We proposed this as an explanation for why prevention of T2D is much easier than reversing it once it is established.

The auxiliary functions in equations (1.10)–(1.16) are described in Table 1.2.

The OGTT flux in (1.10) is modeled by a piecewise linear function similar to [88]. Specifically, the term $OGTT(t)$ is defined as follows:

$$\begin{aligned} OGTT &= \frac{1}{V_G}\left(a_{i-1} + \frac{a_i - a_{i-1}}{t_i - t_{i-1}}(t - t_{i-1})\right), t_{i-1} < t < t_i, i = 1, 2, 3; \\ OGTT &= 0 \text{ elsewhere;} \end{aligned} \tag{1.17}$$

TABLE 1.2 Auxiliary functions (unitless) descriptions

Name	Equation	Description
$M(G)$	1.13	metabolic rate
$ISR(M, \gamma, \sigma)$	1.12	Insulin secretion rate
γ_∞	1.14	Steady state dose-response shift
$\sigma_\infty(ISR, M)$	1.15	Steady state for beta-cell function
$P(ISR)$	1.16	Proliferation rate
$A(M)$	1.16	Apoptosis rate
$\sigma_{ISR\infty}(ISR)$	1.19	ISR component of σ_∞
$\sigma_{M\infty}(M)$	1.19	M component of σ_∞

where $V_G = BW \times \bar{V}$ is the volume of distribution for glucose in dL, BW is body weight in kg, $\bar{V} = 1.569dL/kg$. The parameters are designed assuming BW = 75kg, for a volume of distribution of 11.77 L, but this formulation makes the glucose load 75g independent of those choices. The values for a_i are given in Table 1.3.

The function γ_∞ in (1.14) is given by

$$\gamma_\infty(G) = \frac{\gamma_{max}}{(1 + \exp((G - \gamma_s)/\gamma_n)} - \gamma_0 \tag{1.18}$$

The function σ_∞ in (1.15) is

$$\sigma_\infty(ISR, M) = \sigma_{ISR\infty}(ISR)\sigma_{M\infty}(M) + \sigma_b \tag{1.19}$$

$$\sigma_{ISR\infty}(ISR) = \frac{\sigma_{ISRmax}}{(1 + \sigma_{ISRk} \exp(-(IRS_\sigma - \sigma_{ISRs})/\sigma_{ISRs})} \tag{1.20}$$

$$\sigma_{M\infty}(M) = 1 - \frac{\sigma_{Mmax}}{(1 + \sigma_{Mk} \exp(-(M_\sigma - \sigma_{Ms})/\sigma_{Ms})} \tag{1.21}$$

where $ISR_\sigma = ISR(M_\sigma)$ and $M_\sigma = M(G - G_{\sigma s})$.

TABLE 1.3 Parameter of OGTT

Parameter	Value	Units	Description
a_0	0	mg/min	Glucose flux at t_0
a_1	588.4	mg/min	Glucose flux at t_1
a_2	353	mg/min	Glucose flux at t_2
a_3	0	mg/min	Glucose flux at t_3
t_0	0	min	Initial time of activation of glucose flux
t_1	15	min	First time of activation of glucose flux
t_2	120	min	Second time of activation of glucose flux
t_3	240	min	Third time of activation of glucose flux

TABLE 1.4 Parameter values in differential equations

Parameter	Value	Units	Description
E_{g0}	1.44	$1/d$	Insulin independent glucose disposal rate
S_0	0.23	$ml/\mu U \cdot d$	Initial insulin sensitivity when S_I is dynamic
V	0.01	l	Volume of distribution
k	700	$1/d$	Insulin clearance rate
τ_γ	2.14	d	Time constant of γ
τ_σ	10.71	d	Time constant of σ
τ_β	42.85	d	Time constant of β
τ_{S_I}	16.2	d	Time constant of S_I

The auxiliary functions in the β equation are

$$P(ISR) = P_{max} \frac{ISR^{kP}}{\alpha_P^{kP} + ISR^{kP}} \tag{1.22}$$

$$A(M) = A_{max} \frac{M^{kA}}{\alpha_A^{kA} + M^{kA}} \tag{1.23}$$

$$\frac{dS_I}{dt} = \frac{S_0 - S}{\tau_{S_I}} \tag{1.24}$$

The parameters values for differential equations are shown in Table 1.4. The parameter values in auxiliary functions are shown in Table 1.5.

1.2 INSULIN SECRETION AND OSCILLATIONS

Mathematical modeling of glucose-stimulated pancreatic insulin secretion is a challenging research topic that has involved much work in the last decades. Among the first references, we find the pioneering work of Grodsky [137], who first distinguished a first phase of insulin release, due to the insulin packets immediately releasable as a consequence of a rapid increase in glycemia, from the second phase related to the potentiation effect that occurs during a sustained glucose stimulation.

In the last few decades, many models have been proposed detailing the occurrence of several modes of oscillation of the glucose–insulin system. These models [29, 30, 212, 219–221, 236, 237, 268] have attempted to construct a theoretical description of the mechanisms responsible for this behavior, considering also whether some external (neural) influence is actually needed to coordinate pancreatic islet activity in order to generate macroscopically evident oscillations. What is usually found experimentally are high-frequency pulsatile variations of glycemia and insulinemia with a power spectrum occupying the 5–15 min interval and low-frequency spontaneous oscillations (known as ultradian oscillations in the literature), with a period of approximately 50–150

TABLE 1.5 Parameter values in auxiliary functions

Parameter	Value	Units (unitless if blank)	Description
kM	2		Exponent of metabolic rate M
α_M	150	mg/dl	Half maximum G value for M
$kISR$	2		Exponent of insulin secretion rate
α_{ISR}	1.2		Half maximum M value for ISR
P_{max}	4.55	$1/d$	Maximum proliferation rate
kP	4		Exponent of proliferation rate
α_P	41.77		Half maximum value of ISR for proliferation
A_{max}	3.11	$1/d$	Maximum apoptosis rate
kA	6		Exponent of apoptosis rate
α_A	0.44		Half maximum M value for apoptosis
A_b	0.8	$1/d$	Basal apoptosis rate
γ_{max}	0.2		Maximum value of γ
γ_s	99.9		Horizontal shift of γ_∞
γ_n	1		Slope of γ_∞
γ_0	0.1		Baseline value of γ
σ_{ISRmax}	867.6	$\mu U/\mu g \cdot d$	Maximum value of $\sigma_{ISR\infty}$
σ_{ISRs}	0.1		Horizontal shift of $\sigma_{ISR\infty}$
σ_{ISRn}	0.1		Slope of $\sigma_{ISR\infty}$
σ_{ISRk}	1		Weight of of $\sigma_{ISR\infty}$ exponential
σ_b	3	$\mu U/\mu g \cdot d$	Baseline value of σ
σ_{Mmax}	1		Scale factor of $\sigma_{M\infty}$
σ_{Ms}	0.2		Horizontal shift of $\sigma_{M\infty}$
σ_{Mn}	0.02		Slope of $\sigma_{M\infty}$
σ_{Mk}	0.2		Weight of of $\sigma_{M\infty}$ exponential

min, with their amplitude enhanced upon exogenous glucose administration, from meals, continuous enteral nutrition, or constant intravenous infusions. The models in the literature usually deal with pulsatile insulin secretion as the apparent occurrence, at the level of the portal vein, of a series of partially overlapping insulin pulses, whose period ranges from 5 to 15 min. In fact, at the level of a single beta-cell, insulin is released as discrete granules, leading to the characteristic behavior known as bursting, whose period from spike to spike takes tens of seconds (see [219] and references therein). These simple bursts cluster in compound bursts, with a period of several minutes [9] and intra-islet synchronization leads to consider these compound bursts as produced at the level of a "homogeneous secretory unit". Compound bursting has been supposed to be responsible for overall insulin pulsatility [29]. A group of mathematical models attempts to include, in as much detail as possible, known biochemical mechanisms operating at the beta-cell level. These models entail different biochemical assessments combining electrical and calcium dynamics with the glycolitic oscillator [29, 30] managing to describe the synchronization of intra/inter-islets b-cells and providing the oscillatory response of insulin secretion [219, 268].

The models [31, 63] for insulin granule trafficking reported in this section take place over a fine biological scale, detailing the subcellular mechanism (the insulin granule dynamics) that eventually determines insulin release from the β-cell.

1.2.1 Bursting and Hopf Bifurcation

Pancreatic β-cells are located in cell clusters within the pancreas called the islets of Langerhans. These micro-organs monitor the glucose concentration in the blood and secrete the hormone insulin in response to elevated glucose levels. Since insulin is necessary for the uptake of glucose by other cells in the body, the proper functioning of β-cells is crucial for glucose homeostasis. Malfunctioning β-cells can lead to type II diabetes. Both the average level and temporal pattern of insulin secretion are important for proper glucose homeostasis. In vitro and in vivo data show that insulin secretion is oscillatory with period of several minutes, and in vitro these oscillations have been shown to be in-phase with oscillations in the free cytosolic Ca^{2+} concentration. It has been established in both single β-cells and intact islets that these Ca^{2+} oscillations reflect a bursting pattern in the β-cell electrical activity, which consists of periodic active phases of cell firing followed by silent phases of hyperpolarization. Early mathematical models of β-cells were constructed to describe medium bursting, the type first and most often observed in islets. The first Hodgkin-Huxley type model for β-cells was developed by Chay and Keizer (1983). A simple Chay-Keizer-like model with a single slow variable, the cytosolic Ca^{2+} concentration was introduced by Bertram and Sherman [30]. Because Ca^{2+} changes only moderately slowly this phantom bursting model produces fast bursting and is limited to a small range of burst frequencies. The basic model consists of a Ca^{2+} current, I_{Ca}, a delayed rectifier K^+ current, I_K, a Ca^{2+}-dependent K^+ current, $I_{K(Ca)}$, and a nucleotide- sensitive K^+ current, $I_{K(ATP)}$. In the basic model, the ratio ADP/ATP is constant, so the conductance $g_{K(ATP)}$ is also constant. The differential equations for membrane potential, V, delayed rectifier activation, n, and cytosolic free Ca^{2+}

concentration, c, are as follows:

$$\begin{aligned}\frac{dV}{dt} &= -\left[I_{\mathrm{Ca}} + I_{\mathrm{K}} + I_{\mathrm{K(Ca)}} + I_{\mathrm{K(ATP)}}\right]/C_m \\ \frac{dn}{dt} &= \left[n_\infty(V) - n\right]/\tau_n \\ \frac{dc}{dt} &= f_{\mathrm{cyt}}\, J_{\mathrm{mem}},\end{aligned} \tag{1.25}$$

where C_m is the membrane capacitance, τ_n is the activation time constant for the delayed rectifier channel, $n_\infty(V)$ is the steady state function for the activation variable n, and J_{mem} is the Ca^{2+} flux through the plasma membrane. Since c represents the free Ca^{2+} concentration, we multiply J_{mem} by the fraction of free to total Ca^{2+}, f_{cyt}. Expressions for the ionic currents are as follows:

$$\begin{aligned}I_{\mathrm{Ca}} &= g_{\mathrm{Ca}} m_\infty(V)\left(V - V_{\mathrm{Ca}}\right) \\ I_{\mathrm{K}} &= g_{\mathrm{K}} n\left(V - V_{\mathrm{K}}\right) \\ I_{\mathrm{K(Ca)}} &= g_{\mathrm{K(Ca)}}\omega\left(V - V_{\mathrm{K}}\right) \\ I_{\mathrm{K(ATP)}} &= g_{\mathrm{K(ATP)}}\left(V - V_{\mathrm{K}}\right).\end{aligned} \tag{1.26}$$

The conductance values and reversal potentials, along with other parameters, are listed in Table 1.6. The steady state activation functions have an increasing dependence on voltage and saturate at positive voltages:

$$\begin{aligned}m_\infty(V) &= \left[1 + e^{(v_m - V)/s_m}\right]^{-1} \\ n_\infty(V) &= \left[1 + e^{(v_n - V)/s_n}\right]^{-1}.\end{aligned} \tag{1.27}$$

Since the gating of the Ca^{2+} channel is much faster than the gating of the K^+ channels, we assume rapid equilibrium and incorporate $m_\infty(V)$ directly into I_{Ca}. The variable ω is the fraction of K(Ca) channels activated by cytosolic Ca^{2+}:

$$\omega = \frac{c^5}{c^5 + k_D^5}, \tag{1.28}$$

where k_D is the dissociation constant for Ca^{2+} binding to the channel. The value of the exponent is not critical, other values could be used. Finally, the flux of Ca^{2+} through the membrane is

$$J_{\mathrm{mem}} = -\left(\alpha I_{\mathrm{Ca}} + k_{\mathrm{PMCA}} c\right), \tag{1.29}$$

where α converts units of current to units of flux, and $k_{\mathrm{PMCA}}c$ is the flux through the plasma membrane Ca^{2+} ATPase pumps.

Fast/slow analysis of bursting. The behavior of the basic model is shown in Fig. 1.3. Bursts of action potentials are generated on top of depolarized plateaus, followed by membrane hyperpolarization. The burst period is 2 s

TABLE 1.6 Parameter values for the basic model

Parameter	Value	Parameter	Value
g_{Ca}	1200 pS	g_{K}	3000 pS
$g_{\text{K(Ca)}}$	300 pS	$g_{\text{K}}(\text{ATP})$	230 pS
V_{Ca}	25 mV	V_{K}	−75 mV
C_m	5300 fF	α	4.5×10^{-6} fA^{-1} μM ms^{-1}
τ_n	16 ms	f_{cyt}	0.01
k_{PMCA}	0.2 ms^{-1}	K_D	0.3 μM
v_n	−16 mV	s_n	5 mV
v_m	−20 mV	s_m	12 mV

[Fig. 1(a)]. Action potentials are produced by the interaction of the 'fast' currents I_{Ca} and I_K, while the slow rhythm that packages impulses into bursts is generated by oscillations in $I_{K(Ca)}$. During the active spiking phase, the cytosolic Ca^{2+} concentration rises [Fig. 1(b)], increasing the fraction of activated K(Ca) channels w, thus increasing the K(Ca) conductance [Fig. 1(c)]. Since $I_{K(Ca)}$ is a hyperpolarizing current, when $g_{K(Ca)}$ rises to a sufficiently high level the spiking terminates and the cell enters the hyperpolarized silent phase. During this phase c declines due to pumping of Ca^{2+} out of the cell, so the K(Ca) conductance declines. Eventually, $I_{K(Ca)}$ is small enough to allow the cell to re-enter the spiking phase, and the cycle begins a new.

Another way to view the dynamics of bursting is through a fast/slow analysis, treating the slow variable, c, as a parameter of the subsystem of fast variables (V and n). A bifurcation diagram for this fast subsystem is shown in Fig. 1.4 with w [Eq. (1.28)] as the bifurcation parameter. The variable c could be used as the bifurcation parameter, but the dynamics are clearer with w because total K(Ca) conductance is linear in w. The bifurcation diagram and trajectories were generated with the MATLAB. For large values of w the fast subsystem is at rest at a hyperpolarized voltage. These stable rest states make up the bottom branch of the z-shaped slow manifold ('z-curve') in Fig. 1.4. The lower branch turns and becomes unstable at a saddle node bifurcation (circle point), and then turns again at another saddle node bifurcation. The stationary branch regains stability for w near 0 at a Hopf bifurcation. The branch of periodic solutions emerging from the Hopf bifurcation (diamond point) represents action potentials (not shown in Fig. 1.4). It terminates at an infinite-period homoclinic bifurcation (star point). We now think of w not as a parameter, but as a function of the slowly changing variable c, and superimpose on the bifurcation diagram the c nullcline, transformed according to equation (1.28). We refer to this as the 'w nullcline' (red curve). To perform a fast–slow analysis, one treats the fast-subsystem bifurcation diagram, often referred to as the critical manifold, as a generalized V-nullcline. As with a standard phase plane analysis, one can use the curves to determine the flow of the trajectory in the (c, V) plane, noting that horizontal flow is much

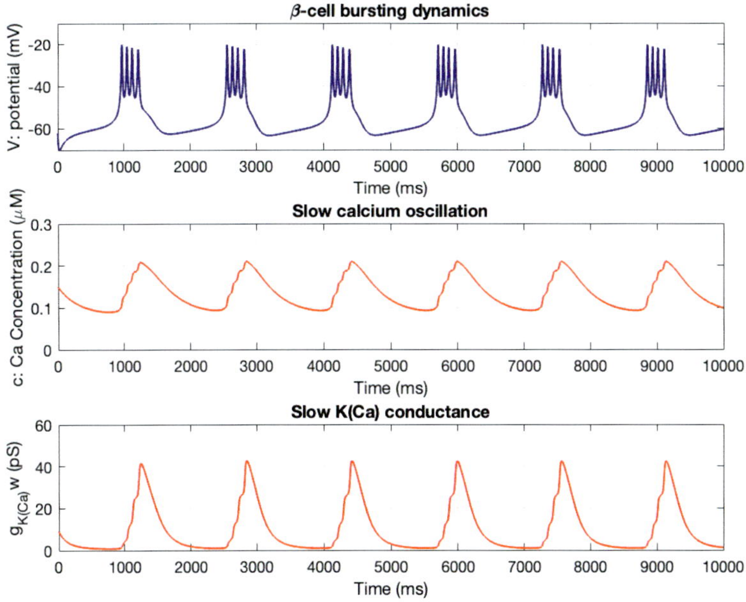

Figure 1.3 Bursting generated by the basic model. (a) Impulses ride on plateaus, with burst period of 2 s. (b) Cytosolic Ca2+ concentration rises during active phases and falls during silent phases. (c) The activity-dependent oscillations in c produce oscillations in the conductance of the K(Ca) channel, driving the bursting.

slower than vertical flow since c changes slowly compared to V. The burst trajectory can then be understood in terms of this flow much in the same way that relaxation oscillations are analyzed in the phase plane. During the silent phase of the burst, the trajectory follows the lower stable branch of the manifold (acting as the nullcline of the fast variable V) until it terminates at a saddle–node bifurcation. From here, the trajectory moves upward to the stable periodic spiking branch. Since it has crossed the c-nullcline, the direction of flow switches from left to right, so the trajectory moves rightward along the spiking branch until it terminates at a homoclinic bifurcation. This is the active phase of the burst. Once the trajectory passes through the homoclinic bifurcation, it moves downward to the stable stationary branch and the flow switches to the left as it begins a new silent phase. The burst is a complex stable limit cycle, but as we see here, it can be clearly understood with the aid of the critical manifold and the slow-variable nullcline. This fast–slow analysis of bursting, pioneered by John Rinzel [232], has been applied to many models of bursting [26, 179, 233].

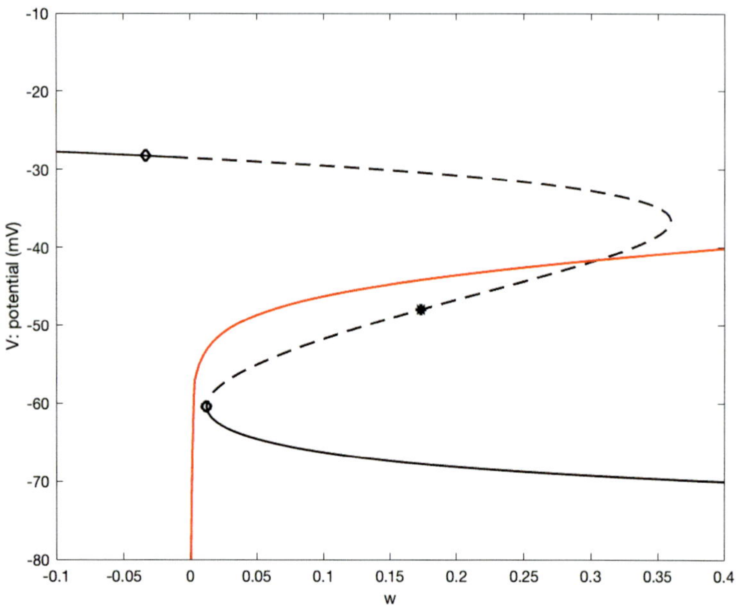

Figure 1.4 Fast/slow analysis of bursting with the basic model. Heavy solid curves represent stable branches, the light dashed curve represents an unstable branch, and the red curve represents the c nullcline transformed according to Eq. (1.28) (the 'w nullcline'). The lower saddle node bifurcation (circle point) terminates the silent phase of bursting and the homoclinic bifurcation (star point) terminates the periodic spiking branch.

Bursting Model with Two Slow Variables (phantom bursting)

Once fluorescent dyes for Ca^{2+} were developed and used with islets, it was clear that the Ca^{2+} traces did not have the sawtooth shape predicted by the Chay–Keizer model (Fig. 1.3B), but instead had more of a square-wave shape, with a slow decline at the end of each burst. By adding a second Ca^{2+} compartment, the endoplasmic reticulum (ER), which acts as an intracellular Ca^{2+} store, one can increase the burst period. During the burst active phase the Ca^{2+} concentration in the ER (c_{ER}) slowly builds up, and during the silent phase, the ER slowly releases Ca^{2+} into the cytosol. This allows the cytosolic Ca^{2+} concentration to be fast, but with slow components due to modulation by the ER Ca^{2+} concentration, which becomes the slow variable dictating the start and end of each burst active phase.

We assume that the Ca^{2+} influx into the ER via SERCA pumps depends linearly on the cytosolic Ca^{2+} concentration:

$$J_{SERCA} = k_{SERCA}c, \tag{1.30}$$

where $k_{SERCA} = 0.4ms^{-1}$.

The efflux out of the ER has two components. The Ca^{2+} leak is taken to be proportional to the gradient between Ca^{2+} concentrations in the cytosol and the ER (c_{er}):

$$J_{leak} = p_{leak}(c_{er} - c), \tag{1.31}$$

where $p_{leak} = 0.0005ms^{-1}$

The net Ca^{2+} efflux from the ER is

$$J_{er} = J_{leak} - J_{SERCA}. \tag{1.32}$$

Since this represents an additional influx term to the cytosolic Ca^{2+} compartment, we modify the differential equation for c:

$$\frac{dc}{dt} = f_{cyt}(J_{mem} + J_{er}). \tag{1.33}$$

For the ER Ca^{2+} concentration, J_{er} must be scaled by the ratio of the volumes of the cytoplasmic compartment (V_{cyt}) and the ER compartment (V_{er}):

$$\frac{dc_{er}}{dt} = -f_{er}(V_{cyt}/V_{er})J_{er}, \tag{1.34}$$

where $f_{er} = 0.01, V_{cyt}/V_{er} = 5$ is the fraction of free Ca^{2+} in the ER.

The Chay–Keizer model with ER represents a departure from previous models in the family because it has two slow variables, c and c_{ER}, instead of one. Both contribute to bursting to different degrees, depending on parameters, so the "slow variable" can be viewed as a composite of the two rather than a single physical variable. This gave rise to the term phantom bursting [25].

The behavior of cytosolic Ca^{2+} time course generated by the phantom model looks very different from Fig. 1.3, with the sawtooth pattern replaced by a square wave [30]. At the end of an active phase, c declines rather than rises, reflecting the exchange of Ca^{2+} from the ER to the cytosol and out of the cell through Ca^{2+} pumps. The Ca^{2+} concentration in the ER is now the variable with a sawtooth time course, since it is the slowest variable of the system. One could perform a fast–slow analysis with either c_{ER} or c as the single slow variable [30].

In addition to providing a more accurate shape for the time course of c, the phantom bursting mechanism allows for a greater range of burst periods, and in particular, burst periods of several minutes. The wide range of burst periods is possible because the period is determined both by the time required for the trajectory to move along a branch of the critical manifold before it stalls, and the time required for the nullcline to move so that the trajectory escapes. In the Chay–Keizer model with an ER, the former reflects the time constant for c, while the latter reflects the much larger time constant for c_{ER}. The deeper the intersection of the nullcline with the periodic or stable stationary branch of the critical manifold, the longer the burst period. Thus, the burst period can be extended to several minutes. In contrast, if the nullcline intersects only the middle, unstable, stationary branch, then the burst will be driven entirely by changes in c (as in Fig. 1.4) and the period will be small, just a few seconds.

The dual oscillator model: Despite the success of phantom bursting in explaining bursting in β-cells, there were data that appeared to defy explanation by the model. These electrophysiology data, from different labs, showed episodes of bursts and cases in which the plateau fraction varied over time in a rhythmic manner. The terms *compound bursting* and *accordion bursting* are given for these two unusual types of electrical behavior. Later electrophysiology and Ca^{2+} imaging data demonstrated that these strange forms of bursting are not so unusual, and compound bursting is commonly seen in islet recordings. Just as with the slow form of bursting, the episode period, and the period of the rhythmic modulation of plateau fraction, is similar to the 5–10 min period of insulin oscillations in the blood; oscillations with that period enhance the efficacy of insulin action. These compelling data suggested that there could be two co-existing oscillators; one oscillator would produce bursts, and the other would group them into episodes or slowly vary the plateau fraction of each burst. The Dual Oscillator Model (DOM) [27,29] was a mathematical realization of that idea. In the DOM, there is an electrical oscillator based largely on the phantom bursting model, and a separate glycolytic oscillator based on [247] that produced a slow oscillation in the ATP/ADP ratio. The oscillations in ATP/ADP affect the cell's electrical activity through K(ATP) channels; an increase in ATP/ADP results in a decrease in $g_{K(ATP)}$, so oscillations in ATP/ADP result in oscillations in $gK(ATP)$.

The integrated oscillator model. Another challenge arose later when a FRET (Fluorescence Resonance Energy Transfer) biosensor was developed to detect oscillations in fructose 1,6-bisphosphate (FBP), called PKAR (Pyruvate Kinase Activity Reporter) [203]. While use of the probe in islets clearly showed slow oscillations in PKAR (and thus FBP), the shape of the oscillations did not match those of the FBP oscillations in the DOM. The correct FBP pattern was achieved by including Ca^{2+}-dependent activation of pyruvate dehydrogenase (PDH) [201] into the model. With this addition to the model, the semi-independence of the electrical and metabolic oscillators was gone. Now, Ca^{2+} influences metabolism both through production and consumption of ATP, and ATP influences electrical activity and thus the Ca^{2+} concentrations through K(ATP) channels. In the revised model, Ca^{2+} can both stimulate phosphofructokinase (PFK) by increasing ATP consumption, which relieves the inhibition of PFK by ATP, and inhibit PFK by removing the stimulation of PFK by FBP. As a consequence, the two oscillators are closely and bidirectionally linked, motivating the name Integrated Oscillator Model (IOM) [27,28].

Mathematical analysis of bursting models. Square-wave that we presented for pancreatic β cell is only one type of bursting. Examples of two other types are commonly known as elliptic and parabolic bursters. Elliptic bursters exhibit small amplitude oscillations during the silent phase and the amplitude of spikes gradually wax and wane. An important feature of parabolic bursters is that the frequency of spikes first increases and then decreases during the active phase. Both elliptic and parabolic bursters arise in models for neuronal activity and other excitable systems. Elliptic bursters arise in models for thalamic neurons, rodent trigeminal neurons, certain neurons within the basal ganglia and 40-Hz oscillations [97]. Rigorous results concerning the existence and stability of bursting oscillations and continuous spiking are presented in [179, 259, 260].

1.2.2 Insulin Granule Dynamics: ODE Models

Insulin granule trafficking in pancreatic β-cells has been investigated in recent years by using fluorescent proteins that are targeted to secretory granules and allow the real-time imaging of granules in living cells. A β-cell contains 10,000–13,000 granules of diameter $\sim$ 350 nm, each containing $\sim$ 1.6 amol of insulin plus other polypeptides and smaller molecules. Most granules belong to a large "reserve pool", around 600 are docked with the plasma membrane, with 50-100 granules in a pool of immediate release, and other $\sim$ 1500 are located close to cell surface. Granule exocytosis requires the fusion of granule membrane with plasma membrane and the formation of a pore that connects granule lumen to extracellular space. Incomplete fusion and kiss-and-run exocytosis may also occur. As found by early observations in vitro and in vivo, stimulation by a rapid and large increase in the extracellular glucose concentration induces a biphasic time course of the insulin secretion rate (ISR) with a 5-10 min peak, the first phase, followed by a more prolonged second phase. Recent experimental data from mouse and rat β-cells showed that only 1-2 granules/min per β-cell are released at a glucose concentration around 3 mM, and 20-30 granules/min per cell are released at the peak of the first phase insulin secretion after a step increase in glucose, with a total secretion of about 680 granules in 50 min. In a first pathway of stimulus-secretion coupling (triggering pathway), the glucose stimulus increases the ATP/ADP ratio, which induces closing of the KATP channels and depolarization of cell membrane. The resulting Ca^{2+} influx through the voltage-sensitive Ca^{2+} channels raises the cytosolic free calcium concentration, $[Ca^{2+}]$c, so promoting the exocytosis of insulin granules.

1.2.2.1 *Dynamic Model Without Ca^{2+} Dynamics*

The model proposed in [31] defines a pool, I, of free proinsulin and a pool, V, of free granule membrane material, not yet enclosing proinsulin. Moreover, four pools of insulin granules were considered: the reserve pool (R), the docked granules (D), the immediately releasable granules (DIR), and the granules fused with cell membrane (F). Model equations are as follows:

$$\frac{dI}{dt} = -kIV - \alpha_I I + b_I; \tag{1.35}$$

$$\frac{dV}{dt} = -kIV - \alpha_V V + b_V + \sigma F(t - \tau_V); \tag{1.36}$$

$$\frac{dR}{dt} = kIV - \gamma(t)R; \tag{1.37}$$

$$\frac{dD}{dt} = \gamma(t)R - k_1^+[C_T - D_{IR}]D + k_1^- D_{IR}; \tag{1.38}$$

$$\frac{dD_{IR}}{dt} = k_1^+[C_T - D_{IR}]D - k_{-1}^- D_{IR} - \rho(t)D_{IR}; \tag{1.39}$$

$$\frac{dF}{dt} = \rho(t)D_{IR} - \sigma F; \tag{1.40}$$

In (1.35) and (1.36), k is an aggregation rate constant, α_I, α_V are degradation rate constants, and b_I, b_V denote, respectively, the rate of proinsulin biosynthesis and the production rate of granule membranes. The last term in the right-hand side of (1.36) accounts for the contribution to granule membrane formation of the recycling of membrane material, with σ the rate constant of the fusion process and τ_V the time interval required for recycling. The variable γ in (1.37) is the rate coefficient of granule externalization and priming, related to the ATP-to-ADP ratio (min^{-1}). γ represents the processes by which granules are irreversibly translocated from trans-Golgi network to plasma membrane, and it is dependent on the glucose concentration, G, according to (1.41). The pool D_{IR} is formed through the binding of docked granules to L-type Ca^{2+} channels, with C_T denoting the pool of total Ca^{2+} channels and k_1^+, k_1^- the rate constants of association and, respectively, dissociation. The variable ρ is the rate coefficient of granule fusion with cell membrane, related to $[Ca^{2+}]$ (min^{-1}). The factors that promote granule fusion are represented by ρ, and σF in (1.40) is the number of granules releasing insulin in the unit time at time t in a single β-cell.

The equations that relate glucose stimulus to the quantities, γ and ρ, that govern granule trafficking are as follows:

$$\frac{d\gamma}{dt} = \eta[-\gamma + \gamma_b + \phi(t) + h_\gamma(G(t - \tau_G))]; \tag{1.41}$$

$$\frac{d\rho}{dt} = \zeta[-\rho + \rho_b + h_\rho(\gamma)]; \tag{1.42}$$

where basal values are indicated by the subscript b; η and ζ are rate constants, and ϕ represents factors that induce ATP and calcium oscillations. Glucose activation is modeled by the saturating function h_γ, with τ_G the time required by glucose metabolism. So γ regulates granule translocation and priming, and through h_ρ regulates granule fusion and the ISR (Insulin secretion rate (pmol/min)). Glucose thus controls the material flux from b_I, b_V to σF.

Glucose activation is modeled by the function h_γ, and the time delay τ_G is the time required by glucose metabolism. Data on isolated β-cells and cell clusters stimulated by glucose show that cell response is maximal and almost constant for $G >$ 10-12 $mmol/l$ and much lower below 6 mmol/l. So h_γ has been chosen equal to zero for G smaller than a threshold G^*, linearly increasing for G in the glucose concentration range $(G^*, \hat{G})$, and then constant. We have:

$$h_\gamma(G) = \begin{cases} 0, & G \leq G^* \\ \frac{\hat{h}}{\hat{G}-G^*}(G - G^*), & G^* < G < \hat{G} \\ \hat{h}, & G > \hat{G} \end{cases} \tag{1.43}$$

where $\hat{h}$ is the maximal value of $h(G)$ and is reached at $G = \hat{G}$.
The function h_ρ, which embodies the action of ATP on Ca^{2+}, is simply defined as

$$h_\rho(\gamma) = \begin{cases} 0, & \gamma < \gamma_b \\ k_\rho(\gamma - \gamma_b), & \gamma \geq \gamma_b \end{cases} \tag{1.44}$$

We remark that, for G below the threshold G^* and $\phi = 0$, the rate coefficients γ and ρ stay at their basal values, and the ISR may be thought to be determined by the "constitutive pathway" of insulin secretion. When G exceeds the threshold, h_γ is no longer equal to zero, and the ISR becomes determined by the "regulated pathway".

In summary, extracellular glucose modulates the mitochondrial signal γ according to Eqs. (1.41)–(1.43), and γ regulates granule translocation and priming. In turn, γ affects ρ, and thus the fusion of DIR granules with cell membrane, according to Eqs. (1.42)–(1.44). So, in the present model, it is the parameter γ that has a major role both in the triggering pathway and in the amplifying pathway. Equations (1.41)–(1.44) represent, in a very rough way, the coupling of glucose metabolism to the signals that activate insulin secretion. In particular, we neglected the dependence of production and degradation rates of ATP on $[Ca^{2+}]_i$, as well as the kinetics of Ca^{2+} stores in the endoplasmic reticulum, which may cause oscillations in the concentrations with a phase shift between γ and ρ.

According to Eq. (1.40), the insulin amount released in the unit time by a single β-cell in the extracellular space is given by $I_0\sigma F$, where I_0 is the insulin amount contained in a granule, if complete emptying of granules that undergo fusion is assumed. To compute the insulin amount released in the unit time by the whole β-cell population (ISR), we must account for both the size of the population (total number of β-cells) and the fraction of cells that actually release insulin in the given experimental situation. Denoting by N_c the average number of β-cells per islet and by N_i the number of islets, the total number

N of β-cells may be written as $N = N_c N_i$. An important factor is the heterogeneous responsiveness of the cell population to glucose (neglecting other secretagogues). The fraction of responsive islet cells and clusters increases with the extracellular glucose, and cell subpopulations with different intrinsic sensitivity to glucose is likely to exist. To keep the model as simple as possible, we adopt a rough description of β-cell recruitment by glucose stimulus, by assuming that only a fraction, f, of the total cell population responds to glucose. This fraction will increase as the glucose concentration G increases, with a time delay for recruitment equal to τ_G, so we have $f(t) = f[G(t - \tau_G)]$. Under the further assumption that β-cells respond to stimulation in a synchronous manner, which may be realistic on a not-too-fast time scale thanks to cell-to-cell electrical and chemical interactions, we may finally write for the insulin secretion rate of the whole cell population at time t, the following expression:

$$\mathrm{ISR}(t) = I_0 \sigma F(t) f(t) N_c N_i. \tag{1.45}$$

Given the time course of glucose concentration G, Eqs. (1.35)–(1.45) predict the time evolution of the control rate coefficients γ and ρ, the evolution of the quantities that describe granule dynamics (I, V, R, D, D_{IR}, F), and the evolution of the recruited cell fraction f and hence of the ISR. The following parameters may be considered constant, independent of the degree of stimulation of the β-cell: $k, \alpha_I, \alpha_V, \tau_V, C_T, k_1^+, k_1^-, \sigma, \tau_G, \eta, \gamma_b, G^*, \hat{G}, \hat{h}, \xi, \rho_b, k_\rho$, and I_0 (parameters of granule dynamics and signaling model); Nc and Ni (parameters of the β-cell population). By contrast, other quantities in the model, namely b_I, b_V, ϕ, and f, may be affected by changes in the concentration of glucose (and other secretagogues) or as a consequence of changes in the experimental conditions. b_V will be taken time and glucose independent and an equation for f as a function of G is given as follows

$$f(G) = \begin{cases} f_b, & G < G^* \\ f_b + (1 - f_b)\frac{G - G^*}{K_f + (G - G^*)}, & G^* \geq G \end{cases} \tag{1.46}$$

where f_b is the fraction of responding cells at glucose concentration smaller than the threshold $G*$ (for simplicity assumed equal to that in Eq. (1.43), and K_f is a constant related to the effectiveness of recruitment. According to Eq. (1.46), $\sim$ 100% of β-cells may be recruited for a large enough G.

For some of the parameters of the model of Eqs. (1.35)–(1.45), we may use experimental measurements or estimates, e.g., $I_0 = 1.6$ *amol* in rat granules and $N_c = 1{,}000$–$2{,}000$ cells for an islet. The granule fusion event plus the insulin cargo release has been reported to require a time of the order of a few seconds, so we may take an estimate for σ in the range 6–30 min^{-1}. Moreover, $C_T = 500$ was reported as an upper estimate for the number of Ca^{2+} channels. We will take $\tau_G = 1\ min$. Other indications about the values of model parameters can be obtained in view of the available experimental data concerning the basal state in isolated islets and steady states of Eqs.

(1.35)–(1.46) that are discussed in next section. The following are the values for the parameters:

$$k = 10^{-2}\ min^{-1},\ \alpha_I = 0.3\ min^{-1},\ \alpha_V = 0.6\ min^{-1},\ \tau_V = 5\ min,$$

$$C_T = 500,\ k_1^+ = 1.447 \times 10^{-5}\ min^{-1},\ k_1^- = 0.10375\ min^{-1},\ \sigma = 30\ min^{-1},$$

$$\tau_G = 1\ min,\ \eta = 4\ min^{-1},\ \gamma_b = 10^{-4}\ min^{-1},\ G^* = 4.58\ mmol/l,$$

$$\hat{G} = 10\ mmol/l,\ \hat{h} = 3.93 \times 10^{-2}\ min^{-1},\ \xi = \eta = 4\ min^{-1},\ \rho_b = 0.02\ min^{-1},$$

$$k_\rho = 350,\ I_0 = 1.6\ amol,\ N_c = 1000,\ N_i = 1,\ b_I = 4\ min^{-1},\ b_V = 6\ min^{-1}.$$

To represent the basal condition (glucose concentration G_b), or a situation in which glucose concentration is kept constant for a long time at a basal or supra-basal value, we may consider the steady-state solution of the model in which b_I, γ, ρ, and f take values corresponding to the assigned value of G, $\phi = 0$, and the pools I, V, R, D, D_{IR}, and F are constant. These constant values are obtained by setting to zero the time derivatives in model equations. We observe that, in the steady state, we have the following chain of equalities:

$$kIV = \gamma R = \rho D_{IR} = \sigma F. \tag{1.47}$$

Taking Eq. (1.47) into account, from Eqs. (1.35) to (1.37), we see that I, V, and R are given in the steady state by the following expressions:

$$I = \frac{b_I \alpha_V}{kb_V I + \alpha_I \alpha_V}, V = \frac{b_V}{\alpha_V}, R = \frac{b_I}{\gamma} \frac{kb_V}{kb_V + \alpha_I \alpha_V}. \tag{1.48}$$

Thus, we have

$$\sigma F = b_I \frac{kb_V}{kb_V + \alpha_I \alpha_V} \tag{1.49}$$

Using Eqs. (1.38)–(1.40), D, D_{IR}, and F can be conveniently expressed in terms of the steady-state value of R:

$$D = \frac{1}{k_1^+} \frac{\rho + k_1^-)\gamma R}{\rho C_T - \gamma R}, D_{IR} = \frac{1}{\rho}\gamma R, F = \frac{1}{\sigma}\gamma R. \tag{1.50}$$

To guarantee the positivity of D in the steady state, the constraint $\rho C_T - \gamma R > 0$ has to be satisfied. For the ISR in the steady state, Eq. (1.49) gives

$$ISR = I_0 \sigma F f N_c N_i = I_0 b_I \frac{kb_V}{kb_V + \alpha_I \alpha_V} N_c N_i, \tag{1.51}$$

showing that, as intuitive, the rate of insulin secretion in the long time is essentially determined by the proinsulin biosynthesis rate, b_I. Because b_I and f depend on G, the above equation is the "dose-response relationship" predicted by the model when glucose levels (and all other quantities) are kept constant for a long time.

Analysis of the model

Analysis of first-phase response: We derive here an approximate expression for the insulin amount released in the first-phase response following a step in glucose concentration. We assume, for the sake of simplicity, that the dynamics of γ and ρ are much faster than granule dynamics (large and values). Although the measured [ATP] and free $[Ca^{2+}]$ in β-cell cytosol after a glucose step show rise times of a few minutes, glucose appears to provoke the formation of sub-plasma membrane ATP micro-domains, where ATP rapidly responds to a glucose increase with a half-time 20 s. The state of nearby K_{ATP} and L-type Ca^{2+} channels is likely to rapidly change, leading to fast Ca^{2+} influx at sites close to the granules of the D_{IR} pool. The transient increase in $[Ca^{2+}]_i$ at these sites, and thus in ρ, may be completed in 1 min. We will take as baseline values $\eta = \xi = 4\ min^{-1}$, so the transient of γ and ρ will require ~ 1 min.

Following the step change in glucose concentration to a supra-basal value G, and after the time delay τ_G, γ and ρ will rapidly attain their steady-state values, denoted as $\tilde{\gamma}$ and $\tilde{\rho}$, respectively. From Eq. (1.41) [with $\psi(t) = 0$] and Eq. (1.43), we have $\tilde{\gamma} = \gamma_b + h_\gamma(G)$ and $\tilde{\rho} = \rho_b + k_\rho h(G)$. Let us take the time origin so that $\gamma(t) = \tilde{\gamma}$ and $\rho(t) = \tilde{\rho}$ for $t > 0$. Assuming that pool D does not change appreciably during the first-phase response, we solve Eq. (1.39) with D(t) held constant at its initial (basal) value D_b, ρ equal to $\tilde{\rho}$, and initial condition $D_{IR}(0) = D_{IR,b}$. The pool D_{IR} will be depleted according to

$$D_{IR}(t) = \frac{b}{a} + \left(D_{IR,b} - \frac{b}{a}\right)\exp(-at), \tag{1.52}$$

where $a = k_1^+ D_b + k^- + \tilde{\rho}$ and $b = k_1^+ D_b C_T$. Then we solve Eq. (1.40) for F, with initial condition at the basal value $F_b, \rho = \tilde{\rho}$ and $D_{IR}(t)$ given by Eq. (1.42), obtaining

$$\begin{aligned} F(t) = F_b \exp(-\sigma t) &- \frac{\tilde{\rho}}{\sigma}\frac{b}{a}[1 - \exp(-\sigma t)] \\ &+ \frac{\tilde{\rho}}{\sigma - a}\left(D_{IR,b} - \frac{b}{a}\right)[\exp(-at) - \exp(-\sigma t)]. \end{aligned} \tag{1.53}$$

We must compute the integral of the ISR over a time interval, say of length T, that just contains the first ISR peak. Recalling Eq. (1.45), we compute the total number of insulin granules released by a single β-cell in the interval T, that is, the integral of $\sigma F(t)$ from t 0 to $t = T$. Assuming a and F_b small, this integral, denoted as Z(G), is given by

$$Z(G) = \frac{b}{a}\left\{bT + \left(D_{IR,b} - \frac{b}{a}\right)[1 - \exp(-aT)]\right\}. \tag{1.54}$$

Thus, the insulin amount, IS(G), released in the first-phase response to a glucose step G can be written as

$$IS(G) = I_0 Z(G) f(G) N, \tag{1.55}$$

where N here is the number of -cells in rat pancreas. The function f was chosen of the form

$$f(G) = \begin{cases} f_b, & G < G^* \\ f_b + (1 - f_b)\frac{G-G^*}{K_f+(G-G^*)}, & G^* \geq G \end{cases} \tag{1.56}$$

where f_b is the fraction of responding cells at glucose concentration smaller than the threshold G^* (for simplicity assumed equal to that in Eq. (1.42), and K_f is a constant related to the effectiveness of recruitment. According to Eq. (1.56), 100% of β-cells may be recruited for a large enough G.

Analysis of second-phase response An approximate expression for the second-phase ISR can be obtained as follows. Let us assume that, during this phase, the pool R decays exponentially from the basal value R_b to a final value R, where R is expressed as in Eq. (1.47) with the final values of γ and b_I, $\tilde{\gamma}$ and b_1, respectively, and the other parameters unchanged. The rate constant of the exponential is, so we have (initial time t = 0)

$$R(t) = \tilde{R} + (R_b - \tilde{R}) \exp(-\gamma t). \tag{1.57}$$

Using the quasi-stationary approximation $D_{IR} = 0$ and summing the equations for D and D_{IR}, we may write

$$\dot{D}(t) = \tilde{\gamma} R(t) - \tilde{\rho} D_{IR}(t), \ D_{IR}(t) = \frac{k_1^+ C_T D(t)}{k_1^+ D(t) + k_1^- + \tilde{\rho}}. \tag{1.58}$$

For $\tilde{\rho} >> k_1^+ D + k_1^-$ (valid when G is large and the concentration of free Ca^{2+} is at its maximum level), the differential equation in (1.58) may be written as a linear differential equation for D that can be solved using Eq. (1.57) and with $D(0) = D_b$, obtaining

$$\begin{aligned} D(t) = D_b \exp(-k_1^+ C_T t) + \frac{\tilde{\gamma}\tilde{R}}{k_1^+ C_T}\left[1 - \exp(-k_1^+ C_T t)\right] \\ + \frac{\tilde{\gamma}(R_b - \tilde{R})}{k_1^+ C_T - \tilde{\gamma}}[\exp(-\tilde{\gamma} t) - \exp(-k_1^+ C_T t)]. \end{aligned} \tag{1.59}$$

By the further quasi-stationary approximation $\dot{F} = 0$, we finally get

$$\sigma F(t) = k_1^+ C_T D(t), \tag{1.60}$$

that may be used with Eq. (1.59) to compute the approximate expression of the second-phase ISR. The derivative of F(t) at $t = 0$ is given by $k_1^+ C_T (\tilde{\gamma} R_b - k_1^+ C_T D_b)$.

If $k_1^+ C_T = 7.24 \times 10^{-3}\ min^{-1}$, and $\tilde{\gamma} \leq \gamma_b + \hat{h} = 3.93 \times 10^{-3}\ min^{-1}$ (baseline parameters), the descending front of second-phase ISR has a large time constant ($1/\tilde{\gamma} >$4 h). The time constant becomes smaller if $\hat{h}$ is larger. With the baseline parameters, the negative term in the above derivative may be neglected for $G > 10$ mmol/l.

Simulation Results

Stimulation by High K^+: The continuous increase in K^+ caused a sustained $[Ca^{2+}]$ rise, whereas the insulin secretion rate exhibited a large initial peak followed by a slow return to the initial value. The impulsive increments in K^+ caused an intermittent rise of $[Ca^{2+}]$ and a sequence of decreasing peaks of the insulin secretion rate. The pattern of the response, but not its basal value, was influenced by the glucose level (0 or 3 mmol/l). This type of stimulation is modeled here by assuming that the time course of reflects the time course of $[Ca^{2+}]$, whereas γ retains its basal value γ_b. Thus, starting from the basal value ρ_b, the time course of ρ in the case of continuous stimulation has been obtained as the response of a linear first-order system with rate constant ζ to a step function (the step increase in K^+). A component increasing linearly with slope s_ρ has been added to mimic more closely the measured $[Ca^{2+}]$ in the time interval 0-50 min.

The function $\rho(t)$ is in this case the input signal for the model of Eqs. (1.35)–(1.40) The model response to this stimulation (taking 1,000-cells in an islet and f = 1) is computed, and the time course of pools D and DIR is computed. The latter pool is seen to be rapidly depleted upon stimulation. The response of I and V shows that these pools are affected after the time lag, τ_V, required for the recycling from the plasma membrane to the pool V, which is in fact transiently increased. The pool R remains virtually unchanged. The predicted ISR is computed. The number of granules released per β cell, given by the integral of F over the time, is equal to 67 granules in the first 5 min of the response. According to this model, this type of stimulation does not affect the steady-state values of I, V, R, F, and ISR, which are recovered in the long time: only the steady-state values of D and DIR are decreased (see Eqs. (1.47) and (1.49)). If a Ca^{2+}-mediated enhancement of microtubule-based granule transport were included in the model, high K^+ stimulation would produce a component of granule translocation to plasma membrane with a decrease in R.

Stimulation by Extracellular Glucose: The second phase of glucose-stimulated insulin secretion had been initially considered to be sustained by proinsulin biosynthesis. Subsequently, this interpretation was refuted. Confirmed by model simulations, an increase in the rate of proinsulin biosynthesis b_I, concomitant with the increase in ρ, does not produce a secondary response if γ is kept at γ_b. As previously discussed, a critical role is played by the increase in the rate coefficient γ modulated by extracellular glucose, because intervenes in both the triggering and the amplifying pathway.

The ISR predicted by the model exhibits both the first and the second phase of insulin secretion. However, the amplifying effect can be "deleted" in the model by letting γ and ρ evolve according to Eqs. (1.41)–(1.44) but imposing that γ is kept to its basal value γ_b in the Eqs. (1.37)–(1.38) that govern granule translocation. In this case, the response only shows a first phase, followed by a decline in the ISR. The ISR patterns are obtained when G has a fast or a slow ramp rise where the delay in the response is because of the time required to reach G^*.

1.2.2.2 A Model with Ca^{2+} Dynamics

Here we present a kinetic model for insulin secretion in pancreatic beta-cells developed in [63]. This model can be used to calculate both the rate of granule fusion and the rate of insulin secretion when the cell is stimulated with an arbitrary electrical potential. First, we highlight some basic assumptions and general properties of the model.

1. The model contains two dynamical systems: i), the set of exocytotic reactions (the exocytosis cascade (EC)) between insulin-containing granules and the cell membrane, including the crucial Ca^{2+}-triggered fusion reaction, that lead to insulin secretion; and ii), the set of voltage-sensitive Ca^{2+}-channels and Ca^{2+}-transporters that handle the dynamics of Ca^{2+} inside the cell when the cell is applied with a depolarizing membrane potential.

2. Insulin-containing granules in the cell model are divided into a large reserve pool and a smaller "exocytosable" pool of "docked" granules, which can be further divided into several pools with different fusion competencies. Granules supplied from the reserve pool to the EC have to undergo some "maturation" or "priming" steps before they can execute the Ca^{2+}-triggered fusion reaction.

3. The model contains both L-type and R-type voltage-sensitive Ca^{2+}-channels to mediate Ca^{2+}-influx when the cell is depolarized and four types of Ca^{2+}-transporters to handle the clearance of Ca^{2+} from the cytosol.

4. Fusion of primed granules is assumed to take place exclusively in the "microdomain" at the inner mouth of an L-type channel (not the R-type), where the concentration of Ca^{2+} is much higher than that in the cytosol when the cell is stimulated. This assumption is based on the finding that insulin-containing granules can form stable complexes with L-type channels and on the realization that localized Ca^{2+}-influx plays an important role in insulin secretion. The R-type channels, on the other hand, contribute to exocytosis by adding to the global calcium signal but are not colocalized with vesicles.

5. The resupply step is assumed to depend on both ATP and bulk cytosolic Ca^{2+}. The ATP dependency derives from the finding that insulin

secretion from single islets drops to a low level after a long depolarization in the absence of glucose. The Ca^{2+} dependency is derived from the finding that insulin secretion in the second phase decreases when the cytosolic $[Ca^{2+}]$ is reduced by blocking the R-type Ca^{2+}-channels.

6. Priming is also assumed to depend on bulk cytosolic Ca^{2+} and, in some simulations, on glucose metabolism.

7. The Ca^{2+} dynamical system is not influenced by the EC.

8. Since fusion involves Ca^{2+}-ions in the microdomain of the L-type channel whereas resupply and priming involve Ca^{2+} the cytosol, the temporal distribution of Ca^{2+} between the two compartments plays an important role in insulin secretion. In this model, this distribution is handled by a two-compartment kinetic model. Microdomains and the two-compartment formalism for $[Ca^{2+}]$.

Microdomains and the two-compartment formalism for $[Ca^{2+}]$ dynamics

As shown schematically in Fig. 1.5, a "functional" micro-domain is defined as a half-sphere surrounding the inner mouth of an L-type channel. The microdomain is referred to as "functional" because it is the place where a primed granule can form a stable complex with the plasma membrane and execute the Ca^{2+}-triggered fusion step. The microdomain at an R-type channel, in contrast, is not functional because granules do not form stable complexes with the channel and therefore very few fusion events will occur there. Although there is not a membrane separating the microdomain and the cytosol, modeling studies have shown that a sharp temporal $[Ca^{2+}]$ gradient can be maintained near the channel. We therefore use the simple two-compartment model illustrated in Fig. 1.6 to describe the temporal and spatial distribution of Ca^{2+} in a stimulated b-cell. When the cell is depolarized, Ca^{2+}-ions passing through the L-type channels first go into the microdomain (flux J_L in Fig. 1.5) and then diffuse to the cytosol, whereas those passing through the R-type channels go directly to the cytosol (flux J_R in Fig. 1.5). Flux between the two phenomenological compartments are assumed to be proportional to the concentration difference.

Let us consider a cell that is supplied with a time-dependent potential $V(t)$ at time 0. Let $C_i(t)$ and $C_{md}(t)$ denote the Ca^{2+}-concentrations in the cytosol and the microdomain compartments, respectively, at time t. Then, they obey the chemical kinetic equations:

$$\frac{dC_{md}(t)}{dt} = f_{md}J_L(t) - f_{md}B[C_{md} - C_i(t)] \tag{1.61}$$

$$\frac{dC_i(t)}{dt} = f_iJ_R(t) + f_V f_i B[C_{md} - C_i(t)] - f_iL(C_i(t)), \tag{1.62}$$

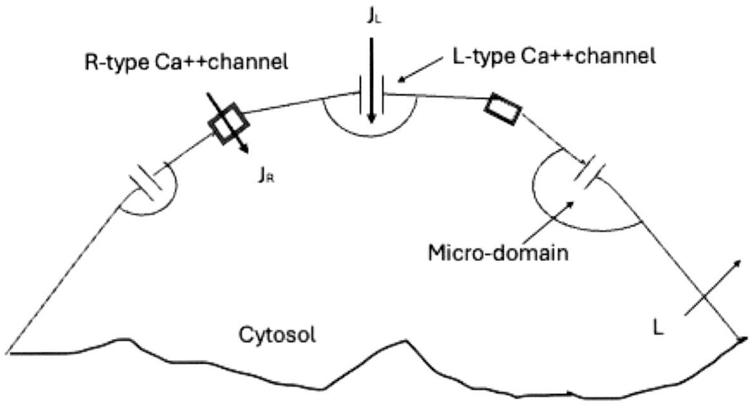

Figure 1.5 Two-compartment model for intracellular calcium ion dynamics. Ca^{2+}-channels and the "microdomain" of a b-cell model. The influx of Ca^{2+} is handled by two types of voltage-gated Ca^{2+}-channels: the L-type and the R-type. A microdomain is defined as the half-sphere surrounding the inner mouth of an L-type Ca^{2+}-channel with a diameter of 0.3 μm to provide a phenomenological compartment with elevated Ca^{2+}; the region of elevated Ca^{2+} in a real cell would in fact be much smaller, perhaps 10 nm. When the cell membrane is depolarized, Ca^{2+} passing through the L-type channel first goes into the microdomain and then diffuses to the cytosol, whereas only the contribution of Ca^{2+} passing through the R-type channel to cytosolic Ca^{2+}-concentration is accounted for.

where $J_L(t)$ and $J_r(t)$ are, respectively, the molar Ca^{2+}-influx through open L-type and open R-type Ca^{2+}-channels at time t; f_{md} and f_i are constants representing the ratio of the free to the bound Ca^{2+} in the microdomain and the cytosol compartments, respectively; B is the transport rate constant of Ca^{2+} between the two compartments (a parameter that is fit); f_V is the ratio of the compartmental volume of the microdomain to that of the cytosol; and $L(C_i)$ is the molar clearance rate of Ca^{2+} out of the cytosol compartment at $C_i(t)$. In Eqs. (1.61) and (1.62), we neglect the change in $[Ca^{2+}]$ caused by the binding of Ca^{2+} to granules. That is, the dynamics of Ca^{2+} is assumed to be independent of the kinetics of granule fusion and exocytosis. This assumption is reasonable, because the number of granules is much smaller than the number of Ca^{2+}-ions in the cell. Values of $J_L(t)$ and $J_R(t)$ at any given membrane potential $V(t)$ can be calculated from the current through open Ca^{2+}-channels:

$$\begin{aligned} J_L(t) &= -\alpha I_L(t)/\nu_{md}, \\ J_R(t) &= -\alpha I_R(t)/\nu_{cell}, \end{aligned} \tag{1.63}$$

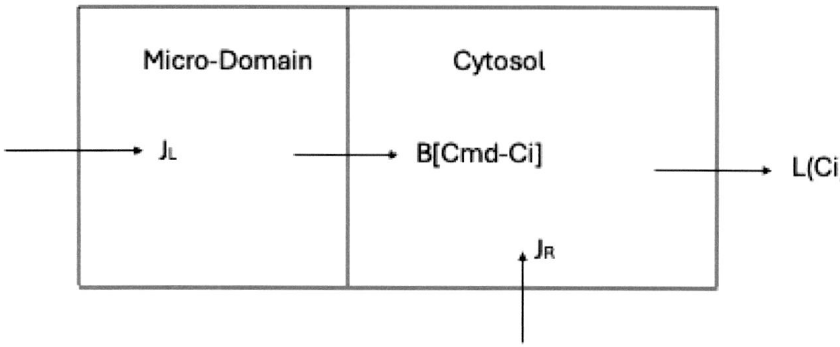

Figure 1.6 The two-compartment kinetic model describing the dynamic distribution of Ca^{2+} between the microdomain and the cytosol compartments. C_{md} and C_i denote the concentration of Ca^{2+} in the microdomain and the cytosol compartment, respectively, B is the rate of exchange between the microdomain and the cytosol, and $L(C_i)$ denotes the rate of Ca^{2+} clearance from the cell, which is handled by four kinds of Ca^{2+}-transporters.

where ν_{md} and ν_{cell} are the volume of the microdomain compartment and the cell, respectively, and a is a constant factor that converts the current into the mole flux of Ca^{2+}-ions. Our microdomain compartment is a phenomenological construct that provides a region functionally specialized to have a Ca^{2+}-concentration elevated by two orders of magnitude over that of the cytosol. In an actual cell, the region of elevated Ca^{2+} would be more like the tall spike indicated by three-dimensional diffusion simulations, and a vesicle would have to be within a few tens of nanometer of a channel to experience concentrations on the order of our C_{md}.

The electrical properties of the L-type and R-type channels are assumed to be identical. However, the number of R-type channels is assumed to be only one-fourth that of the L-type, resulting in the following expressions:

$$\begin{aligned} I_L(t) &= g_L m_\infty(V(t))[V(t) - V_{ca}], \\ I_R(t) &= 0.25 g_L m_\infty(V(t))[V(t) - V_{ca}], \end{aligned} \tag{1.64}$$

$$m_\infty(V(t)) = \left[1 + e^{(V_m - V(t))/s_m}\right]^{-1} \tag{1.65}$$

where g_L is the conductance of the L-type Ca^{2+}-channel, V_{Ca} is the equilibrium potential for the Ca^{2+}-ions across the membrane, and V_m and s_m are constants.

The rate of clearance is assumed to be handled by four types of transporters: the sarcoendoplasmic reticulum ATPase (SERCA), the plasma membrane ATPase (PMCA), the Na-Ca exchanger (NCX), and the leak channel.

TABLE 1.7 Parameter values for the two-compartment model for $[Ca^{2+}]$ dynamics.

Parameter	Value	Source
g_L	250 pS	[63]
B	200 s^{-1}	[63]
V_m	-20 mV	[63]
V_{ca}	25 mV	[63]
ν_{cell}	1.15 pl	[63]
ν_{md}	4.2 fl	[63]
s_m	5 mV	[63]
f_V	0.00365	[63]
f_i	0.01	[63]
f_{md}	0.01	[63]
α	$5.18 \times 10^{-18} \mu\ mol/ms/fA$	[63]
K_{SERCA}	0.27 μ M	[63]
K_{PMCA}	0.5 μ M	[63]
J^{max}_{PMCA}	21 μ M/s	[63]
J^{max}_{SERCA}	41 μ M/s	[63]
J^{0}_{NCX}	18.67 μ M/s	[63]
J^{leak}_{PMCA}	-0.94 μ M/s	[63]

Neglecting the effects of pH and ATP, the clearance rate is then expressed as

$$L(C_i) = J_{SERCA} + J_{PMCA} + J_{NCX} + J_{leak}; \tag{1.66}$$

where

$$\begin{aligned} J_{SERCA} &= J^{max}_{SERCA}/\left[1 + (K_{SERCA}/C_i)^2\right], \\ J_{PMCA} &= J^{max}_{PMCA}/\left[1 + K_{PMCA}/C_i\right], \\ J_{NCX} &= [C_i - 0.25], \\ J_{leak} &= -0.94\ \mu M/s. \end{aligned} \tag{1.67}$$

Table 1.7 lists the values of the parameters of the two-compartment model.

The exocytosis cascade and the kinetic model

The EC that describes the interaction between the insulin-containing granules and the plasma membrane inside a beta-cell leading to insulin secretion is divided schematically into seven steps, as shown in Fig. 1.7. We assume that a granule has to dock to the membrane from a reserve pool, be primed, and move to the micro-domain at an L-type Ca^{2+}-channel before it can bind with Ca^{2+} and fuse with the cell membrane. Recent evidence points to the existence of an additional pool of granules, called the highly calcium-sensitive pool (HCSP) with high affinity for Ca^{2+} that can presumably fuse outside a channel micro-domain, but we leave this as an extension for future versions of the model. After fusion, the pore between the granule and the extracellular space has to expand before insulin can be released. Both the resupply and priming steps are also assumed to involve Ca^{2+}.

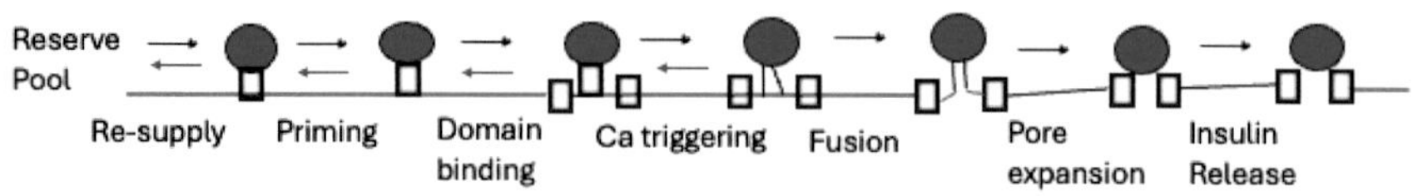

Figure 1.7 Schematic drawing of the EC proposed for pancreatic b-cells. The thick long line represents the plasma membrane of the cell, and the two shaded blocks on the membrane represent an L-type Ca^{2+}-channel where a micro-domain is formed. The state of the granule-membrane complex is schematically represented by the shape of the drawing between the granule and the membrane: state 6 consists of vesicles "docked" but not yet primed for fusion; state 5 is the primed vesicles outside the micro-domain; state 1 is the primed vesicles bound to the micro-domain; state 4 is the pre-fusion state; F represents the fused state; and R represents the insulin releasable state. The Ca^{2+}-triggering step involves the Ca^{2+} in the micro-domain, whereas both the resupply and the priming steps involve the Ca^{2+} in the cytosol.

The Ca dependency of the priming step comes from the fusion kinetic studies on chromaffin cells by Voets and colleagues, whereas that for the resupply step comes from the finding that reduction of cytosolic Ca^{2+}-concentration reduces the second phase of the insulin secretion rate (see below). The resupply and priming steps are further assumed to be modulatable by the amplifying signal or signals generated from glucose metabolism or other cellular reactions. Thus, the rate of granule fusion and insulin secretion in a beta-cell is determined not only by the Ca^{2+} surrounding L-type Ca^{2+}-channels but also by the bulk cytosolic Ca^{2+}-concentration and one or more amplifying signals from glucose metabolism. At the resting state, C_{md} is very small and all the docked granules exist essentially only in the first three pools (1, 5, and 6) in the cascade (see Table 3). The sum of the granules in these three pools is related to the total amount of insulin released in the first phase measured in a single islet. In contrast, the sum of the granules in pools 1 and 5 alone determines the total amount of fusion in the first phase measured in briefer single-cell capacitance experiments.

The simplest kinetic scheme for this EC is given in Fig. 1.8, where each step in the cascade is represented by a single chemical reaction except the Ca^{2+}-triggering step, which is described by three Ca^{2+} binding reactions as proposed for chromaffin cells. Note that the "micro-domain binding" step here corresponds to the "priming" step in the kinetic model of Voets and the "priming" step here corresponds to their "resupply" step. The kinetics of the cascade is regulated by the concentration of Ca^{2+} in the cytosol through the forward rate constant of the resupply and the priming step, as indicated in the equations $r_2 = r_2^0 C_i/[C_i + K_p]$, $r_3 = r_3^0 C_i/[C_i + K_p]$.

The three pre-triggering steps are assumed to be reversible, whereas the three post-triggering steps are assumed to be irreversible. Refinements such

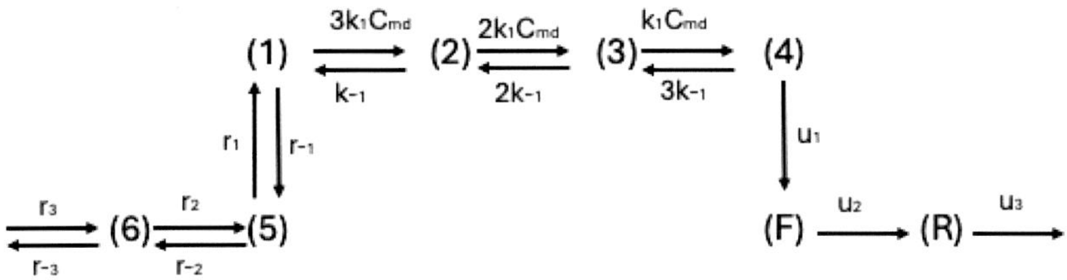

Figure 1.8 Kinetic scheme proposed for the EC in Fig. 1.7. C_{md} is the concentration of Ca^{2+} in the micro-domain.

as vesicles that bypass the docking step and go directly to fusion, the aforementioned HCSP, and kiss-and-run secretion are deferred to future iterations of the model. Note that some reports indicate that the contribution of kiss-and-run is small. Narrowing the focus results in a single feed-forward pathway that is easier to analyze and clarifies how much can be explained with the simplest model.

Due to the existence of these irreversible steps in the kinetic scheme, the model is not an equilibrium system. That is, the rates of fusion and insulin secretion of the system, defined respectively as $J_F = u_1 N_4$ and $J_{IS} = u_3 N_R$ with N_i representing the number of granules in pool i, are always nonzero, even at the resting steady state, as long as C_{md} is not 0.

The time-dependent distribution of the pool population in Fig. 1.8 after the cell is depolarized can be described by the differential equations:

$$
\begin{aligned}
\frac{dN_1}{dt} &= -[3k_1 C_{md}(t) + r_{-1}]N_1 + k_{-1}N_2 + r_1 N_5 \\
\frac{dN_2}{dt} &= 3k_1 C_{md}(t)N_1 - [2k_1 C_{md} + k_{-1}]N_2 + 2k_{-1}N_3 \\
\frac{dN_3}{dt} &= 2k_1 C_{md}(t)N_2 - [k_1 C_{md}(t) + 2k_{-1}]N_3 + 3k_{-1}N_4 \\
\frac{dN_4}{dt} &= k_1 C_{md}(t)N_3 - [3k_{-1} + u_1]N_4 \\
\frac{dN_5}{dt} &= r_{-1}N_1 - [r_1 + r_{-2}]N_5 + r_2 N_6 \\
\frac{dN_6}{dt} &= r_3 + r_{-2}N_5 + [r_{-3} + r_2]N_6 \\
\frac{dN_F}{dt} &= u_1 N_4 - u_2 N_F \\
\frac{dN_R}{dt} &= u_2 N_F - u_3 N_R
\end{aligned}
\tag{1.68}
$$

where N_i represents the number of granules in pool i in Fig. 1.8, and C_{md} is the concentration of Ca^{2+} in the microdomain compartment as described

TABLE 1.8 Kinetic Parameter values for the EC model

Parameter	Value	Parameter	Value
k_1	20 μMs^{-1}	k_{-1}	100 s^{-1}
r_1	0.6 s^{-1}	r_{-1}	1.0 s^{-1}
r_2^0	0.006 s^{-1}	r_{-2}	0.001 s^{-1}
r_3^0	1.205 s^{-1}	r_{-3}	0.0001 s^{-1}
u_1	2000 s^{-1}	u_2	3.0 s^{-1}
u_3	0.02 s^{-1}	K_p	2.3 μM

in Eq. (1.61). The resting values of the pool population as well as the Ca^{2+}-concentration in the two compartments can be obtained by solving the algebraic equations obtained by setting the left-hand side of Eqs. (1.61), (1.62), and (1.68) to 0; those equations are linear because V_m is fixed at rest. With these initial values, the time-course of the pool population can be calculated from Eqs. (1.61), (1.62), and (1.68) when an arbitrary time-dependent depolarization (such as a single pulse or a train of pulses) is applied at time 0. The rate of granule fusion and the rate of insulin secretion (in units of granules) at time t can then be evaluated from these $N_i(t)$ as

$$\begin{aligned} J_F(t) &= u_1 N_4(t) \\ J_{IS} &= u_3 N_R(t). \end{aligned} \tag{1.69}$$

Similarly, the accumulated total number of granules fused and the total amount of insulin secreted (in units of granules) can be evaluated as

$$\begin{aligned} M_F(t) &= \int_0^t u_1 N_4(t')dt' \\ M_R &= \int_0^t u_3 N_R(t')dt'. \end{aligned} \tag{1.70}$$

Both the resupply and the priming steps are assumed to depend on C_i using the simple equilibrium binding formulae

$$\begin{aligned} r_2 &= r_2^0 C_i(t)/[C_i(t) + K_p] \\ r_3 &= r_3^0 C_i(t)/[C_i(t) + K_p] \end{aligned} \tag{1.71}$$

where K_p is a constant and C_i is the concentration of Ca^{2+} in the bulk cytosol. We use the same value of K_p(=2.3 μM). There are 11 rate constants in the EC, which were determined by fitting the cell model to experimental exocytosis and secretion data, as in Table 1.8.

1.3 PATHWAYS TO DIABETES

Diabetes is by definition a state of hyperglycemia, but its natural history is diverse. For example, some individuals experience fasting hyperglycemia first

TABLE 1.9 Granule populations in different states at the steady state in Fig. 4

State	Number of granules	State	Number of granules
1	14.71	2	0.612
3	0.008	4	0
5	24.54	6	218.02
F	0.003	R	0.51

(impaired fasting glucose, IFG), followed by hyperglycemia at the 2 h time point (2hPG) of an oral glucose tolerance test (OGTT), defined as impaired glucose tolerance (IGT), and some experience these in the opposite order. Eventually, all people with diabetes will have both IFG and IGT (combined glucose impairment, CGI), so we refer to these two pathways as "IGT-first" and "IFG-first," respectively. An important implication of these observations is that the best period for determining differences in the underlying physiology of these pathways is during the prediabetic stage, when the phenotypes are still distinct.

Prediabetes is also the stage in which progression to type 2 diabetes (T2D) can be markedly delayed or prevented, and interventions can plausibly be made even more effective by targeting the specific metabolic defects of the patient. For example, IFG is generally thought to reflect insulin resistance at the liver, resulting in elevated hepatic glucose production (HGP), whereas IGT is thought to reflect peripheral insulin resistance, mainly in muscle, resulting in reduced glucose disposal. One would like to know whether using drugs that primarily affect hepatic or peripheral insulin resistance makes a material difference for patients on the IFG-first or IGT-first pathway and whether any such benefit carries over once T2D has begun.

Blood glucose levels are regulated by two negative feedback loops. In the short term, hyperglycemia stimulates a rapid increase in insulin release from the pancreatic β-cells. Chronic hyperglycemia may contribute to a second negative feedback loop by increasing the mass of insulin secreting β-cells through changes in the rates of β-cell replication and death. Type 2 diabetes has been associated with defects in components of both the short-term and chronic negative feedback loops. Minimal models of glucose regulation incorporate only glucose and/or insulin dynamics. Here we discuss a model of β-cell mass, insulin, and glucose dynamics, which consists of a system of three nonlinear ordinary differential equations, where glucose and insulin dynamics are fast relative to β-cell mass dynamics [265].

Diabetes is not a state that one enters and exits, like an infection, but a chronic condition that is the culmination of a series of gradual changes. Understanding of this progression is best obtained by longitudinal studies over a period of years or decades. A good question to ask is whether CGI is an obligatory stage between IFG and T2D and between IGT and T2D. These features of diabetes suggest that a longitudinal mathematical model for disease progression could be a valuable adjunct to clinical studies. Here we discuss such a model developed in [142] and demonstrate that it can distinguish hepatic and peripheral insulin resistance and can simulate the IGT-first and IFG-first pathways to T2D over a period of years.

1.3.1 A Model of β-Cell Mass, Insulin, and Glucose Kinetics (The βIG Model)

Although type 2 diabetes is associated with insulin resistance, insulin secretory defects, and insufficient β-cell mass, each of these defects can also be found in people without diabetes. This suggests that multiple defects are required for the onset of type 2 diabetes, it is unclear if these defects have a single but causal origin or if they occur independently. Experimental data support hypothesis that insulin resistance can cause β-cell defects, and hence diabetes, either by overworking the β-cells (β-cell exhaustion) or by toxic effects of hyperglycemia on the β cells (glucose toxicity. However, the existence of normoglycemia in humans and animals highly resistant to insulin suggests independent defects in insulin sensitivity and β-cell function are required for type 2 diabetes. Finally, hyperglycemia is known to induce insulin resistance and this supports the hypothesis that a primary insulin secretory defect that causes hyperglycemia could lead to insulin resistance and diabetes via increased glucose levels.

Minimal models and their variants have focused predominately on the dynamics of a single variable, usually blood glucose or insulin level, on a time-scale measured in minutes. Generally, these models are used as tools for measuring either rates (such as glucose production and uptake rates or insulin secretion and clearance rates) or sensitivities (such as insulin sensitivity, glucose effectiveness, or the sensitivity of insulin secretion rates to glucose). Some models have examined coupled glucose and insulin dynamics. In each of these studies, multiple parameter changes, representing multiple physiological defects, were required to simulate glucose and insulin dynamics observed in humans with diabetes. However, neither of these efforts incorporated β-cell mass dynamics. Here, we present a mathematical model of β-cell mass dynamics as a component of a coupled model of β-cell mass, insulin, and glucose dynamics. This model was developed in [265] and allows us to examine the normal behavior of the system and to investigate the effects of a single defect or a combination of defects on the behavior of the whole system. In doing so, we can find three distinct pathways to the diabetic state: regulated hyperglycemia, bifurcation and dynamical hyperglycemia.

GLUCOSE DYNAMICS: glucose dynamics are modeled with a single-compartment mass balance equation

$$\frac{dG}{dt} = \text{Production} - \text{Uptake}, \tag{1.72}$$

where G is the concentration of glucose in the blood (measured in $mgdl^{-1}$), and t the time (measured in days). The rates of glucose production and uptake are normalized by the volume of glucose distribution to obtain the proper units ($mgdl^{-1}d^{-1}$). The rates of glucose production and uptake depend on blood glucose and insulin levels. These relationships have been defined experimentally with the glucose clamp technique, which allows for the measurement of glucose production and uptake rates at various steady-state blood glucose and insulin levels (Bergman et al., 1985). At constant insulin levels, glucose production decreases while uptake increases, both linearly with respect to glucose levels. The slopes of these linear dependences are the "glucose effectiveness" parameters. Hyperinsulinemic clamp studies have shown that the glucose effectiveness parameters are linearly related to blood insulin levels. The slope of the glucose effectiveness vs. insulin curve is referred to as insulin sensitivity. Thus,

$$\text{Production } = P_0 - (E_{G0P} + S_{IP}I(t))G(t) \tag{1.73}$$

$$\text{Uptake } = U_0 - (E_{G0U} + S_{IU}I(t))G(t) \tag{1.74}$$

where P_0 and U_0 are the rates of glucose production and uptake at zero glucose ($mgdl^{-1}d^{-1}$), E_{G0P} and E_{G0U} (d^{-1}) are glucose effectiveness at zero insulin for production and uptake, S_{IP}, S_{IU} ($\mu U^{-1}mld^{-1}$) are insulin sensitivity for production and uptake, and I represents blood insulin concentrations ($\mu U/ml$). Using Eqs. (1.72)–(1.74), we arrive at

$$\frac{dG(t)}{dt} = R_0 - (E_{G0} + S_I I(t))G(t) \tag{1.75}$$

where R_0 is the net rate of production at zero glucose, E_{G0} is the total glucose effectiveness at zero insulin, and S_I is the total insulin sensitivity.

INSULIN DYNAMICS: Insulin is secreted by pancreatic b cells, cleared by the liver, kidneys, and insulin receptors, and distributed into several compartments (e.g. portal vein, peripheral blood, and interstitial fluid). Our main concern is the long-time evolution of fasting insulin levels in peripheral blood. Since the dynamics of fasting insulin levels on this time-scale are slow, we use a single-compartment equation given by

$$\frac{dI}{dt} = \text{Secretion} - \text{Clearance}, \tag{1.76}$$

where Secretion and Clearance are rates normalized by insulin's volume of distribution ($kUml^{-1}d^{-1}$). The rate of insulin clearance is proportional to blood insulin levels when the system is near steady state. Given the relatively slow dynamics in the present model, we assume

$$\text{Clearance } = kI, \tag{1.77}$$

where k is a clearance constant which represents the combined insulin uptake at the liver, kidneys, and insulin receptors (d^{-1}). The in vitro relationship determined by existing literature indicate that the net insulin secretion rate can be modeled as a sigmoidal function of glucose level. Hence, we assume

$$\text{Secretion } = \frac{\beta\sigma G^2}{\alpha + G^2}, \tag{1.78}$$

where β is the mass of pancreatic β-cells (measured in mg). All β cells are assumed to secrete insulin at the same maximal rate σ ($\mu Uml^{-1}day^{-1}$), and $G^2/(\alpha + G^2)$ is a Hill function with coefficient 2 that describes a sigmoid ranging from 0 to 1 which reaches half its maximum at $G = \alpha^{1/2}$. Substituting Eqs. (1.76) and (1.77) into Eq. (1.78), we obtain the equation governing insulin kinetics,

$$\frac{dI(t)}{dt} = \beta\sigma \frac{G^2(t)}{a^2 + G^2(t))} - kI(t). \tag{1.79}$$

β-CELL MASS DYNAMICS: Despite a complex distribution of pancreatic β cells throughout the pancreas, β-cell mass dynamics have been successfully quantified with a single-compartment model

$$\frac{d\beta}{dt} = \text{Formation} - \text{ Loss}, \tag{1.80}$$

where Formation and Loss represent the rates at which β-cell mass is added to or removed from the population, respectively. New β cells can be formed by the replication of existing b cells, neogenesis (replication and differentiation) from stem cells, and transdifferentiation of other cells. Presently, it is not possible to quantify rates of neogenesis and transdifferentiation. However, calculations suggest indirectly that they make a negligible contribution to β-cell mass dynamics except during development and in response to extreme physiological or chemically induced trauma. For these reasons, neogenesis and transdifferentiation are not incorporated into the present model, and Formation is assumed to be equal to replication. In vitro studies show that the percentage of β cells undergoing replication varies as a nonlinear function of glucose level in the medium. Replication rates for b cells increase with increasing glucose. levels; however, at extreme hyperglycemia, β cell replication may be reduced. We modeled this behavior with a simple second-degree polynomial (patterned after logistic growth),

$$\text{Replication } = (r_{1r}G(t) - r_{2r}G^2(t))\beta \tag{1.81}$$

where $r_{1r}(mg^{-1}dlday^{-1})$ and $r_{2r}(mg^{-2}dl^2day^{-1})$ are rate constants.

Cells can be lost from the b-cell mass by apoptosis (regulated cell death), necrosis (unregulated cell death), or possibly transdifferentiation into other types of endocrine cells. For the model presented here, the rate of transdifferentiation is assumed to be negligible. In vitro, β-cell Death has been shown to vary nonlinearly with glucose. Increasing the glucose level from 0 to approximately 11 mM in the medium surrounding cultured β cells reduced the rate of β-cell death. Above 11 mM glucose, the rate of β-cell death either remained low or increased. We have modeled this behavior with a simple second degree polynomial,

$$\text{Death } = (-d_0 + r_{1a}G(t) - r_{2a}G^2(t))\beta \tag{1.82}$$

TABLE 1.10 Normal parameter values

Parameter	Value	Units	Reference
S_I	0.72	$ml\mu U^{-1}d^{-1}$	Finegood (1997)
E_{G0}	1.44	d^{-1}	Bergman et al. (1981)
R_0	864	$mgdl^{-1}d^{-1}$	Bergman et al. (1981)
σ	43.2	$\mu Uml^{-1}d^{-1}$	Bergman et al. (1981)
α	20000	mg^2dl^{-2}	Malaise et al. (1967)
k	432	d^{-1}	Toffolo (1997)
d_0	0.06	d^{-1}	Bergman et al. (1981)
r_1	0.84×10^{-3}	$mg^{-1}dld^{-1}$	Bergman et al. (1981)
r_2	0.24×10^{-5}	$mg^{-2}dl^2d^{-1}$	Bergman et al. (1981)

where $d_0(d^1)$ is the death rate at zero glucose and $r_{1a}(mg^{-1}dld^{-1})$ and $r_{2a}(mg^{-2}dl^2d^{-1})$ are constants. Substituting eqns (1.81) and (1.82) into eqn (1.80), we obtain the equation for b-cell mass dynamics,

$$\frac{d\beta(t)}{dt} = (-d_0 + r_1G(t) - r_2G^2(t))\beta \tag{1.83}$$

where $r_1(= r_{1r} - r_{1a})$ and $r_2(= r_{2r} - r_{2a})$ are constants. In summary, the βIG model is comprised of eqns (1.75), (1.79), and (1.83). Parameter values assumed for the normal human physiological state are given in Table 1.7. Below, we examine both the behavior of solutions of the βIG model in the phase space of the variables using the standard parameter values (Table 1.10), and the change in geometrical structure of the solutions in the phase space as the parameter values are varied. Finally, we postulate some plausible pathways that lead from a normal physiological state to a pathological diabetic state.

1.3.2 Long-Term Models

In this section, we introduce a longitudinal mathematical model [142] that is capable of representing the metabolic state of an individual at any point in time during their progression from normal glucose tolerance to type 2 diabetes (T2D) over a period of years. This long term model is built on the previous OGTT model in section 1.1.3 and the kinetic model for insulin secretion in section 1.2.2.2.

The core element, retained in the new version, is a glucose-insulin feedback loop, represented by two differential equations:

$$\frac{dG(t)}{dt} = MEAL + HGP - (E_{G0} + S_I I(t))G(t)) \tag{1.84}$$

$$\frac{dI(t)}{dt} = \left(\frac{\beta}{V}ISR - kI(t)\right) \tag{1.85}$$

TABLE 1.11 Parameter values for MEAL

Parameter	Value	Description	Units
$meal_{max}$	11.055	Maximum meal rate	$mg/dl/min$
mk	4	degree of polynomial	unitless
α_{meal}	40	half activation rate	unitless
η	0.3	exponet of rise for meal flux	unitless
μ	−0.015	rate of decay for meal flux	*unitless*

Modeling glucose flux during daily meals and glucose tolerance tests. In the previous version of the OGTT model, G represented average daily glucose and insulin levels in response to steady glucose input. To address IFG and IGT, we need to be able to dissociate fasting glucose from post-challenge glucose. The first step is to introduce variable glucose influx from meals, represented by the term MEAL in Eq. (1.84). Timing of meals is standardized to 6:00 AM, 12:00 noon, and 6:00 PM. The expression we use is

$$MEAL = \text{meal}_{max} \left(\frac{t^{mk}}{\alpha_{meal} + t^{mk}} \right)^{\eta} \exp(-\mu t). \tag{1.86}$$

Parameters values in (1.86) are listed in Table 1.11.

We do not yet account for other nutrients (amino acids, fats). Flux during an OGTT is modeled with a more rapid rise and decay of flux. Flux during an IVGTT rises and decays still more rapidly.

Modeling hepatic glucose production. To distinguish peripheral and hepatic insulin resistance and describe how they are related to each other, we need to refine the model description of hepatic glucose production (HGP in Eq. (1.84)). In the OGTT version of the model (1.10), HGP was assumed to be constant, which is an acceptable approximation as long as fasting plasma insulin is adequate to compensate completely for any hepatic insulin resistance. To study the failure of compensation, however, we need to make HGP a decreasing function of I:

$$HGP = \frac{hepa_{max}}{\alpha_{HGP} + hepa_{S_I} I} + HGP_{bas}. \tag{1.87}$$

This is sufficient to give the typical drop and recovery of HGP after a meal. Less obvious, but also important, we need to account for the correlation between hepatic and peripheral insulin resistance, which we do by making two of the parameters in Eq. (1.87) $hepa_{max}$ and α_{HGP}, functions of S_I:

$$hepa_{max} = \frac{hepa_{bar}}{hepa_k + S_I} + hepa_{sh} \tag{1.88}$$

$$\alpha_{HGP} = \frac{\alpha_{bar}}{\alpha_k + S_I} + \alpha_{sh}. \tag{1.89}$$

TABLE 1.12 Parameter values for HGP

Parameter	Value	Description	Units
HGP_{bas}	0.104	Basal HGP rate	$mg/dl/min$
$hepa_{bar}$	15.443	Coefficient of $hepa_{max}$	$10^{-4}min(mg/dl/min)$
$hepa_k$	0.27	Translation of $hepa_{max}$	$10^{-4}ml/\mu U/min$
$hepa_{sh}$	−3.542	shift of $hepa_{max}$	$(\mu U/ml)(mg/dl/min)$
α_{bar}	6	Coefficient of α_{max}	$10^{-4}/min$
α_k	0.4	Translation of α_{max}	$10^{-4}ml/\mu U/min$
α_{sh}	−0.5	shift of α_{max}	$\mu U/ml$

Both $hepa_{max}$ and α_{HGP} decrease with S_I, and the net effect is that HGP decreases as S_I increases.

If this, or something like this, is not done, then severe peripheral resistance combined with strong compensatory insulin secretion can result in fasting hypoglycemia, which is not the typical pattern.

In more typical cases of progression to prediabetes or diabetes, the relative impairment in insulin secretion would mask this effect: the level of glycemia would be reduced, but hypoglycemia would not result. We chose the parameters such that HGP remains normal when insulin is elevated unless there is a defect in beta-cell mass or function.

To represent hepatic insulin resistance over and above the component related to peripheral insulin resistance, we decrease the parameter $hepa_{SI}$ in Eq. (1.87), which increases HGP at any value of I. Equations (1.87)–(1.89) are phenomenological expressions that achieve the goals of making HGP decrease with I and increase when insulin resistance is present, but other expressions could also possibly work. One considered making the value of $hepa_{S_I}$ depend on I as an alternative way to avoid hypoglycemia, but this did not work well. It is also possible that glucagon, which is not in the model, would help to prevent hypoglycemia.

Parameter values in (1.87)–(1.89) are listed in Table 1.12.

To study the dynamics of glucose and insulin under glucose challenges such as meals, OGTT, and IVGTT, the model needs to account for the multiple kinetic components of insulin secretion. We adapted an existing model of insulin granule exocytosis discussed in section 1.2.2.2, which was designed to capture the biphasic pattern of ISR in response to a glucose step in vitro or a hyperglycemic clamp in vivo. The first phase is characterized by a sharp peak of ISR during the first 10 min and the second phase by a steady increase of ISR over the next hour.

The exocytosis model requires as input the cytosolic Ca^{2+} concentration, which is modeled as a sigmoidal function of the beta-cell metabolic rate M (Eq. (1.90)), and the much higher Ca^{2+} concentration in the microdomains of Ca^{2+} channels, which is modeled as a function of cytosolic Ca^{2+} (Eq. 1.91). The dose-response curve shift, previously included in (1.12), represents the

TABLE 1.13 Parameter values for Ca^{2+} and Microdomain

Parameter	Value	Description	Units
$C_{i,max}$	2	maximum Ca^{2+}	μM
kC_i	4	Exponent of sigmoidal function	unitless
α_{C_i}	0.62	half activation value	unitless
$C_{i,b}$	0.07	Basal calcium	μM
$C_{md,max}$	150	maximum C_{md}	μM
kC_{md}	4	Exponent of sigmoidal function	unitless
$\alpha_{C_{md}}$	1	half activation value	unitless
$C_{md,b}$	0.0635	Basal microdomain calcium	μM

TABLE 1.14 Parameter values for amplifying factor

Parameter	Value	Description	Units
$G_{F,max}$	4.45	maximum value	unitless
kG_F	16	Exponent of sigmoidal function	unitless
α_{G_F}	260	half activation value	mg/dl
$G_{F,sh}$	−89	Shift of glucose	$/mg/dl$
$G_{F,b}$	1.78	Basal G_F	unitless

dynamic changes in KATP channel density as before but now explicitly alters cytosolic Ca^{2+} at a given level of M (Eq. 1.90):

$$C_i = \frac{C_{i,max}(M+\gamma)^{kC_i}}{\alpha_{C_i}^{kC_i} + (M+\gamma)^{kC_i}} + C_{i,b} \tag{1.90}$$

M and γ are as in (1.12) and (1.13).

$$C_{md} = \frac{C_{md,max}(C_i)^{kC_{md}}}{\alpha_{C_{md}}^{kC_{md}} + (C_i)^{kC_{md}}} + C_{md,b} \tag{1.91}$$

The parameters in (1.90) and (1.91) are listed in Table 1.13.

The amplifying effect of glucose is incorporated as a multiplicative factor in the rate of vesicle mobilization (G_F in Eq. (1.92)):

$$G_F = \frac{G_{F,max}(G - G_{F,sh})^{kG_F}}{\alpha_{G_F}^{kG_F} + (G - G_{F,sh})^{kG_F}} + G_{F,b} \tag{1.92}$$

The effect of the incretin GLP-1 and drugs that mimic it to increase insulin secretion is modeled as enhancing the amplifying effect of glucose by increasing the parameter G_{Fmax} in Eq. (1.92). This is in accord with a key feature of these agonists, that they have little or no effect on secretion in the absence of glucose, minimizing the risk of hypoglycemia that plagues sulfonylureas. Modeling the effect of incretins on glucose is more difficult, as it would require including their effects to inhibit glucagon secretion or promote weight loss, which is not feasible in the present model.

Modeling insulin granule exocytosis. We adapt the model discussed in section 1.2.2.2, which was designed to capture the biphasic pattern of ISR in response to a glucose step in vitro or a hyperglycemic clamp in vivo. The first phase is characterized by a sharp peak of ISR during the first 10 min and the second phase by a steady increase of ISR over the next hour. These phases are mediated by progression of vesicles through a sequence of stages culminating in exocytosis (fusion with the plasma membrane and release of insulin to the circulation). A large reserve pool, treated as an inexhaustible reservoir, feeds the docked pool (vesicles at binding sites on the plasma membrane). Once docked, vesicles are primed and enter the readily releasable pool (RRP). Primed vesicles join the immediately releasable pool by becoming closely associated with voltage-dependent Ca^{2+} channels. First-phase secretion depends mainly on the size of the RRP at basal glucose, and second-phase secretion is controlled by the rate of mobilization of vesicles to the docked pool.

$$
\begin{aligned}
N_{1C} &= \frac{km_1}{3k_1C_{md} + rm_1} \\
N_{1D} &= \frac{r_1}{3k_1C_{md} + rm_1} \\
N_{2E} &= \frac{3k_1C_{md}}{2k_1C_{md} + km_1} \\
N_{2F} &= \frac{2km_1}{2k_1C_{md} + km_1} \\
N_{3L} &= \frac{2k_1C_{md}}{k_1C_{md} + 2km_1} \\
N_{3N} &= \frac{2km_1}{k_1C_{md} + 2km_1} \\
C_{N4} &= \frac{k_1C_{md}}{3km_1 + u_1} \\
C_{N3} &= \frac{N_{3L}}{1 - N_{3N}C_{N4}} \\
C_{N2} &= \frac{N_{2E}}{1 - N_{2F}C_{N3}} \\
C_{N1} &= \frac{N_{1D}}{1 - N_{1C}C_{N2}} \\
\frac{dN_5}{dt} &= t_s(rm_1C_{N1}N_5 - (r_1 + rm_2)N_5 + r_2N_6) \\
\frac{dN_6}{dt} &= t_s(r_3 + rm_2N_5 - (r_2 + rm_3)N_6)
\end{aligned}
\tag{1.93}
$$

where the rate of mobilization of insulin granules, r_3, is modified to include a component of β-cell function, σ, and a glucose amplifying factor G_F that is

TABLE 1.15 Kinetic Parameter values for the exocytosis model

Parameter	Value	Parameter	Value
k_1	20 μMs^{-1}	km_1	100 s^{-1}
r_1	0.6 s^{-1}	rm_1	1.0 s^{-1}
r_2^0	0.006 s^{-1}	rm_2	0.001 s^{-1}
r_3^0	1.205 s^{-1}	rm_3	0.0001 s^{-1}
u_1	2000 s^{-1}	u_2	3.0 s^{-1}
u_3	0.02 s^{-1}	k_{p2}	2.3 μM
t_s	60 $s \cdot min^{-1}$	ρ	9 $\mu M/mg$

modeled by a Hill function (1.92);

$$r_3 = \sigma G_F r_3^0 \frac{C_i}{C_i + k_{p2}} \tag{1.94}$$

and σ is determined by (1.15).

Equations of the exocytosis model, simplified from section 1.2.2.2 by setting fast steps N1 – N4 to steady state:

$$\begin{aligned} N_1 &= C_{N1} N_5 \\ N_2 &= C_{N2} N_1 \\ N_3 &= C_{N3} N_2 \\ N_4 &= C_{N4} N_3 \\ N_F &= u_1 N_4 / u_2 \\ N_R &= u_2 N_F / u_3 \\ r_2 &= r_2^0 \frac{C_i}{C_i + k_{p2}} \\ ISR &= \rho t_s u_3 N_R \end{aligned} \tag{1.95}$$

The insulin secretion rate ISR is in the long term version no longer a function of glucose but is calculated as an output of the exocytosis model ISR thus now depends on the history of exposure to G, as it should, not just the current value. The parameters for the exocytosis model are listed in Table 1.15.

Dynamics of peripheral and hepatic insulin resistance. Both peripheral insulin sensitivity, S_I, and hepatic insulin resistance, $hepa_{S_I}$, are modeled as decreasing exponentially to target levels tar_{S_I} and $tar_{hepa_{SI}}$ with time constants τ_{SI} and $\tau_{hepa_{SI}}$, respectively.

$$\frac{dS_I}{dt} = \frac{tar_{S_I} - S_I}{\tau_{S_I}} \tag{1.96}$$

$$\frac{dhepa_{S_I}}{dt} = \frac{tar_{hepa_{SI}} - hepa_{S_I}}{\tau_{hepa_{SI}}} \tag{1.97}$$

Insulin Resistance Induced by Insulin

TABLE 1.16 Parameter values for induced insulin resistance

Parameter	Value	Units
τ_E	2880	min(2 days)
$\bar{E}$	0.5	unitless
I_{sh}	5	$\mu Ug/ml$
kE	4	
α_E	$5 - 300$	$\mu Ug/ml$
E_b	0.5	unitless

We model the hypothesized effect of insulin to induce insulin resistance beyond the core component governed by intrinsic insulin signaling in the target tissues by the following equations:

$$S_I = S_{I,0}E$$

where

$$\frac{dS_{I,0}}{dt} = \frac{tar_{S_I} - S_{I,0}}{\tau_{S_I}}$$

and

$$\frac{dE}{dt} = \frac{E_\infty(I) - E}{\tau_E}$$

where $E_\infty(I)$ takes the form:

$$E_\infty(I) = \bar{E}\left(I - \frac{(I - I_{sh})^{kE}}{\alpha_E^{kE} + (I - I_{sh})^{kE}}\right) + E_b$$

The parameter values are listed in Table 1.16.

1.3.3 Mathematical Analysis and Simulation of the βIG Model and Long-Term Models

In this section, we are going to analyze the βIG model and present results of the Long-Term model.

1.3.3.1 *Analysis of the βIG Model*

The βIG model consisting of Eqs. (1.75), (1.79), and (1.83) is the special case of the stochastic model (1.117) proposed in section 1.6.2 with $\alpha_1 = 0$ and $\alpha_2 = 0$, hence the existence and uniqueness of solution for the βIG model follows from Theorem 1.25 in section 1.6.2.

The βIG model can be decomposed into fast (G, I) and slow β subsystems. The fast subsystem describes acute changes of glucose and insulin levels on a time-scale of minutes while the slow subsystem describes evolution of the β-cell mass on a time-scale of days. We will examine the behavior of these subsystems independently and then analyze the system as a whole, while all parameters are assumed to be the normal values listed in Table 1.10.

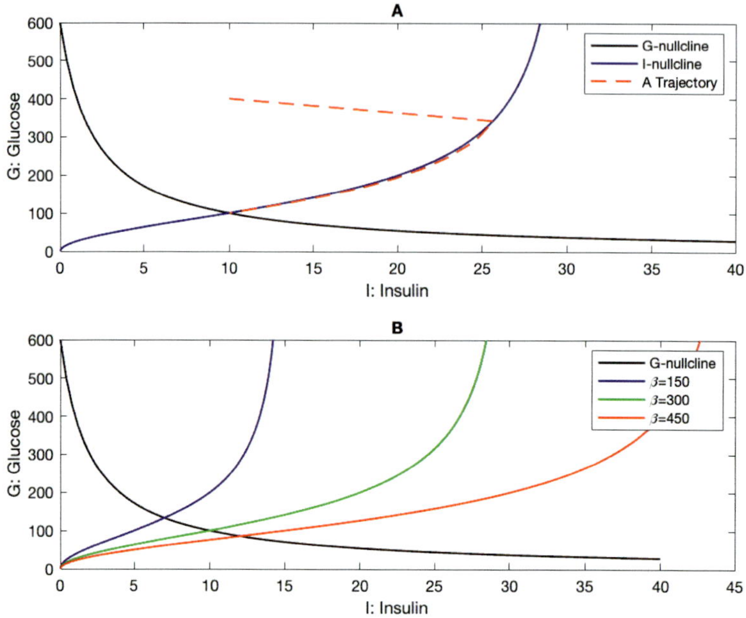

Figure 1.9 Global behavior of the fast subsystem. (A) β cell mass is fixed at 300 $mg\ dl^{-1}$. Shown are the glucose nullcline, the insulin nullcline, and a simulation of the response of the fast subsystem to a bolus injection of glucose (red dashed curve). Stability analysis shows that the fixed point, located at the intersection of the glucose and insulin nullclines, is a globally attractive stable spiral. (B) The glucose nullcline and three insulin nullclines are shown for $\beta = 150, 300$, and 450. As the β cell mass increases, the fixed point of the fast subsystem moves to lower glucose and higher insulin levels, but the global behavior remains unchanged.

Due to its slow dynamics, β-cell mass will be treated as a parameter when analyzing the fast subsystem. From the nullclines (dG/dt=0 and dI/dt=0) for a given normal β-cell mass value and a local and global stability analysis of the steady-state solution, we find that the fast subsystem has a single globally attracting stable spiral point [Fig. 1.9(a)]. The effect of β-cell mass on the behavior of the fast subsystem is demonstrated in Fig. 1.9(b). For each β-cell mass value, there is a single globally attracting fixed point. This fixed point is shifted to lower glucose and higher insulin level as increases. In summary, for any initial condition, blood glucose and insulin levels will undergo a damped oscillation in time settling down to a steady which is dependent on the β-cell mass.

To study the slow subsystem, we assume that the fast subsystem is at a steady state and changes in the β-cell mass slowly shift that steady state.

The one-dimensional slow subsystem (1.83), has three steady-state solutions, which we index by $\beta = 0, G = 100$, and $G = 250$. These three steady states will be referred to as the pathological, physiological, and unstable steady states, respectively.

The behavior of the slow subsystem is best described using a plot of the β-cell replication and death rates, eqns (1.81) and (1.82), as functions of glucose levels as shown in Fig. 1.10. This graph can be divided into three zones of behavior. In Zone I (hypoglycemia), death rates are greater than replication rates and the -cell mass decreases which causes glucose levels to rise. Thus, glucose is regulated back to the physiological fixed point. In Zone II (mild hyperglycemia), replication rates are greater than death rates, and the -cell mass increases, causing glucose levels to decrease. Thus, glucose is again regulated back to the physiological steady state. Taken together, Zones I and II constitute a basin of regulation to the physiological steady state. However, in Zone III (extreme hyperglycemia), death rates exceed replication rates, thereby driving glucose levels even higher. This positive feedback loop drives the system to the pathological steady state corresponding to zero -cell mass and extreme hyperglycemia. For this reason, Zone III is referred to as a basin of dysregulation or a basin of regulation to a pathological state. In summary, the slow subsystem has two stable steady states and an unstable steady state that divides the basins of attraction for the two stable points.

Analyzing the system as a whole, the βIG model has three steady-state solutions in (β, I, G): a stable spiral (300, 10, 100) at which the eigen values of the Jacobian matrix are $\lambda_1 = -421.9669, \lambda_2 = -18.6588$, and $\lambda_3 = -0.01422$,a saddle point (37, 2.8, 250) at which the eigenvalues of the Jacobian matrix are $\lambda_1 = -431.01196, \lambda_2 = -4.484590$, and $\lambda_3 = 0.04055$, and a stable node (0, 0, 600) at which the eigenvalues of the Jacobian matrix are $\lambda_1 = -0.42, \lambda_2 = -1.44$, and $\lambda_3 = -432$. These points correspond to the physiological fixed point, the saddle point, and the pathological fixed point of the slow subsystem, respectively. The two-dimensional glucose and insulin null surfaces are attractive and their intersection forms a one-dimensional slow manifold. All solutions move quickly along trajectories which are approximately perpendicular to the β-cell mass axis onto the slow manifold, and then move along this slow manifold according to the β-cell mass dynamics. There are three β -cell mass null surfaces, namely, the planes defined by $G = 100, 250\ mg\ dl^{-1}$, and $\beta = 0$. A projection of the slow manifold and the β-cell mass nullsurfaces onto the G and β-plane is given in Fig. 1.11. For all points above $G = 250\ mg\ dl^{-1}$ and below $G = 100\ mg\ dl^{-1}$, the β-cell mass is decreasing and for all points between these planes, the mass is increasing. The steady-state saddle point solution divides this slow manifold into two parts. In the upper part, β is decreasing and all solutions move toward the pathological fixed point, whereas in the lower part the β-cell mass dynamics drive all solutions toward the physiological fixed point (Fig. 1.11). Due to the fast glucose and insulin dynamics, the global separatrix can be approximated by a plane that is perpendicular to the β-cell axis and passes through the saddle point.

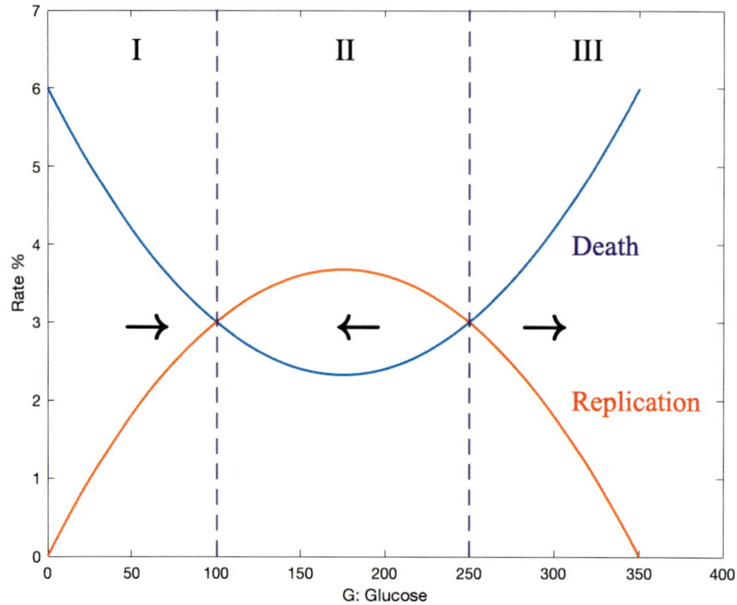

Figure 1.10 Global behavior of the slow subsystem. Replication and death rates are plotted against blood glucose levels. These curves intersect at two non-trivial steady states, a physiological fixed point and a saddle point. In addition, there is a pathological, trivial steady state at $\beta = 0$. In Zone I, death rates exceed replication rates, driving β-cell mass down and causing the steady-state glucose level to rise. In Zone II, replication rates exceed death rates driving β-cel mass up and the blood glucose level down. Zones I and II constitute a basin of attraction for the physiological fixed point. In Zone III, death exceeds replication, causing a decrease in -cell mass and driving the glucose level even higher. This is a zone of pathological regulation, in which the system is driven to the trivial steady state of zero-β-cell mass.

This plane then divides the phase space into two basins of attraction, one for the physyioogical fixed point and one for the pathological fixed point. The fast subsystem solution quickly comes to a steady state at the initial β-cell mass, then this steady-state solution is driven by the β-cell mass dynamics to either the physiological or pathological steady state.

Effects of Parameter Changes on Global Behavior: The number of non-trivial steady-state solutions is determined by the parameters of the β-cell mass equation, while the position of these fixed points is determined by all nine-dimensional parameters. The trivial steady-state solution is fixed at zero

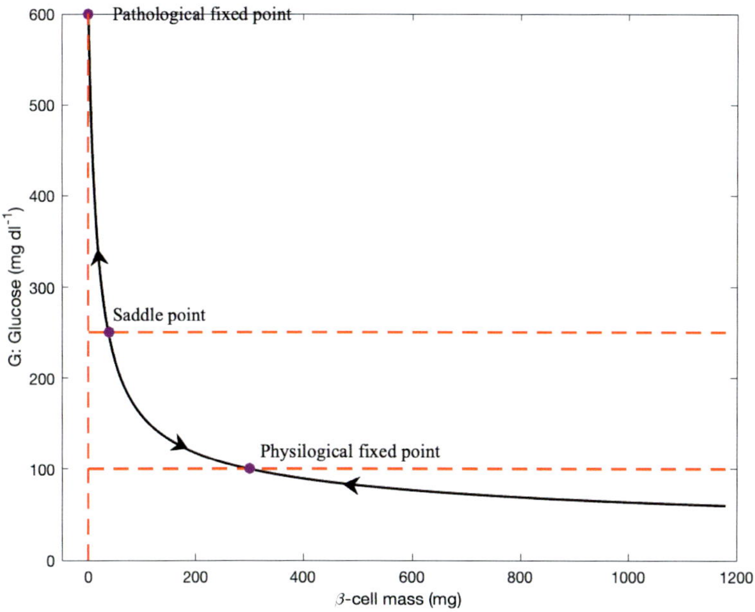

Figure 1.11 Global behavior of the βIG model. Plotted here is a projection of the slow manifold and the β-cell mass null surfaces onto the G and β plane. In terms of the variables (β, I, G), the system has three steady states: physiological (300, 10, 100) and pathological (0, 0, 600) fixed points, and a saddle point at (37, 2.8, 250). All solutions travel on trajectories approximately perpendicular to the -cell mass axis onto the slow manifold, then move along the slow manifold according to β-cell mass dynamics. The derivative dβ /dt is negative for all points below the G=100 null surface, and above the G=250 null surface and it is positive between the non-trivial β-cell mass null surfaces. The saddle point divides the slow manifold into two basins of attraction, one for each of the physiological and pathological fixed points.

β-cell mass and insulin, but has a steady-state glucose level that is dependent on the glucose parameters (R_0, E_{G0}).

(1)*DEFECTS IN GLUCOSE DYNAMICS*: Defects in insulin sensitivity, represented by a reduced S_I, decrease the curvature of the glucose nullcline and thus, the slow manifold. This forces the physiological and saddle points to shift to higher β-cell mass and insulin levels, but does not affect the number of fixed points or the glucose levels at any of these fixed points. Thus, the long-term effects of non-progressive insulin resistance are hyperinsulinemia, β-cell hyperplasia, and normoglycemia.

(2) *DEFECTS IN INSULIN DYNAMICS*: An increase in the insulin clearance rate or a decrease in the insulin secretion rate per active cell, modeled by an increase in k or a decrease in σ, respectively, compresses the insulin null surface along the direction of the insulin axis. This changes the curvature of the slow manifold, thereby shifting the physiological and saddle points to higher -cell mass values.

(3) *DEFECTS IN β-CELL MASS DYNAMICS*: Defects in β-cell replication and/or death rates, represented by an increase in d_0 or r_2 or by a decrease in r_1, cause the non-trivial β-cell mass null surfaces ($G = 100$ and $250\ mg\ dl^{-1}$) to move closer together along the direction of the glucose axis. The physiological fixed point shifts to a point with higher glucose, lower insulin, and lower β-cell mass, while the saddle point shifts to a point with lower glucose, higher insulin, and higher β-cell mass, increasing the volume of the basin of pathological attraction. If a defect in the β-cell mass parameters progresses to the point where death rates exceed replication rates at all glucose levels, then there is only one steady-state solution, namely the globally attractive pathological steady state with zero-cell mass. Although the relationship between plasma glucose levels and mild defects in β-cell replication and/or death rates has not been determined in vivo, a large increase in the β-cell death rate has been shown to drive β-cell mass toward zero and generate extreme hyperglycemia. In summary, the -cell mass parameters determine the number of fixed points, as well as the glucose levels at the physiological and saddle points, when they exist.

Pathways into Diabetes: If we define diabetes as persistent hyperglycemia, then there are three general pathways into diabetes according to the βIG model: (1) move the physiological fixed point to a hyperglycemic level, (2) eliminate the physiological and saddle points, and (3) drive a trajectory across the separatrix. These pathways into diabetes will be referred to as regulated hyperglycemia, bifurcation, and dynamical hyperglycemia (or catch and pass), respectively.

(1) *REGULATED HYPERGLYCEMIA*: Defects in β-cell mass regulation can shift the physiological fixed point to a hyperglycemic level. Since steady-state glucose levels are determined by β-cell mass dynamics, there are two possible ways to shift the physiological fixed point to a hyperglycemic level: (1) a defect in β-cell mass regulation, or (2) a loss of β-cell mass regulation combined with a defect in glucose and/or insulin dynamics. Small defects in any of the β-cell mass parameters, for example a decrease in the response of replication and/or an increase in the response of death rates to glucose, cause the physiological fixed point to shift to a hyperglycemic level [Fig. 1.12]. The β-cell mass is responsive to changes in plasma glucose concentrations and has a basin of physiological attraction, but the physiologically regulated glucose level is now hyperglycemic. A second way to shift the physiological fixed point to a hyperglycemic level is to couple a loss of β-cell mass regulation to an abnormality in glucose and/or insulin dynamics. Setting each of the β-cell mass parameters to zero yields equal replication and death rates at all

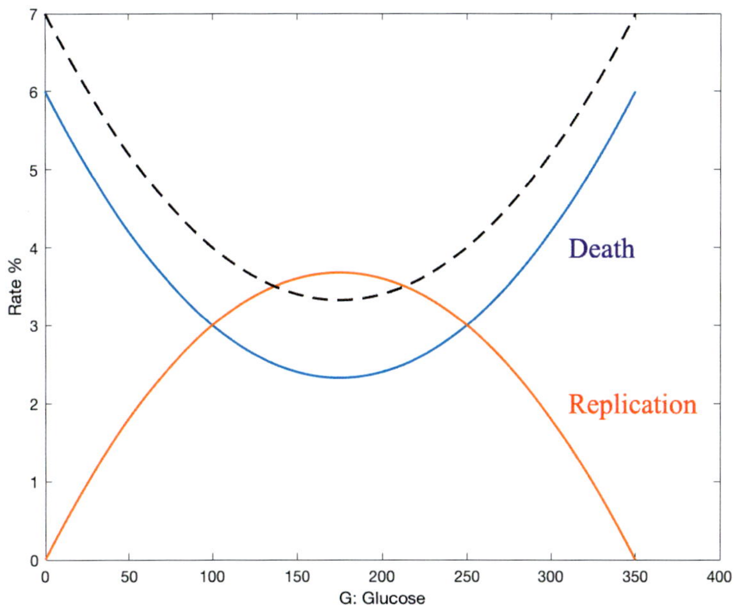

Figure 1.12 A small upward shift of the death rate curve (——-) moves the physiological fixed point to a higher glucose level and shrinks the basin of physiological attraction.

glucose levels, and as a result, the β-cell mass becomes non-responsive. In this situation, the βIG model reduces to the two-dimensional fast subsystem, and defects in any of the glucose or insulin parameters can generate hyperglycemia.

(2)*BIFURCATION*: The bifurcation pathway consists of any combination of parameter changes that result in the elimination of the physiological and saddle fixed points. Large defects in β-cell mass dynamics cause a saddle-node bifurcation, resulting in the single globally attractive pathological fixed point at zero β-cell mass. This occurs when death rates exceed replication rates at all glucose levels (Fig. 1.13). A bifurcation diagram is shown in Fig. 1.14. The dashed line in Fig. 1.14 represents the saddle point while the solid lines represent the two stable fixed points. As r_1 decreases to r_{1c}, the saddle and physiological points move closer together, eventually meeting at a saddle-node bifurcation; so for values of $r_1 < r_{1c}$, there only exists the pathological fixed point. At $r_1 = 0.0015 dlmg^{-1}$, a transcritical bifurcation occurs, involving the saddle point and the pathological fixed point. For larger r_1, the basin of physiological attraction grows to encompass all physiological initial conditions, while the basin of pathological attraction encompasses initial conditions with negative insulin and β-cell mass. Similar bifurcation diagrams can be generated

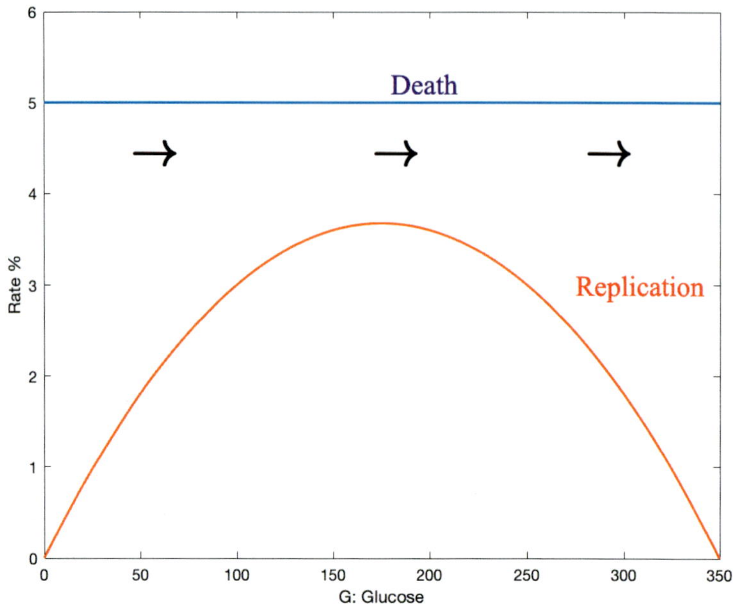

Figure 1.13 Bifurcation. Large changes in the replication and/or death curves results in a situation where the death rate exceeds the replication rate for all glucose levels. Here the physiological and saddle points are eliminated. As the -cell mass falls, insulin levels fall, and glucose levels are driven up. Under these conditions the system has a single globally attractive pathological fixed point at zero β-cell mass.

for r_2 and d_0. The saddle-node bifurcation pathway outlined above resembles type 1 diabetes mellitus. An autoimmune attack on the pancreatic cells increases death rates above replication rates for all glucose levels, and the β-cell mass alls toward zero.

(3) *DYNAMICAL HYPERGLYCEMIA*: Dynamical hyperglycemia, also referred to as the "catch and pass" pathway, is a race between the actual β-cell mass and the location of the β-cell mass required to maintain normal glucose levels as parameters change. Defects in glucose and/or insulin dynamics increase the β-cell mass required to maintain the glucose level at the physiological fixed point. A defect manifests itself as a change in one of these parameters which generates a transient state where the β-cell mass is unable to secrete enough insulin to maintain normal blood glucose levels. Hyperglycemia persists while the β -cell mass adapts. A time-dependent shift in one or more of these parameters results in a race between a progressive defect, which drives glucose levels up, and β-cell mass adaptation, which drives glucose levels down.

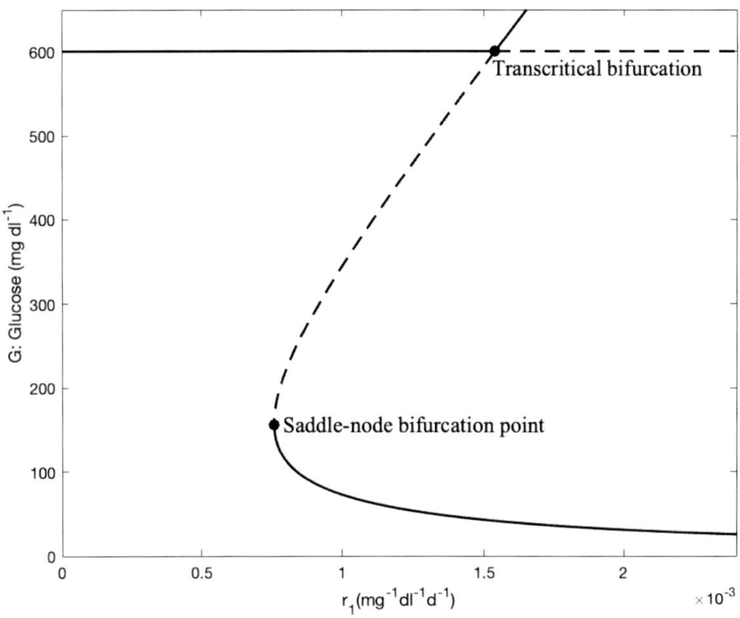

Figure 1.14 Bifurcation diagram. The glucose levels of the stable fixed points and the saddle point (- - - - -) are plotted as functions of the parameter r_1. Keeping all other parameters fixed, a saddle-node bifurcation occurs at the critical value $r_{1c} = 0.00076$. The βIG model has a pathological fixed point for $r_1 < r_{1c}$ and three fixed points (a physiological stable spiral, a saddle, and a pathological stable node) for $r_1 > r_{1c}$. A transcritical bifurcation occurs at $r_1 = 0.0015$. To the right of this point, the fixed point with a glucose level greater than 600 $mg\ dl^{-1}$ is not physiologically interesting as it has negative β-cell mass.

Figure 1.15 shows the β-cell mass at the physiological and saddle points (solid curves) as a function of insulin sensitivity. In zone I, above the curve of physiological fixed points, glucose levels are below 100 $mg\ dl^{-1}$ and the -cell mass is decreasing. In zone II, between the solid curves, glucose levels range from 100 to 250 $mg\ dl^{-1}$ and the β-cell mass increases. The points in zones I and II constitute the basin of physiological attraction. In zone III, below the lower solid curve, glucose levels are above 250 $mg\ dl^{-1}$ and the β-cell mass decreases. The points below the lower solid curve constitute the basin of pathological attraction. Note that at large values of S_I, large changes in insulin sensitivity can be offset by relatively small changes in β-cell mass. However, at small values of S_I a dramatic change in β-cell mass is needed to balance any change in S_I.

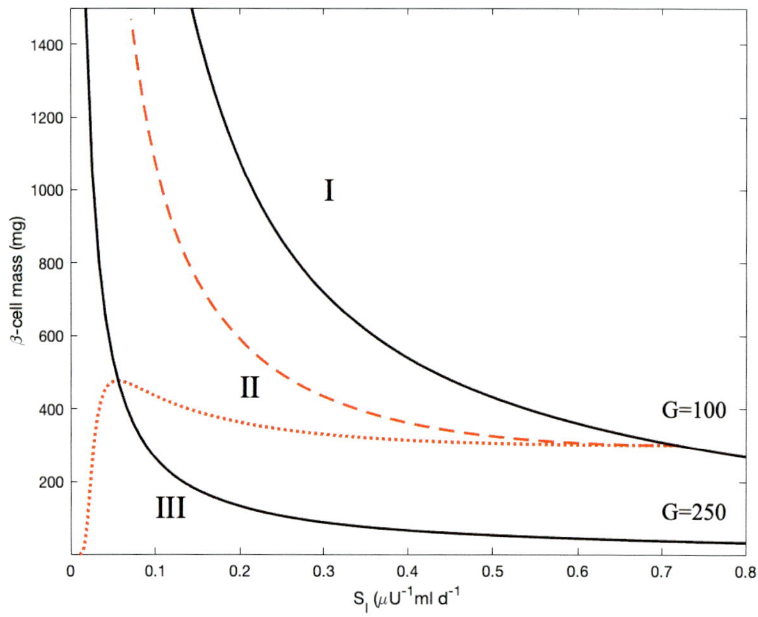

Figure 1.15 Dynamical hyperglycemia. The solid cures represent the β-cell mass of the physiological (upper) and saddle fixed points (lower) as functions of insulin sensitivity, S_I. The derivative dβ/dt is negative in Zone I (above the upper curve), and III (below the lower curve), but is positive in Zone II (between the solid curves). If S_I is reduced slowly (c=0.01), then the -β-cell mass can adapt and maintain mild hyperglycemia (- - - - -). However, if S_I is reduced too quickly (c=0.05), then the β-cell mass adapts for some period of time, but eventually glucose levels are driven above 250 mg dl^{-1} and the β-cell mass begins to decrease (........).

We now investigate the adaptation of the β-cell mass in response to a continuous change in S_I, which is modeled by

$$\frac{dS_I}{dt} = -cS_I, \tag{1.98}$$

where c is the rate constant (d^{-1}). Two trajectories are superimposed on Fig. 1.15: normal adaptation (c=0.01, dashed curve) and the catch and pass pathway (c=0.05, dotted curve). Note that both trajectories start at the physiological steady state of $G = 100mgdl^{-1}$ for $S_I = 0.72\mu U\ ml\ d^{-1}$ and that simulations are run for a period of 120 days. In the first case (c=0.01), the actual β-cell mass adapts at roughly the same rate as the increase in β-cell mass of the physiological fixed point. Thus, the trajectory remains in Zone II, close to the curve of physiological fixed points and mild hyperglycemia is maintained throughout the simulation via increases in β-cell mass and blood insulin levels. In the case of the catch and pass pathway, however, the decrease in S_I is too fast. The β-cell mass and generates a transient state where the β-cell mass blood insulin levels for this trajectory increase too slowly, so that the trajectory moves away from the curve of physiological fixed points and toward the curve of saddle points. Eventually, the trajectory crosses the curve of saddle points into Zone III, where the -cell mass and blood insulin levels begin to decrease, accelerating the rise in blood glucose levels. Note that the catch and pass pathway also can be realized with a slowly decreasing S_I.

1.3.3.2 Simulation results for the long-term model

In [142], longitudinal simulations of the long-term model (1.84)–(1.96) over a period of 5 yr were carried out starting in the normal glucose tolerance (NGT) state in which either peripheral insulin resistance is dominant, in which case the first stage of hyperglycemia is IGT, or hepatic insulin resistance is dominant, in which case the first stage of hyperglycemia is IFG.

(1) *Impaired glucose tolerance (IGT)-first pathway to diabetes.*

As strong decrease in peripheral insulin sensitivity S_I combined with a mild decrease in hepatic insulin sensitivity $hepa_{SI}$, 2hPG increases rapidly while FPG increases more slowly, resulting in progression from normal glucose tolerance (NGT) to IGT, CGI, and ultimately T2D. Fasting plasma insulin (FPI) and 2 h plasma insulin (2hPI) rise as the beta cells initially compensate partially for the insulin resistance, then fall, following the classic "Starling law" of the pancreas. The initial rise in secretion results from an increase in beta-cell sensitivity to glucose (the variable γ increases), and the decline results from a fall in the slower component of beta-cell function σ. Beta-cell mass (β) also rises and falls, but the variation is limited because of the slowness, and the fall occurs only after T2D is already underway.

A subtle but important point of this simulation is that insulin resistance in both the liver and peripheral tissues reaches saturation well before the advent of T2D. It is rather the continuing fall in beta-cell function, σ, that drives conversion to T2D. The fall in σ is triggered by the hyperglycemia and glucotoxicity that follow the early loss of insulin sensitivity (Fig. 1D) but would not lead to T2D if the preexisting capacity of beta-cell function to compensate were stronger. This is illustrated by a simulation with the same degree of insulin resistance, but a milder beta-cell defect, which mimics a nondiabetic subject with insulin resistance. FPG and 2hPG increase modestly in response to insulin resistance and reach a plateau in the IGT state as levels off and plasma insulin plateaus. The limitation of the rise in glucose reduces the effects of glucotoxicity and buys time for beta-cell mass to increase and stabilize the IGT state.

Not only is a combination of insulin resistance and impaired secretion necessary for T2D but insulin resistance develops and saturates first and T2D develops only if the beta cells fail. Some defect in beta-cell function is required even for prediabetes. Conversely, a preexisting defect in insulin secretion would be silent in the absence of insulin resistance, unless it were severe.

(2) *Impaired fasting glucose (IFG)-first pathway to diabetes.*

Contrasted to IGT-First pathway, we look at the case where dominant hepatic insulin resistance with minor peripheral resistance; the same beta-cell function defect is assumed as in IGT. Hepatic insulin resistance drives FPG across the threshold for IFG, whereas 2hPG remains below the threshold for IGT. After the initial threshold crossing, however, FPG and 2hPG continue to rise, and IFG progresses to CGI as in IGT. Insulin again rises with the help of γ and falls when the drop in σ becomes too great. As in the IGT-first pathway, the conversion to T2D is driven mainly by reduced beta-cell function, σ, because insulin resistance in both the liver and peripheral tissues saturates well before T2D (or even CGI) begins. Beta-cell mass again plays a minor role.

In a longitudinal study cited in [142] some subjects who had progressed from NGT to IGT went on to T2D at the next follow-up, which prompted one to ask whether CGI could be skipped. Simulation demonstrates that this can happen if peripheral insulin resistance is made much greater than hepatic resistance. Extreme loss of peripheral insulin sensitivity causes 2hPG to rise dramatically, whereas FPG remains in the normal range, converting NGT to IGT. 2hPG continues to deteriorate without a substantial increase in FPG, resulting in progression of IGT to T2D without passing through CGI. Eventually, FPG crosses the thresholds for IFG and T2D, but after the individual has already reached T2D based on 2hPG

1.4 MODELS IN THE FORM OF DELAY DIFFERENTIAL EQUATIONS

Several IVGTT models have been proposed and some are widely used [22, 134, 182, 184, 213, 215]. All these models incorporate the insulin secretion delay implicitly in ordinary differential equation (ODE) model by using compartment-split technique or explicitly in delay differential equation (DDE) models. However, most of above work has not discussed the reasonable range for the time delay and how to estimate the reasonable value of the delay according to the sampled data. Instead, the length of delay is often set to be larger than 20 min, which is in contrast to that the delay is between 5 and 15 min for normal subjects in normal environment [184]. Intuitively, the length of the delay in glucose tolerance test should not be longer than that in normal environment. In addition, several attempts have been made to obtain the conditions for the global stability of the equilibrium point of the models [134, 182, 184, 213, 215]. Unfortunately, all the conditions are delay-independent. For the information about the delay $\tau > 0$, it is only known that there exists a $\tau_0 > 0$ such that the equilibrium point is locally stable if $\tau < \tau_0$; and unstable otherwise (thus a periodic solution is bifurcated out). To reveal the insight regarding the time delay, it would be very helpful to know an estimate of the upper bound $\bar{\tau}$ so that the equilibrium point is globally stable when $\tau < \bar{\tau}$. Applying the Liapunov function approach, the delay dependent conditions for the global stability of the single delay IVGTT model proposed in [213] were obtained. Estimated upper bounds can be derived from these conditions explicitly or implicitly. One can also improve the numerical simulations by using functional initial conditions in the delay differential equation model. To simulate the bolus glucose infusion and the abrupt insulin secretion, constant initial conditions with adjustments at time t = 0 are applied in [134, 182, 184, 213, 215]. This is neither natural to the design of the test, nor appropriate for a functional differential equation system. In [185], the starting time of glucose infusion to $-2'$ was shifted and a non-constant function as initial value in $[-\tau, 0]$ was used.

We introduce the model in IVGTT which is a single delay differential equation model (SDM) (Model (1.99)) proposed in [185, 213] with specific function forms, which, even though it is a special case of the model proposed in [182], motivates its ease in application, parameter choice physiologically and qualitative properties. A study of the obtained parameter estimates showed advantages in robustness and precision with the SDM compared with the Minimal Model [215].

Denote the plasma concentrations of glucose and insulin at time $t \geq \tau$ by $G(t) > 0$ (mg/dl) and $I(t) > 0$ (lU/ml), respectively. The single delay model in [215] is given by

$$\begin{aligned} G'(t) &= b - eG(t) - aG(t)I(t) \\ I'(t) &= df(G(t-\tau)) - cI(t) \end{aligned} \tag{1.99}$$

with initial conditions $G(t) \equiv G_b$ for $t \in [-\tau, 0), G(0) = G_b + G_\Delta$ and $I(0) = I_b + I_\Delta$, where $G_b > 0$ and $I_b > 0$ are basal levels of glycemia and insulinemia after overnight fast (also called baseline), and G_Δ and I_Δ are the theoretical increase over basal concentrations. The parameter $b > 0$ (mg/dl/min) is the rate of the constant glucose input; $e \geq 0$ (1/min) is the parameter for the insulin independent glucose utilization by, e.g., brain cells; $a > 0$ (ml/lU/min) is the parameter for the insulin dependent glucose utilization; $c > 0$ (1/min) is the rate of the insulin degradation; and the term $df(G(t-\tau))$ is the insulin secretion responded to the glucose stimulation with time delay τ

$$f(x) = \frac{x^\gamma}{x^\gamma + \alpha^\gamma}$$

with $d > 0$ (lU/mg/min) as the maximum secretion rate, $\alpha > 0$ as the half-saturation and $\gamma > 0$. If $\gamma \leq 1$, $f(x)$ is in the shape of Michaelis-Menten kinetics; if $\gamma > 1$, $f(x)$ is in sigmoidal shape. Model (1) has a unique equilibrium and the equilibrium point is at (G_b, I_b), so that after a perturbation the glucose and insulin blood levels will return back their basal value, which implies that

$$b = G_b(e + aI_b), d = cI_b/(1 + (\alpha/G_b)^\gamma). \tag{1.100}$$

It must be noticed that the SDM also falls in the general class of models proposed and studied in [182].

The main determinants of glucose uptake from plasma in the body are brain glucose consumption (essentially constant, therefor represented as a zero-order kinetics) and muscle and adipose tissue consumption and storage (insulin and glucose-concentration dependent, hence second-order kinetics). Therefore, first-order, insulin-independent glucose utilization has often been considered negligible [134, 213, 215] i.e., $e = 0$. Therefore Model (1.99) can be further simplified as follows

$$\begin{aligned} G'(t) &= b - aG(t)I(t) \\ I'(t) &= df(G(t-\tau)) - cI(t) \end{aligned} \tag{1.101}$$

In [215], the Akaike Information Criterion (AIC) was applied in model selection by comparing Model (1.101) with Model (1.99), and it was determined that Model (1.101) is more suitable for representing observed IVGTTs. Moreover, impaired insulin-dependent glucose disposal is one of the reasons of insulin resistance that is typical in type 2 diabetes. Decreased insulin-dependent glucose transport by GLUT4 also occurs, for example, in chronic alcohol users. Low insulin sensitivity may also occur in type 1 diabetes and could be caused by impaired GLUT4 (Glucose Transporter type 4) translocation [213]. This indicates that insulin independent GLUT1 (Glucose Transporter type 1) may be dominant in translocation of glucose molecules at least in some disease states. These considerations, as well as potential concentration effects shifting (at least in the short term) glucose to the interstitial space, prompt a cautious reevaluation of the role of insulin-independent tissue glucose uptake and therefore of the generally positive, even small, value of the parameter e.

We are going to present some analytic results of Model (1.99) and (1.101), these analytical results were obtained in [134, 182, 184, 185, 213, 215].

The system (1.99) is called persistent if the solutions are eventually uniformly bounded by positive constants from both above and below. A fastly oscillated solution is defined as a solution $(G(t), I(t))$ that oscillates around the equilibrium (G_b, I_b) and within two consecutive zeros $t_0 < t_1$ of $I(t) - I_b$, $I(t)$ attains its maximum or minimum at $t_* < t_0 + 2\tau$.

Let $(G(t), I(t))$ be a solution of Model (1.99) or Model (1.101), we define

$$\bar{G} = \limsup_{t\to\infty} G(t), \underline{G} = \liminf_{t\to\infty} G(t);$$

and

$$\bar{I} = \limsup_{t\to\infty} I(t), \underline{I} = \liminf_{t\to\infty} I(t).$$

Theorem 1.7 *[182] Model (1.99) and Model (1.101) are persistent. Thus, the limits defined above are finite.*

Theorem 1.8 *[182, 213] Following inequalities hold:*

$$df(\underline{G}) \le c\underline{I} \le c\bar{I} \le df(\bar{G}); (e + a\underline{I})\bar{G} \le b \le (e + a\bar{I})\underline{G}.$$

Theorem 1.9 *[182, 213] The necessary condition and sufficient conditions for global stability of Model (1.99) and Model (1.101) is*

$$\frac{\gamma a I_b}{1 + \left(\frac{G_b}{\alpha}\right)^{\gamma}} \leq e + a I_b. \tag{1.102}$$

Theorem 1.10 *[182] If $\gamma \leq 1$, the unique equilibrium Model (1.99) or the model (1.101) is globally asymptotically stable.*

Theorem 1.11 *[213] If the inequality in (1.102) does not hold, then there is a $\tau_0 > 0$ such that (i) when $\tau < \tau_0$, the equilibrium (G_b, I_b) is locally stable; (ii) when $\tau \geq \tau_0$, the equilibrium is unstable. In other words, Model (1.99) and Model (1.101) undergo a Hopf bifurcation at $\tau = \tau_0$ when τ increases from $\tau = 0$.*

Theorem 1.12 *[134] In Model (1.99), the equilibrium is a global attractor if*

$$\frac{adG_b}{ce}\sqrt{\sup_{[0,G_b]} f'(G) \sup_{[G_b,\infty]} f'(G)} < 1.$$

Notice that the conditions for the globally asymptotical stability of the equilibrium in Theorems 1.9, 1.10 and 1.12 are delay-independent. But Theorem 1.9 is a necessary and sufficient condition, so the result in Theorem 1.11 shall be either a weaker condition or equivalent to Theorem 1.9. Nevertheless, only 3% of clinical data satisfy the condition in Theorem 1.9 [213]. So, to ensure the global attractive behavior of the tolerance test, analysis on delay dependent global stability is necessary.

Lemma 1.13 *[185] If $(G(t), I(t))$ is a solution with positive initial conditions of Model (1.99), then*

$$m_I = \min\{I(0), \frac{k_2}{c}\} \leq I(t) \leq M_I = \max\{I(0), \frac{d}{c}\}$$

and

$$m_G = \min\{G(0), \frac{b}{k_1}\} < G(t) \leq M_G = \max\{G(0), \frac{b}{k_3}\}$$

where $k_1 = e + aM_I, k_2 = df(m_G)$ and $k_3 = e + am_I$.

For the sake of convenience, we denote for $\gamma > 1$

$$L = d\frac{\gamma + 1)^2}{4\gamma\alpha}\left(\frac{\gamma - 1}{\gamma + 1}\right)^{\frac{\gamma-1}{\gamma}}, \tag{1.103}$$

which is the maximum value of the derivative of $df(G)$ for $G > 0$, and

$R = e + aI_b$; and $K = aM_G$. By Lemma 1.13, L, R and K are independent of τ. When consider Model (1.101), $R = aI_b$.

When $\tau = 0$, Model (1.99) and Model (1.101) become a two-dimensional ordinary differential equation system. It is easy to show that the unique equilibrium (G_b, I_b) is globally asymptotically stable by Poincaré-Bendixson theorem. When $\tau > 0$, the models are functional differential equations. Poincare-Bendixson Theorem does not apply. To establish a criterion of delay dependent global stability, one construct a Liapunov function and prove that the solutions of Model (1.99) or Model (1.101) are attracted to the equilibrium (G_b, I_b).

Theorem 1.14 *[185] If there exists a positive constant $u > 0$ such that*

$$\tau < \min\{\frac{2u}{L}, \frac{2c}{L(R+2K)}\} \tag{1.104}$$

and

$$\Delta = M_u^2 - 4R(u - \tau L/2)(c - \tau L(R+2K)/2) < 0, \tag{1.105}$$

where $M_u = \max\{L, Ku\}$, then the equilibrium (G_b, I_b) of Model (1.99) is globally and asymptotically stable.

1.5 MODELS IN THE FORM OF INTEGRO-DIFFERENTIAL EQUATIONS

An integro-differential model is the dynamical model proposed in [92, 202]. The model is as follows

$$\begin{aligned} \frac{dG(t)}{dt} &= -b_1G(t) - b_4I(t)G(t) + b_7, \\ G(t) &= G_b \forall t \in [-b_5, 0], G(0) = G_b + b_0 \qquad (1.106) \\ \frac{dI(t)}{dt} &= -b_2I(t) + \frac{b_6}{b_5}\int_{t-b_5}^{t} G(s)ds, I(0) = I_b + b_3b_0 \qquad (1.107) \end{aligned}$$

where the parameters are as follows:
t [min] is time; G [mg/dl] is the glucose plasma concentration;
G_b [mg/dl] is the basal (preinjection) plasma glucose concentration;
I [pM] is the insulin plasma concentration;
I_b [pM] is the basal (preinjection) insulin plasma concentration;
b_0 [mg/dl] is the theoretical increase in plasma concentration over basal glucose concentration at time zero after instantaneous administration and redistribution of the I.V. glucose bolus;
b_1 [min^{-1}] is the spontaneous glucose first order disappearance rate constant;
b_2 [min^{-1}] is the apparent first-order disappearance rate constant for insulin;

b_3 [pM/(mg/dl)] is the first-phase insulin concentration increase per (mg/dl) increase in the concentration of glucose at time zero due to the injected bolus;
b_4 [min^{-1} pM^{-1}] is the constant amount of insulin-dependent glucose disappearance rate constant per pM of plasma insulin concentration;
b_5 [min] is the length of the past period whose plasma glucose concentrations influence the current pancreatic insulin secretion;
b_6 [min^{-1} pM/(mg/dl)] is the constant amount of second-phase insulin release rate per (mg/dl) of average plasma glucose concentration throughout the previous b_5 minutes;
b_7 [(mg/dl) min^{-1}] is the constant increase in plasma glucose concentration due to constant baseline liver glucose release.

Next, we will provide a proof for the stability of the dynamical model. To do so we will be providing multiple lemmas which will be used throughout the proofs to help guide us to the conclusion.
Now suppose $(G^*,\ I^*)$ is some equilibrium point for the system, then

$$\begin{cases} 0 = -b_1G^* - b_4I^*G^* + b_7 \\ 0 = -b_2I^* + b_6G^* \end{cases}$$

From the system we can form the equation $\frac{b_4b_6}{b_2}G^{*2}+b_1G^*-b_7 = 0, I^* = \frac{b_6}{b_2}G^*$. There is only one solution to the quadratic equation with $G^* > 0$, so there is only one equilibrium point of the system.

Lemma 1.15 *If* $(G(t), I(t)) \in C^1([0,\infty))$ *is a solution of the dynamical model, then*
(1) $0 < G(t) < \max(G(0), \frac{b_7}{b_1})$*, for all* $t \in [0,\infty)$ *and* $\limsup_{t\to\infty} G(t) \leq \frac{b_7}{b_1}$.
If $G(T) < \frac{b_7}{b_1}$ *for some* $T \geq 0$*, then* $0 < G(t) < \frac{b_7}{b_1}$*, for all* $t \in [T,\infty)$.
(2) $0 < I(t) < \max\left(I(0), \frac{b_6}{b_2}\max\left(G(0), \frac{b_7}{b_1}\right)\right)$ *for all* $t \in [0,\infty)$ *and*
$\limsup_{t\to\infty} I(t) \leq \frac{b_6}{b_2}\frac{b_7}{b_1}$.
If $I(T) < \frac{b_6}{b_2}\frac{b_7}{b_1}$ *for some* $T \geq 0$*, then* $0 < I(t) < \frac{b_6}{b_2}\frac{b_7}{b_1}$*, for all* $t \in [T,\infty)$.

Proof. First $G(t) > 0$ can easily be seen when solving for $G(t)$ directly using the integrating factor method.

$$G(t) = G(T)e^{-b_1t-b_4\int_T^t Idt} + \frac{b_7}{e^{b_1t+b_4\int_T^t Idt}}\int_T^t e^{b_1\tau+b_4\int_T^\tau I(s)ds}d\tau \qquad (1.108)$$

Solving (1.107) for $I(t)$, we have

$$I(t) = e^{-b_2t}I(T) + e^{-b_2t}\left[\frac{b_6}{b_5}\int_T^t e^{b_2\tau}\int_{\tau-b_5}^{\tau} G(s)dsd\tau\right]. \qquad (1.109)$$

which implies $I(t) > 0$. Using $I(t) > 0$ and (1.108) we have

$$G(t) \leq G(0)e^{-b_1t} + \frac{b_7}{b_1}(1-e^{-b_1t}) \leq \max(G(0), \frac{b_7}{b_1}). \qquad (1.110)$$

substituting the above into (1.109) we have the lemma. ■

Theorem 1.16 *There exists a unique solution* $(G(t), X(t), I(t)) \in C^1[0,\infty)$ *to the system of (1.106), (1.107).*

Proof. As in the proof the classical local existence theorem, using Newton's approximation we can show that there exists a solution $(G(t), I(t)) \in C^1[0,T]$ for some $T > 0$, the local solution interval $[0,T]$ can be extended indefinitely since $G(t), I(t)$ are bounded from the above lemma. ∎

So we see here that we have an upper bound for $G(t)$ on $[T,\infty)$ for sufficiently large T. Let us denote this upper bound for G as $M_0 = \frac{b_7}{b_1}$ and an upper bound for $I(t)$ as N_0 such that $N_0 = \frac{b_6}{b_2}\frac{b_7}{b_1}$. This will prove to be useful in our next lemmas.

Lemma 1.17 *If* $I(t) \leq N_0$ *on* $[T,\infty)$*, then* $G(t) \geq \frac{b_7}{b_1+b_4N_0}, \forall t \in [T,\infty)$.

Proof. From lemma 1.15 we know $I(t) \leq N_0$ thus we know $\frac{dG}{dt} \geq -b_1G - b_4N_0G + b_7$. From here we can solve for $G(t)$ in a similar fashion as lemma 1.15 for $I(t)$ and see that $G(t) \geq \frac{b_7}{b_1+b_4N_0}$. ∎

From here we see that we have a lower bound for $G(t)$. Let us denote this lower bound as m_0.

Lemma 1.18 *If* $G(t) \geq m_0$ *on* $[T,\infty)$*, then* $I(t) \geq \frac{b_6}{b_2}m_0$. *on* $[T,\infty)$.

Proof. If $G(t) \geq m_0$, then by equation (1.109) we have $\frac{dI}{dt} \geq -b_2I + b_6m_0 \Rightarrow \frac{dI}{dt} + b_2I \geq b_6m_0$. From here we can solve for $I(t)$ similar to lemma 10 and see $I(t) \geq \frac{b_6}{b_2}m_0$. ∎

Here we see that we have a lower bound for $I(t)$. Let us denote this lower bound of $I(t)$ as n_0 such that $n_0 = \frac{b_6}{b_2}m_0$. This notation will be useful in the next lemmas.

Lemma 1.19 *If* $I(t) \geq n_0$ *on* $[T,\infty)$*, then* $G(t) \leq \frac{b_7}{b_1+b_4n_0}$ *on* $[T,\infty)$

Proof. If $I(t) \geq n_0$, then by equation (1.108), $\frac{dG}{dt} \leq -b_1G - b_4n_0G + b_7 \Rightarrow \frac{dG}{dt} + (b_1 + b_4n_0)G \leq b_7$. From here we can solve for $G(t)$ in the same fashion as lemma 11. Therefore we have $G(t) \leq \frac{b_7}{b_1+b_4n_0}$. ∎

From here we once again have an upper bound for $G(t)$. We can denote this new upper bound as M_1. We can see that continuing this process will result in a sequence of finding upper or lower bounds for functions $I(t)$ and $G(t)$. We notice that as this sequence continues each subsequent upper bound of $G(t)$ is decreasing while each subsequent lower bound of $G(t)$ is increasing. We can see this as we continue the sequence described by the lemmas. The sequence is as follows $M_0 \to N_0 \to m_0 \to n_0 \to M_1 \to ...$ So we understand that the sequence continues so let us analyze M_0 and M_1. Clearly $M_0 = \frac{b_7}{b_1} > \frac{b_7}{b_1+b_4n_0} = M_1$. Thus following the sequence we will have $N_1 < N_0 \to m_1 > m_0 \to n_1 > n_0 \to ...$ Therefore we have sequences for upper and lower bounds of $G(t)$ such that each $M_i > M_{i+1}$ and each $m_i < m_{i+1}$. Since each sequence

is monotone it is not far fetched to believe $G(t)$ converges in $\mathbb{R}$ to some finite value.
Let

$$h(x) = \frac{b_7}{b_1 + \frac{b_4 b_6 b_7}{b_1 b_2 + b_4 b_6 x}} \tag{1.111}$$

and defined $M_{k+1} = h(M_k)$ and $m_{k+1} = h(m_k), k = 0, 1, 2 \cdots$.
By straight computation we have

Lemma 1.20 *(1) $h(x)$ is increasing in x*
(2) $\{M_k\}$ is decreasing and $\{m_k\}$ is increasing, both sequences are bounded.
(3) The equation is equivalent to $\frac{b_4 b_6}{b_2} x^2 + b_1 x - b_7 = 0$.

Theorem 1.21 $\lim_{t\to\infty} G(t) = G^*, \lim_{t\to\infty} I(t) = I^*$ *and G^* is the positive fixed point of $h(x) = x$, i.e.$h(G^*) = G^*$.*

Proof. Applying Lemmas 1.17–1.20 successively, we have a sequence T_k with $T_k \to \infty$ such that on $[T_k, \infty)$,

$$G(t) \in [m_k, M_k], I(t) \in [\frac{b_6}{b_2} m_k, \frac{b_6}{b_2} M_k].$$

Since both M_k and m_k converge to the positive fixed point of $h(x) = x$, we have the lemma. ■

1.6 STOCHASTIC MODELS

Applying stochastic models to diabetes research and management represents a promising approach that leverages probabilistic and random variables to understand and predict the disease's dynamics. Stochastic models provide a framework to simulate the complex progression of diabetes, accounting for inherent uncertainties and variability in biological processes. They can incorporate factors such as genetic predisposition, lifestyle choices, and environmental influences that contribute to the development and progression of diabetes.

One significant application of stochastic models is in predicting complications associated with diabetes, such as cardiovascular diseases, neuropathy, and retinopathy. By integrating probabilistic elements, these models can estimate the likelihood and timing of these complications, thereby guiding preventive strategies and personalized treatment plans. Stochastic models are instrumental in evaluating the effectiveness of different treatment strategies. They allow researchers to simulate the response of individuals or populations to interventions like medication, lifestyle changes, or surgical procedures. This simulation-based approach helps optimize treatment protocols and improve patient outcomes.

With the growing emphasis on personalized medicine, stochastic models enable the customization of diabetes management plans based on individual characteristics and risk profiles. By considering variability in patient data and disease progression, these models facilitate tailored interventions that maximize therapeutic benefits while minimizing adverse effects.

On a broader scale, stochastic models contribute to public health policy by predicting diabetes prevalence trends, assessing the impact of policy interventions (e.g., sugar taxes, health education programs), and allocating resources effectively. These models provide insights into population-level health outcomes and guide decision-making to mitigate the burden of diabetes on healthcare systems.

While stochastic models offer valuable insights, they are not without challenges. Model complexity, data availability, and the need for validation against real-world outcomes are critical considerations. Improving data quality and refining model parameters are ongoing efforts to enhance the reliability and applicability of these models in diabetes research and clinical practice.

1.6.1 Stochastic IVGTT Glucose-insulin Model

In this section, we discuss a stochastic IVGTT model proposed in [242]. In the deterministic model (1.99), we consider the stochastic disturbance on the glucose effectiveness index e and insulin degradation rate c for the sake of simplicity. More specifically, at a given time t, the glucose effectiveness index e and insulin degradation rate c are perturbed as

$$e + \alpha_1 \frac{dB_1(t)}{dt} \text{and } c + \alpha_2 \frac{dB_2(t)}{dt},$$

respectively, where $B_i(t), i = 1, 2$, are two independent standard Brownian motions, and $\alpha_i (i = 1, 2)$ are positive constants with α_i^2 representing the intensity of the white noise $B_i(t)$. As a result, we formulate following stochastic system

$$\begin{aligned} dG(t) &= (b - eG(t) - aG(t)I(t))dt + \alpha_1 dB_1(t) \\ I(t) &= (df(G(t-\tau)) - cI(t))dt + \alpha_2 dB_2(t) \end{aligned} \tag{1.112}$$

with the same initial conditions as (1.99).

Let $(\Omega, \mathcal{F}, \{\mathcal{F}\}_{\sqcup \geq \prime}, \mathcal{P})$ be a complete probability space with a filtration $\{\mathcal{F}\}_{\sqcup \geq \prime}$ satisfying the usual conditions that $\mathcal{F}_\prime$ contains all P null sets and $\mathcal{F}_{\sqcup_\infty} \subset \mathcal{F}_{\sqcup_\in}$ if $t_1 \leq t_2$. Let $B_i(t), i = 1, 2$ denote two scalar Brownian motions defined on the complete probability space Ω.

Definition 1.1 *A stochastic system is said to be almost surely stochastically permanent if for any initial value* $x_0 \in \mathbf{R}_+^2$, *the solution* $x(t) = (x_1(t), x_2(t), ..., x_n(t))$*satisfies*

$$0 < \liminf_{t\to\infty} x_i(t) \leq \limsup_{t\to\infty} x(t) \leq \infty, a.s.i = 1, 2, ...n.$$

Theorem 1.22 *[242] For an initial value problem (1.112), there exists a unique global positive solution in $\mathbf{R}_+^2$ on time interval $t \geq 0$ almost surely, that is, the solution will remain in $\mathbf{R}_+^2$ with probability 1.*

Theorem 1.23 *[242] System (1.112) is almost surely stochastically permanent, i.e, the solution (G(t),I(t)) to Eq (1.112) satisfies*

$$\begin{aligned} 0 < \phi_m &:= \inf_{t\in[0,\infty)} G(t) \leq \Phi_M := \sup_{t\in[0,\infty)} G(t) \\ 0 < \psi_m &:= \inf_{t\in[0,\infty)} I(t) \leq \Psi_M := \sup_{t\in[0,\infty)} I(t) \end{aligned} \tag{1.113}$$

From section 1.4, the deterministic system (1.99) has a fixed point (G_b, I_b); but it is not a fixed point of Eq. (1.112). Noting that $f(x) = \frac{x^\gamma}{x^\gamma+\alpha^\gamma}$, we have

$$0 < M := \sup_{t\in[0,\infty)} f'(t) < \infty. \tag{1.114}$$

Theorem 1.24 *[242] If there exist $u > 0$ and $\epsilon > 0$ such that*

$$\frac{1}{2}dM(e+aI_b)\tau + \frac{1}{2}u\alpha_1^2 < ue + uaI_b - \frac{\epsilon}{2}M_u$$

and

$$\frac{1}{2}dM(2a\Phi_M + e + aI_b)\tau + \frac{1}{2}\alpha_1^2 < c - \frac{1}{2\epsilon}M_u,$$

then the following results holds:

$$\begin{aligned} \limsup_{t\to\infty} \frac{1}{t}\mathbf{E}\int_0^t \Bigg\{ &\left(G(s) - \frac{ue + uaI_b - \frac{\epsilon}{2}M_u - \frac{dM}{2}(e+aI_b)\tau}{ue + uaI_b - \frac{\epsilon}{2}M_u - \frac{dM}{2}(e+aI_b)\tau - \frac{1}{2}\alpha_1^2} G_b \right)^2 \times \\ &\left(I(s) - \frac{c - \frac{1}{2\epsilon}M_u - \frac{dM}{2}(2a\Phi_M + e + aI_b)\tau}{c - \frac{1}{2\epsilon}M_u - \frac{dM}{2}(2a\Phi_M + e + aI_b)\tau - \frac{1}{2}\alpha_2^2} I_b \right)^2 \Bigg\} ds \leq \frac{H_1}{H_2}, \end{aligned}$$

where $M_u = \max\{dM, ua\Phi_M\}$, and

$$\begin{aligned} H_1 = &\frac{\left(ue + uaI_b - \frac{\epsilon}{2}M_u - \frac{dM}{2}(e+aI_b)\tau\right)\frac{1}{2}u\alpha_1^2}{ue + uaI_b - \frac{\epsilon}{2}M_u - \frac{dM}{2}(e+aI_b)\tau - \frac{1}{2}u\alpha_1^2} G_b^2 \\ &+ \frac{\left(c - \frac{1}{2\epsilon}M_u - \frac{dM}{2}(2a\Phi_M + e + aI_b)\tau\right)\frac{1}{2}\alpha_2^2}{c - \frac{1}{2\epsilon}M_u - \frac{dM}{2}(2a\Phi_M + e + aI_b)\tau - \frac{1}{2}\alpha_2^2} I_b^2, \end{aligned}$$

and

$$\begin{aligned} H_2 = \min\Bigg\{ &ue + uaI_b - \frac{\epsilon}{2}M_u - \frac{dM}{2}(e+aI_b)\tau - \frac{1}{2}u\alpha_1^2, \\ &c - \frac{1}{2\epsilon}M_u - \frac{dM}{2}(2a\Phi_M + e + aI_b)\tau - \frac{1}{2}\alpha_2^2 \Bigg\}. \end{aligned}$$

The stochastic system (1.112) does not have a positive equilibrium point, but the solutions of the system perturbs around a point near the positive equilibrium point of its corresponding deterministic system. The above theorem shows that the smaller the stochastic disturbance is, the closer the point is to the positive equilibrium point, and the vibration amplitude decreases as the disturbance decreases.

The parameters estimation

Although the stochastic system (1.112) is constructed based on the deterministic system (1.99), it can be identified directly from the clinical data without the necessity of finding (1.99) in advance. One can estimate the parameters in (1.112) by a maximum likelihood estimation (MLE) method. Let $\theta = (b, e, a, c, d, \tau, \alpha, \gamma, \alpha_1, \alpha_2)$ be the collection of parameters in the system (1.112) , Let $Y(t) = (G(t), I(t))^T$, $h(Y(t), \theta) = (b - eG(t) - aG(t)I(t), df(G(t-\tau)) - cI(t))$, $B(t) = (B_1(t), B_2(t))^T$, and $\phi(Y(t), \theta) = (\alpha_1 G(t), \alpha_1 I(t))^T$. Then the system (1.3) can be represented as

$$dY(t) = h(Y(t), \theta)dt + \phi(Y(t), \theta)dB(t)Y(0) = y_0.$$

As $\Delta t \to 0$,the Euler scheme produces the following discretization:

$$Y(t + \Delta t) - Y(t) = h(Y(t), \theta)\Delta t + \phi(Y(t), \theta)(B(t + \Delta t) - B(t)).$$

Since B_i, $i = 1, 2$ are independent Brownian motions, $Y(t + \Delta t) - Y(t)$ are a five-dimensional Gaussian independent variables with mean $h(Y(t), \theta)\Delta t$ and covariance matrix.

$$\Sigma(Y(t_{i-1}, \theta)\Delta t = \begin{bmatrix} \alpha_1^2 G^2(t) & 0 \\ 0 & \alpha_2^2 I^2(t) \end{bmatrix}$$

Let $\delta_i(\theta) = Y(t_i) - Y(t_{i-1}) - h(Y(t_{i-1}), \theta)(t_i - t_{i-1})$, where $Y(t_0) = y_0$. We obtain the following log-likelihood function:

$$\begin{aligned} \ln(\theta|Y(t_1), ..., Y(t_n)) = -\frac{1}{2}\sum_{i=2}^{n}(\delta_i(\theta)^{\intercal}(\Sigma(Y(t_{i-1}, \theta)(t_i - t_{i-1}))^{-1}\delta_i(\theta) \\ + ln(|\Sigma(Y(t_{i-1}, \theta)(t_i - t_{i-1}))|)). \end{aligned}$$

By maximizing the above log-likelihood function with respect to θ, we obtain a consistent estimator, denoted by $\hat{\theta}$ under some mild conditions.

Simulation results

In [242], MLE was performed to estimate (α_1, α_2) based on the clinical data while the other parameters were fixed as the experiment data listed in [92]. The simulation results suggest that the intensity of stochastic components in the system (1.112) needs to be carefully chosen. On one hand, if the intensity is too small, the improvement of model fitness is not sufficient. On the other hand, the over-large intensity may fail to improve the model fitness. In addition, the simulation results also indicate that given a reasonable set of values of the parameters $(b, e, a, d, \tau, c, \alpha, \gamma)$, the MLE method can provide satisfactory estimates of (α_1, α_2) and the solution of the proposed system (1.112) can significantly improve the model fitness with certain probabilities.

Simulations also show as the values of α_1 and α_2 get larger, the disturbance amplitudes of the solution curves of the stochastic system (1.112) are enlarged and consequently depart further away from the positive equilibrium point of system (1.99). This phenomena is expected as α_2's control the intensity of disturbance, and confirms our theoretical findings in Theorem 1.23. In the process of IVGTT, there may be many disturbance of human activity that are hard to control such as psychological pressure, emotions, excessive morning exercises and so on. Simulations suggest that if the disturbances of human activity are enough large, there may be larger error in diagnostic results provided by a deterministic model.

1.6.2 Stochastic β Cell-Insulin-Glucose Model (βIG Model)

The deterministic βIG model studied in section 1.3.1 is as follows:

$$\begin{cases} \frac{dG(t)}{dt} = R_0 - (E_{G0} + S_I I(t))G(t) \\ \frac{dI(t)}{dt} = \beta\sigma \frac{G^2(t)}{a^2+G^2(t))} - kI(t) \\ \frac{d\beta(t)}{dt} = (-d_0 + r_1 G(t) - r_2 G^2(t))\beta \end{cases} . \tag{1.115}$$

With initial conditions

$$(G(0), I(0), \beta(0)) \in \mathbb{R}^3_+. \tag{1.116}$$

The model has three equilibrium points (two stable points and one saddle point). In addition, the normal parameters from Table 1.10 are assumed.

In the following, we propose a stochastic generalization of that model [18]; more specifically, at a given time t, the glucose effectiveness E_{G0}, the insulin degradation k, and the linear coefficient of the sum of the replication and death rate of β-cell mass zero glucose concentration are perturbed as follows

$$E_{G0} + \alpha_1 \frac{dB_1(t)}{dt}$$

$$k + \alpha_2 \frac{dB_2(t)}{dt}$$

and

$$-d_0 + \alpha_3 \frac{dB_3(t)}{dt}$$

where $B_i(t)$, $i = 1, 2, 3$ are three independent Brownian motions, and

α_i, $i = 1, 2, 3$ are three positive constants with α_i^2 representing the intensity of the white noise $B_i(t)$.

Thus we have the stochastic system,

$$\begin{cases} dG(t) = (R_0 - (E_{G0} + S_I I(t))G(t))dt + \alpha_1 G(t)dB_1(t) \\ dI(t) = (\beta\sigma\frac{G^2(t)}{a^2+G^2(t))} - kI(t))dt + \alpha_2 I(t)dB_2(t) \\ d\beta(t) = (-d_0 + r_1 G(t) - r_2 G^2(t))\beta(t)dt + \alpha_3 \beta(t)dB_3(t) \end{cases} . \tag{1.117}$$

With the initial conditions (1.116).

1.6.2.1 Positive Global Solutions

The following result shows that the stochastic system is well posed.

Theorem 1.25 *For any given initial value $(G(0), I(0), \beta(0)) \in \mathbb{R}^3_+$ and $t \geqslant 0$ The system (1.117) has a unique global positive solution $(G(t), I(t), \beta(t)) \in \mathbb{R}^3_+$ almost surely, i.e. the solution will remain in $\mathbb{R}^3_+$ with probability 1.*

Proof. Since all functions on the right side of (1.117) are all function of class C^1 and thus locally Lipschitz, for any given initial value $(G(0), I(0), \beta(0) \in \mathbb{R}^3_+)$, there is a unique maximal solution $(G(t), I(t), \beta(t))$ for $t \in [0, \tau)$, where τ is the explosion time.

Let's show that the solution is positive. Treating each equation of (1.117) as a linear SDE, we obtain,

$$G(t) = G(0)e^{\left[\int_0^t -(E_{G0}+S_I I(s)\ +\ \frac{\alpha_1^2}{2})ds\ +\ \alpha_1 B(t)\right]}$$
$$+ \int_0^t R_0 e^{\left[\int_s^t -(E_{G0}+S_I I(u)\ +\ \frac{\alpha_1^2}{2})du\ +\ \alpha_1 \int_s^t dB(u)\right]} ds;$$

$$I(t) = I(0)e^{\left[(-k-\frac{\alpha_2^2}{2})t+\alpha_2 B_2(t)\right]}$$
$$+ \int_0^t \beta\sigma \frac{G^2(s)}{a^2 + G^2(s)} e^{\left[(-k-\frac{\alpha_2^2}{2})(t-s)+\alpha_2(B_2(t)-B_2(s))\right]} ds;$$

$$\beta(t) \ = \ \beta(0)e^{\int_0^t \left(-d_0+r_1 G(s)-r_2 G^2(s)-\frac{\alpha_3^2}{2}\right)ds\ +\ \alpha_3 B(t)};$$

it is clear that $G(t) > 0$, $I(t) > 0$, and $\beta(t) > 0$.

Unfortunately, the coefficients of the system do not satisfy a linear growth condition, so we have to prove that $\tau = \infty$. This follows from the following lemmas that give upper bounds for $G(t)$, $I(t)$ and $\beta(t)$. The bounds show that the local solution can not blow up at any finite time, hence $\tau = \infty$. ∎

Lemma 1.26 *If $(G(t), I(t), \beta(t)$ is a solution of (1.117) on $[0, \tau)$, then there exists a positive constant Φ_M such that $G(t) \leqslant \Phi_M$ for all $t \in [0, \tau)$ a.s.*

Proof. From the first equation of the system (1.117), we have

$$dG(t) \leqslant (R_0 - E_{G0}G(t))dt + \alpha_1 G(t)dB_1(t).$$

Let consider the equation

$$\begin{cases} d\Phi(t) = (R_0 - E_{G0}\Phi(t))dt + \alpha_1\Phi(t)dB_1(t) \\ \Phi(0) = G(0) \end{cases};$$

which has a solution

$$\Phi(t) = e^{\left[\int_0^t -(E_{G0}+\frac{\alpha_1^2}{2})ds+\ \alpha_1 B(t)\right]} G(0) + \int_0^t R_0 e^{\left[\int_s^t (E_{G0}+\frac{\alpha_1^2}{2})du\ -\ \alpha_1 \int_s^t dB(u)\right]} ds.$$

By comparison principle for stochastic differential equations [158, 159], we obtain that

$$G(t) \leqslant \Phi(t), t \in [0, \tau);$$

which implies that there exists a positive constant Φ_M satisfying $\Phi(t) \leqslant \Phi_M$ for all $t \in [0, \tau)$ a.s. ■

Lemma 1.27 *If $(G(t), I(t), \beta(t))$ is a solution of (1.117) on $[0, \tau)$, then there exists a positive constants Φ_1 and ϕ_1 such that $\beta(t) \leqslant \Phi_1 e^{\phi_1 t}$ for all $t \in [0, \tau)$ a.s.*

Proof. The quadratic function $Q(G) = -d_0 + r_1 G - r_2 G^2$ on $[0, \Phi_M]$ has a maximum Q_M such that $q(G) \leq Q_M$. From (1.117), we have $d\beta(t) \leq Q_m\beta(t)+ \alpha_3\beta(t)dB_3(t)$. Hence by comparison theorem $\beta(t) \leq \beta(0)e^{Q_m - \frac{\alpha_3^2}{2} + \alpha_3 B(t)}$ which implies the lemma. ■

Lemma 1.28 *If $(G(t), I(t), \beta(t))$ is a solution of (1.117) on $[0, \tau)$, then there exists a positive constants Φ_2 and ϕ_2 such that $I(t) \leqslant \Phi_2 e^{\phi_2 t}$ for all $t \in [0, \tau)$ a.s.*

Proof. From (1.117), we have

$$dI(t) \leqslant (\sigma f(\Phi_M)\Phi_1 e^{\phi_1 t} - kI(t))dt + \alpha_2 I(t)dB_2(t),$$

since $f(x) = \frac{x^2}{\alpha+x^2}$; $f'(x) = \frac{2\alpha x}{(\alpha+x^2)^2} > 0$, for $x > 0$, f is an increasing function on $(0, \infty)$.

Let $\Psi(t)$ be the solution of the equation

$$\begin{cases} d\Psi(t) = (\sigma f(\Phi_M)\Phi_1 e^{\phi_1 t} - k\Psi(t))dt + \alpha_2\Psi(t)dB_2(t) \\ \Psi(0) = I(0) \end{cases}.$$

Then,

$$\Psi(t) = I(0)e^{[(-k-\frac{\alpha_2^2}{2})t+\alpha_2 B_2(t)]} + \int_0^t \beta\Phi_1\sigma f(\Phi_M)e^{[(\phi_1-k-\frac{\alpha_2^2}{2})(t-s)+\alpha_2(B_2(t)-B_2(s))]}ds;$$

which implies by comparison

$$I(t) \leqslant \Psi(t) \leqslant \Phi_2 e^{\phi_2 t}, t \in [0,\tau) \quad a.s.$$

where Φ_2, ϕ_2 are positive constants. ∎

1.6.2.2 Asymptotic Behavior

In [265], for normal parameters, the model has two stable fixed points: the physiological fixed point (G,I,β) $= P_1 =$ (100,10,300), the pathological fixed point $P_2 =$ (600,0,0), and a saddle point S = (250, 2.8, 37).

However, those points are no longer equilibrium points for the stochastic model. Yet, we will study the long term behavior of solutions of the stochastic system around those points. In so doing, we will use the following linearized system for both $P_1 = (100, 10, 300)$ and $S = (250, 2.8, 37)$.

Let $(G(0), I(0), \beta(0)) \in \mathbb{R}_+^3$ be the initial condition of the system and (G^*, I^*, β^*) be the stable fixed point (100,10,300) of the corresponding deterministic system (1.115). Linearizing (1.117) about (G^*, I^*, β^*), we can write (1.117) as

$$d\Upsilon = [N\cdot\Upsilon + O(\Upsilon^2)]dt + A_1\Upsilon dB_1 + A_2\Upsilon dB_2 + A_3\Upsilon dB_3 + D_1 dB_1 + D_2 dB_2 + D_3 dB_3, \quad (1.118)$$

where $\Upsilon = (G-G^*, I-I^*, \beta-\beta^*)^T$,

$$N = \begin{bmatrix} -E_{G0} - S_I I^* & -S_I G^* & 0 \\ 2\beta^*\sigma\alpha\frac{G^*}{(\alpha^2+G^{*2})^2} & -k & \sigma\frac{G^{*2}}{\alpha^2+G^{*2}} \\ (r_1 - 2r_2 G^*)\beta^* & 0 & -d_0 + r_1 G^* - 2r_2 G^{*2} \end{bmatrix} \quad (1.119)$$

$$\begin{cases} O(\Upsilon^2) = (O_1(\Upsilon^2), O_2(\Upsilon^2), O_3(\Upsilon^2))^T \\ O_1(\Upsilon^2) = -S_I(G-G^*)(I-I^*) \\ O_2(\Upsilon^2) = \frac{\beta^0\sigma\alpha^2(\alpha^2+G^{02}-2G^0)}{(\alpha^2+G^{02})^4}(G-G^*)^2 + \frac{2\sigma\alpha^2 G^0}{(\alpha^2+G^{02})^2}(G-G^*)(\beta-\beta^*) \\ O_3(\Upsilon^2) = -r_2\beta^1(G-G^*)^2 + (r_1 - 2r_2 G^1)(G-G^*)(\beta-\beta^*) \end{cases};$$

(1.120)

here G^0 and G^1 are some values between G^* and G, and β^0 and β^1 are some values between β^*, and β;

$$A_1 = \begin{bmatrix} \alpha_1 & 0 & 0 \\ 0 & 0 & 0 \\ 0 & 0 & 0 \end{bmatrix} \quad A_2 = \begin{bmatrix} 0 & 0 & 0 \\ 0 & \alpha_2 & 0 \\ 0 & 0 & 0 \end{bmatrix} \quad A_3 = \begin{bmatrix} 0 & 0 & 0 \\ 0 & 0 & 0 \\ 0 & 0 & \alpha_3 \end{bmatrix}; \tag{1.121}$$

$$D_1 = \begin{bmatrix} \alpha_1 G^* \\ 0 \\ 0 \end{bmatrix} \quad D_2 = \begin{bmatrix} 0 \\ \alpha_2 I^* \\ 0 \end{bmatrix} \quad D_3 \begin{bmatrix} 0 \\ 0 \\ \alpha_3 \beta^* \end{bmatrix}. \tag{1.122}$$

Note that the matrix N has eigenvalues

$$\lambda_1 = -0.01422, \ \lambda_2 = -18.6588 \ \textit{and} \ \lambda_3 = -421.9669 \tag{1.123}$$

which implies that there exists constant $K_1 > 0$, for any $t \geqslant 0$,

$$\|e^{Nt}\| \leqslant K_1 e^{\lambda_1 t} \tag{1.124}$$

Using variation of constant formula, we can write (3.1) as

$$\Upsilon(t) = e^{M(t)}\Upsilon(0) + \int_0^t e^{M(t)-M(s)} O(\Upsilon^2)(s)ds + D(t); \tag{1.125}$$

where

$$M(t) = N(t) - \frac{1}{2}\begin{bmatrix} \alpha_1^2 & 0 & 0 \\ 0 & \alpha_2^2 & 0 \\ 0 & 0 & \alpha_3^2 \end{bmatrix} t + \begin{bmatrix} \alpha_1 B_1(t) & 0 & 0 \\ 0 & \alpha_2 B_2(t) & 0 \\ 0 & 0 & \alpha_3 B_3(t) \end{bmatrix} \tag{1.126}$$

$$\begin{aligned} D(t) = [\int_0^t e^{M(t)-M(s)} \begin{bmatrix} \alpha_1^2 G^{*2} \\ \alpha_2^2 I^{*2} \\ \alpha_3^2 \beta^{*2} \end{bmatrix} + \int_0^t e^{M(t)-M(s)} D_1 dB_1(t) \\ + \int_0^t e^{M(t)-M(s)} D_2 dB_2(t) + \int_0^t e^{M(t)-M(s)} D_3 dB_3(t)]. \end{aligned} \tag{1.127}$$

Note that for Brownian motion $B_k(t),\ \ k = 1, 2, 3$ we have

$$\begin{cases} \limsup_{t\to\infty} \frac{B_k(t)}{\sqrt{2tloglogt}} = 1 \ \liminf_{t\to\infty} \frac{B_k(t)}{\sqrt{2tloglogt}} = -1 \\ \limsup_{t\to 0^+} \frac{B_k(t)}{\sqrt{2tloglogt}} = 1 \ \liminf_{t\to 0^+} \frac{B_k(t)}{\sqrt{2tloglogt}} = -1. \end{cases} \tag{1.128}$$

In light of (1.125), (1.127), and (1.118) we can derive that

$$\|e^{M(t)}\| \leqslant K_2 e^{-\lambda_1 t} \tag{1.129}$$

for any $\lambda_1 < \lambda < 0$, and $t > 0$ a.s, and

$$\|e^{M(t)-M(s)}\| \leqslant K_2 e^{-\lambda(t-s)} \tag{1.130}$$

for any $\lambda_1 < \lambda < 0$, and $t > s$ a.s.

From (1.127)–(1.130) we can derive that

$$lim_{t\to\infty} D(t) = k_0 \begin{bmatrix} \alpha_1^2 G^{*2} \\ \alpha_2^2 I^{*2} \\ \alpha_3^2 \beta^{*2} \end{bmatrix} + k_1 D_1 + k_2 D_2 + k_3 D_3 =: D^*; \tag{1.131}$$

where $k_0,\ and\, k_1, ..., k_3$ are some constants; and $lim_{t\to\infty} e^{M(t)}\Upsilon(0) = 0$.

Let $C_1 = sup_{t\in[0,\infty)}(\|e^{M(t)}\Upsilon(0)\| + \|D(t)\|)$. In order to obtain the solution $\Upsilon(t)$'s asymptotic behavior, we introduce a ball in a Banach space.

$$\mathcal{B} = \{\Upsilon(t) \in C^0([0,\infty), \mathbb{R}^3_+) \mid \|\Upsilon(t)\| \leqslant 2C_1\}$$

and operator $\mathcal{L} : \mathcal{B} \to \mathcal{B}$

$$\mathcal{L}(\Upsilon)(t) = e^{M(t)}\Upsilon(0) + \int_0^t e^{M(t)-M(s)} O(\Upsilon^2)(s)ds + D(t) \tag{1.132}$$

Lemma 1.29 *For sufficiently small $\Upsilon(0)$ α_1 α_2, and α_3, the operator $\mathcal{L}$ defined by (1.132) is a contraction from $\mathcal{B}$ to $\mathcal{B}$.*

Proof.

From (1.132) and (1.130), we have

$$\|\mathcal{L}(\Upsilon)(t)\| \leqslant C_1 + K_2\|O(\Upsilon^2)\|,$$

and from (1.121)

$$\|O(\Upsilon^2)\| \leqslant K_3\|\Upsilon\|^2 \leqslant 4C_1^2 K_3,$$

we have

$$\|\mathcal{L}(\Upsilon)(t) \leqslant C_1 + 4K_2K_3C_1^2 \ \leqslant\ C_1(1 + 4K_2K_3C_1) \ \leqslant\ 2C_1,$$

since $1 + 4K_2K_3C_1 \ \leqslant\ 2$ when $\Upsilon(0)$ α_1, α_2, *and* α_3 are sufficiently small, consequently C_1 is sufficiently small.

Now let $\Upsilon_1,\ \Upsilon_2\ \in\ \mathcal{B}$, then

$$\|\mathcal{L}(\Upsilon_2) - \mathcal{L}(\Upsilon_1)\| \ \leqslant\ \|\textstyle\int_0^t e^{M(t)-M(s)}(O(\Upsilon_2^2) - O(\Upsilon_1^2))ds\|$$

$$\leqslant\ \textstyle\int_0^t K_3\|e^{M(t)-M(s)}\|\|\Upsilon_2 - \Upsilon_1\|(\|\Upsilon_1\| + \|\Upsilon_2\|)ds$$

$$\leqslant\ 4C_1K_3K_2\|\Upsilon_2 - \Upsilon_1\|\ .$$

We have for sufficiently small $\Upsilon(0)$ α_1, α_2, *and* α_3, C_1 is sufficiently small $4C_1K_3K_2 < 1$, which implies that $\mathcal{L}(\Upsilon)$ is a contraction. ■

Theorem 1.30 *There exists a unique solution of* Υ *in* $\mathcal{B}$ *if* $\Upsilon(0)$, α_1 α_2, *and* α_3 *are sufficiently small.*

Proof. Applying Banach fixed point theorem, we have the theorem.
■

From the above theorem, we have the asymptotic behavior of system (1.117).

Theorem 1.31 *If* $|G(0) - G^*| + |I(0) - I^*| + |\beta(0) - \beta^*|$ *and* $\alpha_1^2 + \alpha_2^2 + \alpha_3^2$ *are sufficiently small, then*

$$\begin{aligned}|G(t) - G^*| + |I(t) - I^*| + |\beta(t) - \beta^*| \ &\leq \ 2(|G(0) - G^*| \\ &+ |I(0) - I^*| + |\beta(0) - \beta^*|)e^{\lambda t} + 2\|D(t)\| \quad a.s\end{aligned}$$

for $\lambda_1 < \lambda < 0$ *and* $t \geqslant 0$.

Remark 1.32 *The fixed point* $P_2 = (600, 0, 0)$ *is a stable point of the system (1.115), the Jacobian matrix has three negative eigen values* $\lambda_1 = -432, \lambda_2 = -\frac{36}{25}, \lambda_3 = -0.42$. *The above theorem is also true for* $(G^*, I^*, \beta^*) = (600, 0, 0)$.

1.6.2.3 Numerical simulation

We proceed to the numerical simulation of the system (1.117) by the method of Monte-Carlo. The objective is to observe the behavior of the solution around the equilibrium points of the deterministic system. The parameters in the deterministic system are used as in Table 1.10.

We first take $\alpha_1 = 0.05$, $\alpha_2 = \alpha_3 = 0.01$ in the following *case 1- case3.*
Case 1. Around the deterministic physiological stable point $(G^*, I^*, \beta^*) = (100, 10, 300)$, the initial point (101,9,299) is taken. While the trajectories oscillate around the deterministic stable fixed point (see Fig. 1.16), the histograms show a roughly Gaussian distribution around the point $(G^*, I^*, \beta^*) = (100, 10, 300)$. This confirms Theorem 1.31.
Case 2. Around the deterministic pathological equilibrium point $(G^*, I^*, \beta^*) = (600, 0, 0)$, The initial point chosen is (599,1,1). Figure 1.17 captures the respective behavior of glucose, insulin and β-cells. Although there is no equilibrium point for the stochastic system, we observe the asymptotic convergence toward $(600, 0, 0)$. The histogram suggests a Gaussian distribution of G around the mean 600. The same trends are also noticed for both insulin and β-cells. This confirms Remark 1.32
Case 3. Around the saddle point $(G^*, I^*, \beta^*) = (250, 2.8, 37)$ for the deterministic system (1.115). This case is interesting because the asymptotic behavior depends on the position of the starting point. If we take (245,2.8,36) as a starting point, the solution tends to the point (600, 0, 0). If the initial value (260,3.0,38) is taken, then the solution goes to (100, 10, 300) as Fig. 1.18 shows.

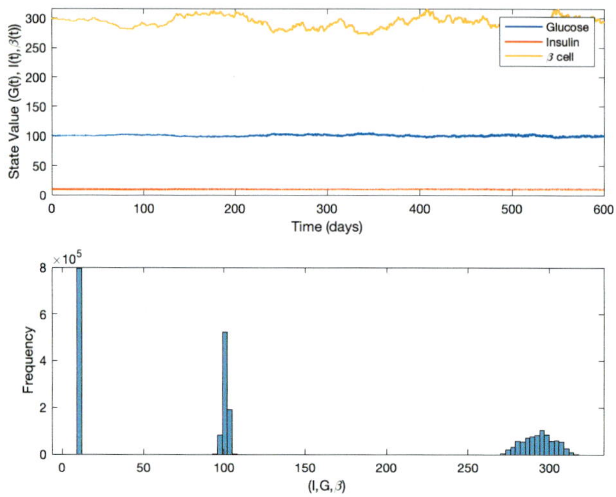

Figure 1.16 (a)The local asymptotic behavior of the stochastic βIG system around the point $(G^*, I^*, \beta^*) = (100, 10, 300)$ with $\alpha_1 = 0.05,\ \alpha_2 = \alpha_3 = 0.01$ and the initial point (101,9,299). (b) Histograms of the local asymptotic behavior of the stochastic βIG system around the point $(G^*, I^*, \beta^*) = (100, 10, 300)$.

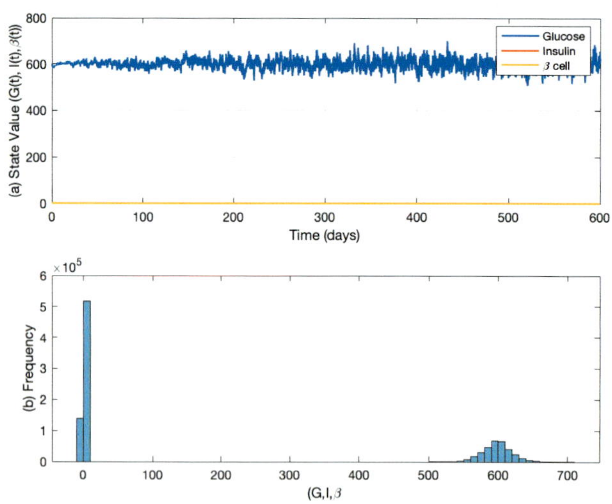

Figure 1.17 (a) The local asymptotic behavior of the stochastic βIG system around the point $(G^*, I^*, \beta^*) = (600, 0, 0)$ with $\alpha_1 = 0.05,\ \alpha_2 = \alpha_3 = 0.01$ and the initial point (599,1,1). (b) Histograms of the local asymptotic behavior of the stochastic βIG system around the point $(G^*, I^*, \beta^*) = (600, 0, 0)$.

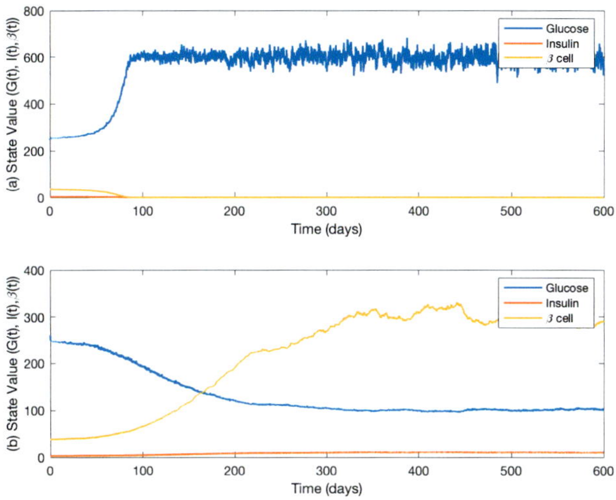

Figure 1.18 (a) The local asymptotic behavior of the stochastic βIG system around the point $(G^*, I^*, \beta^*) = (250, 2.8, 37)$ with $\alpha_1 = 0.05,\ \alpha_2 = \alpha_3 = 0.05$ and the initial point (245,2.8,36). (b) The local asymptotic behavior of the stochastic βIG system around the point $(G^*, I^*, \beta^*) = (250, 2.8, 37)$ with the initial value (260,3.0,38).

Now we increase the stochastic intensity by taking $\alpha_1 = 0.05$, $\alpha_2 = \alpha_3 = 0.05$, and we consider the problem (1.117) with initial condition $(G_0, I_0, \beta_0) = (101, 9, 299)$. Figure 1.19 shows that the solution is not close to the deterministic stable point $(100, 10, 300)$ in contrast of *Case 2* (Fig. 1.16). This indicates that if the stochastic intensity is not small enough, the asymptotic property in Theorem 1.31 no longer holds.

CHAPTER 2

Mathematical Modeling of Atherosclerosis

Some of the large and moderate arteries, such as the aorta and coronary artery, are composed of three layers: the tunica intima, the tunica media and the tunica adventitia. The tunica intima consists of the endothelium, connective tissue, and a basal layer of elastic tissue called internal elastic lamina that separates the tunica intima from tunica media. The endothelium is a thin monolayer of cells that serves as the contact surface with blood. The tunica media is circumferentially composed of vascular smooth muscle cells and elastin-rich extracellular matrix. The tunica adventitia is the outermost layer of the vascular wall. Atherosclerosis is a progressive vascular disease characterized by lipid accumulation in the arterial intima, recruitment of inflammatory cells, smooth muscle cell (SMC) migration and proliferation, extracellular matrix (ECM) remodeling, and, in advanced stages, fibrous cap thinning, necrotic core formation, calcification, and possible plaque rupture with thrombotic complications. The disease processes span molecular signaling (oxidation, cytokine networks), cellular events (monocyte recruitment, macrophage foam-cell formation, apoptotic clearance), tissue-level reModeling (cap formation, calcification), and haemodynamic influences (wall shear stress patterns). As atherosclerosis is a cardiovascular condition that affects critical circulatory systems, studying human atheroma poses logistical and ethical problems, as access to live atherosclerotic tissue is limited and disturbances risk triggering plaque rupture. As a result, the appropriate framework to consider emergent dynamical behavior of this type of disease is mathematical and computational modeling. Mathematical modeling brings a mechanistic framework to test hypotheses, perform in silico experiments, and-ideally-support clinical translation via patient-specific simulations.

The mathematical modeling of atherosclerosis has progressed through distinct stages, reflecting growing understanding of the disease's mechanisms. Early models [51, 128, 174], dating back to the 1970s, were influenced by the "response to injury" hypothesis, which emphasized endothelial damage

DOI: 10.1201/9781003376675-2

due to hemodynamic stresses like wall shear stress (WSS). Initial efforts focused on basic processes such as intimal thickening and low-density lipoprotein (LDL) transport, often using ordinary differential equations (ODEs) to describe particle adhesion and endothelial permeability. By the 1990s and 2000s, models incorporated spatial dynamics through partial differential equations (PDE), including reaction-diffusion systems to simulate inflammation and plaque growth. This period saw the integration of fluid mechanics, with computational fluid dynamics (CFD) used to analyze blood flow and its impact on plaque formation. The 2010s marked a shift toward multiscale and patient-specific models, leveraging advances in imaging technologies (e.g., high-resolution MRI and RNA sequencing) to couple biomechanical, biochemical, and microenvironmental factors. Recent developments emphasize predictive capabilities, such as forecasting plaque vulnerability and regression, with a focus on interdisciplinary approaches combining mathematics, biology, and clinical data.

Mathematical models of atherosclerosis can be broadly categorized based on their focus and methodology. Haemodynamic or CFD models [53, 132, 152, 157] employ incompressible Navier-Stokes (often Newtonian approximation for large arteries). CFD provides velocity, pressure, and derived quantities like WSS, OSI (oscillatory shear index), and particle residence time. Continuum reaction-diffusion PDE models [1, 39, 67, 103, 104, 147, 172, 214, 234, 288, 289] model cellular interactions (e.g., monocytes, macrophages, foam cells) and cytokines. Spatial gradients and diffusion/advection are naturally represented in continuum reaction-diffusion PDE models which are amenable to analysis and uncertainty quantification (UQ) when reduced to simpler forms. Compartmental ODE models [50, 68, 160, 250] use low-dimensional models of averaged plaque variables and are good for parameter estimation, therapy optimization, and conceptual insight. Agent-based and cellular automata models represent discrete cells/agents with rules for movement, signaling, phenotype switching, proliferation, death; capture stochasticity and heterogeneity; can represent non-continuum effects (e.g., local necrotic core formation). Hybrid & multiscale models [47, 71, 101, 151, 180, 240, 261, 267, 269, 272, 293, 296], (examples: PDE (chemicals) + ABM (cells) + finite-element mechanics (tissue stress, with CFD-driven boundary conditions for WSS)), bridge molecular/cellular processes to tissue and vessel scales; enable prediction of mechanical failure (rupture) as an emergent outcome. Biomechanical models [234] predict stress/strain distributions in fibrous cap and plaque components under blood pressure; assess vulnerability via peak cap stress or strain energy density; models nonlinear hyperelastic constitutive laws; anisotropic models accounting for collagen fiber orientation. Stochastic models and probabilistic frameworks [244, 245] model intrinsic randomness (cell fate), extrinsic uncertainty (parameters), and event probabilities (rupture prediction under uncertain inputs). Bayesian model inversion and Monte Carlo UQ are common. Data-driven & Machine Learning (ML) approaches [180, 248] use surrogate modeling (emulate expensive mechanics/biochemistry), feature extraction from imaging, and hybrid mechanistic-data models for risk stratification.

2.1 RISK OF HIGH CHOLESTEROL

A phospholipid molecule has a phosphate compound "head", and a fatty acid "tail". The head is hydrophilic and the tail is hydrophobic. The plasma membrane of a cell consists of a continuous double-layer of phospholipids, where both heads face the water, which is inside and outside the cell, and the two tails point inward toward each other. Cholesterol is a compound found in every cell of our body; it is especially abundant in the plasma membrane of cells. Cholesterol adds firmness to the plasma membrane; it helps maintain its fluidity without becoming overly fluid.

Plasma membrane contains many proteins that perform various tasks, including pumping substances into and out of the cell, and responding to extracellular or intracellular signaling. These proteins are secured in many lipid rafts, locations that are maintained by high concentration of cholesterol, which secure proper housing and function for membrane proteins.

Cholesterol is waxy, fat-like substance, produced in the liver. The liver produces more cholesterol when we eat a diet high in saturated fat. Cholesterol, in small packages, travels from the liver through the blood stream, in order to reach all the cells in our body. These packages are called lipoproteins. They are made of fat (lipo) from the inside and protein on the outside. There are two kinds of lipoprotein: Low density lipoprotein (LDL) and high density lipoprotein (HDL). The main structural difference between LDL and HDL is in their composition. Approximately 50% of the weight of an LDL particle is cholesterol and 20% is protein. With HDL, 20% is cholesterol and 50% is protein accumulated in the artery and carries it back into the liver, where it is either recycled or remove from the body.

The buildup of cholesterol in the artery may initiate the formulation of a plaque; the plaque is made up of cholesterol, fat, calcium, and cells from the blood and the artery wall. Atherosclerosis is a condition where a plaque builds up in the artery. It is a condition viewed as the "hardening of the artery." The plaque may rapture and a loose piece traveling with the blood flow may then completely block an artery downstream. Coronary heart disease is a condition in which a plaque builds up inside the coronary artery. If the flow of arterial blood to the heart muscles is reduced or blocked, a heart attack may occur. A plaque which develops in the carotid artery that brings oxygen-rich blood to the brain may cause a stoke. Plaques can also develop in arteries that bring oxygen rich blood to other organs or limits of body.

2.1.1 A Simplified Model

In this section, we discuss a simplified model presented in [112].

When a lesion develops in the inner surface of the arterial wall, LDL and HDL circulating in the blood may enter the arterial wall and become oxidized by the radicals that are always available in the tissue. Oxidized LDL triggers endothelial cells that form the inner surface of blood vessels to secrete chemoattractant proteins that begin to attract inflammatory macrophages, M1, from the blood into the arterial wall at the site of the oxidized cholesterol. The macrophages ingest the oxidized LDL and become, so called, foam cells. The build up of a plaque in the arterial vessel is enhanced by influx of additional cells including smooth muscle cells from the media (an inner layer in the arterial wall) and T cells from the blood; these cells are attracted by, and activated by, proteins produced by macrophages and endothelial cells. The effect of the (oxidized) LDL on plaque growth, however, is reduced by the good cholesterol,HDL. The HDL molecules attach to foam cells and initiate a process that transfers the oxidized LDL out from the foam cells and into the liver, a process called Reverse Cholesterol Transport (RCT) [111]. The foam cells that have been cleared of the LDL revert back to become macrophages, more precisely, non-inflammatory macrophages. But in addition to clearing oxidized LDL from foam cells, HDL also competes with LDL in becoming oxidized by radicals: it thus decreases the amount of radicals available to oxidize the LDL.

We introduce the following variables:

$$
\begin{aligned}
L &= \text{ LDL concentration in g/cm}^3, \\
H &= \text{ HDL concentration in g/cm}^3, \\
M &= \text{ macrophage density in g/cm}^3, \\
F &= \text{ foam cells density in g/cm}^3.
\end{aligned}
$$

The interplay among cholesterol, macrophages and foam cells is shown schematically in Fig. 2.1, where we have merged LDL with its oxidized form. We further simplify the model by not distinguishing between the M_1 and M_2 macrophages, setting $M = M_1 = M_2$. The artery is assumed to be a long circular cylinder, its diameter, 2B, will be taken to be 2cm, and all variables are functions of (r, t) only. The plaque is given by $R(t) < r < 1$, where r is measured in unit of cm, and t is measured in unit of days. The variables L, H, M, F satisfy the following equations in the region $\{(r, t); R(t) < r < 1, t > 0\}$,

$$\frac{\partial L}{\partial t} - \Delta L = -r_1 L - k_1 \frac{ML}{K_1 + L}, \tag{2.1}$$

$$\frac{\partial H}{\partial t} - \Delta H = -r_2 H - k_2 \frac{HF}{(K_2 + H)}, \tag{2.2}$$

$$\begin{aligned}\frac{\partial M}{\partial t} + \nabla \cdot (\mathbf{u}M) - D\Delta M &= -k_1 \frac{ML}{K_1 + L} \\ &\quad + k_2 \frac{HF}{(K_2 + H)} + \lambda \frac{ML}{\delta + H} - \mu_1 M,\end{aligned} \tag{2.3}$$

$$\frac{\partial F}{\partial t} + \nabla \cdot (\mathbf{v}F) - D\Delta F = k_1 \frac{ML}{K_1 + L} - k_2 \frac{HF}{(K_{HF} + H)} - \mu_2 F, \tag{2.4}$$

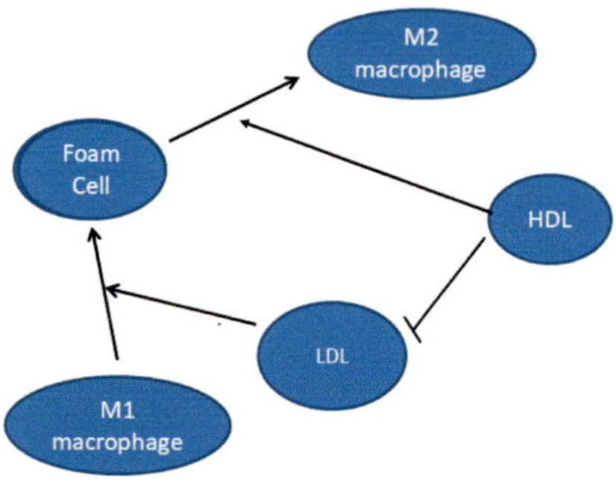

Figure 2.1 Interplay among cholesterol, macrophages and foam cells; the blocked arrow indicates inhibition.

The first term on the right-hand side of (2.1) represents ingestion of L_{ox} by macrophages. The second term represents degradation of L as it combines with radicals. In Eq. (2.2), the first term on the right-hand side is the consumption of H as it combines with membrane proteins on foam cells in a process which removes bad cholesterol from foam cells, thereby changing these cells into non-inflammatory macrophages M_2; we have also merged proinflammatory macrophages M_1 with non-inflammatory macrophage M_2. The last term in Eq. (2.2) is degradation of H as it becomes oxidized. In Eqs. (2.3)and (2.4) we included the transition between M and F: when L molecules are ingested by a macrophage, the macrophage becomes a foam cell, and when H combines with membrane protein on a foam cell in a process that clears it from the bad cholesterol the foam cell turns into a macrophage. Both Eqs. (2.3) and (2.4) include death rates, but in Eq. (2.3) we have added the extra term $\lambda ML/(\delta + H)$. This term is phenomenological: The factor ML accounts for a sequence of reactions, stemming from oxidized L, which results in the activation of inflammatory macrophages, while the inhibition factor $1/(\delta + H)$ is introduced to account for the fact that by oxidizing with radicals, H removes some of the radicals available to oxidize L.
We assume that the combined densities of macrophages and foam cells in the plaque is constant, and take, for $R(t) < r < 1, t > 0$,

$$M + F = M_0 \text{ for } R(t) < r < 1, t > 0. \tag{2.5}$$

However, the total combined mass of M and F generally varies in time, due to the generation term $\lambda M/(\delta + H)$ and the death terms $\mu_1 M, \mu_2 F$. This change in total mass combined with (2.5) gives rise to a velocity field $F\mathbf{v}$ which was incorporated into Eqs. (2.3) and (2.4).

The boundary conditions on the free boundary $r = R(t)$ are:

$$-\frac{\partial L}{\partial n} + \alpha(L - L_0) = 0, \quad -\frac{\partial H}{\partial n} + \alpha(H - H_0) = 0, \tag{2.6}$$

$$-\frac{\partial M}{\partial n} + \beta(M - \bar{M}_0) = 0, \quad -\frac{\partial F}{\partial n} + \beta F = 0, \tag{2.7}$$

where n is the outward normal; these flux conditions are based on the fact that the concentrations of L and H in the blood are L_0 and H_0, respectively, and the density of macrophages in the blood is M_0; there are no foam cells in the blood. We assume a no flux condition on the blood vessel wall $r = 1$ for all variables:

$$\frac{\partial L}{\partial n} = \frac{\partial H}{\partial n} = \frac{\partial M}{\partial n} = \frac{\partial F}{\partial n} = 0. \tag{2.8}$$

By combining Eqs. (2.3)(2.4), and using (2.5) , we get an equation for $\mathbf{v} = v\mathbf{e}_r$, where v is the radial velocity,

$$M_0 v_r = \lambda\frac{ML}{\delta + H} - \mu_1 M - \mu_2 F, v(1) = 0. \tag{2.9}$$

The equation for the free boundary is

$$\frac{dR(t)}{dt} = v(R(t), t). \tag{2.10}$$

All parameters in this simplified model are listed in the Table 2.1.

TABLE 2.1 Parameters' description and value

Parameters	Value
k_1	$144.5\ day^{-1}$ [112]
k_2	$10\ day^{-1}$ [112]
K_1	$10^{-2}\ g\ cm^{-3}$ [112]
K_2	$0.5\ g\ cm^{-3}$ [112]
r_1	$2.24 \times 10^{-5}\ day^{-1}$ [112]
r_2	$5.45 \times 10^{-7}\ day^{-1}$ [112]
μ_1	$0.015\ day^{-1}$ [112]
μ_2	$0.03\ day^{-1}$ [112]
α	1 [112]
β	0.01 [112]
D	$8.64 \times 10^{-7}\ cm^2\ day^{-1}$ [112]
λ	$2.573 \times 10^{-3}\ day^{-1}$ [112]
δ	$-2.541 \times 10^{-3}\ g\ cm^{-3}$ [112]
M_0	$5 \times 10^{-5}\ g\ cm^{-3}$ [112]

2.1.2 Mathematical Analysis of the Simplified Model

In this section, we give some rigorous results regarding the simplified model. First there exists a unique radially symmetric stationary plaque in a small ring-region $1-\epsilon<r<1$. Dropping t-derivative terms, a stationary solution satisfies:

$$-\Delta L=-r_1 L-k_1\frac{ML}{K_1+L}, \tag{2.11}$$

$$-\Delta H=-r_2 H-k_2\frac{HF}{(K_2+H)}, \tag{2.12}$$

$$\nabla\cdot(\mathbf{u}M)-D\Delta M=-k_1\frac{ML}{K_1+L} + k_2\frac{HF}{(K_2+H)}+\lambda\frac{ML}{\delta+H}-\mu_1 M, \tag{2.13}$$

$$\nabla\cdot(\mathbf{v}F)-D\Delta F=k_1\frac{ML}{K_1+L}-k_2\frac{HF}{(K_{HF}+H)}-\mu_2 F, \tag{2.14}$$

with the boundary conditions at $r=1$,

$$\frac{\partial L}{\partial n}=\frac{\partial H}{\partial n}=\frac{\partial M}{\partial n}=\frac{\partial F}{\partial n}=0. \tag{2.15}$$

and at $r=1-\epsilon$,

$$-\frac{\partial L}{\partial n}+\alpha(L-L_0)=0,\quad -\frac{\partial H}{\partial n}+\alpha(H-H_0)=0, \tag{2.16}$$

$$-\frac{\partial M}{\partial n}+\beta(M-\bar{M}_0)=0,\quad -\frac{\partial F}{\partial n}+\beta F=0. \tag{2.17}$$

For the solution to be stationary, we must also have

$$v=0 \text{ at } r=1-\epsilon. \tag{2.18}$$

Theorem 2.1 *[112] Given any $H_*>0$ and small $\epsilon_*>0$, there exists a K_* such that the following holds: For any $0<H_0<H_*$ and $0<\epsilon<\epsilon_*$, there is a unique $L_0>0$ and correspondingly a unique solution of (2.11)-(2.18); furthermore,*

$$|\lambda L_0-\mu_1(H0+\delta)|<K_*\epsilon. \tag{2.19}$$

Let

$$S_1=\frac{\lambda}{\delta+H_0}\frac{1}{\alpha}\left(\frac{k_1M_0L_0}{K_1+L_0}+r_1L_0\right)-\frac{\mu_1}{\delta+H_0}\frac{r_2H_0}{\alpha}+\frac{mu_2}{\beta D}\frac{k_1L_0}{K_1+L_0} \tag{2.20}$$

Theorem 2.2 *[112] For fixed $\epsilon>0$, the stationary solution established in Theorem 2.1 is linearly asymptotically stable if $S_1>0$, and linearly asymptotically unstable if $S_1<0$.*

Theorem 2.3 *[112] Assume that*

$$\frac{\lambda L_0}{\delta + H_0} - \mu_1 < 0,$$

and that for some constants A, ϵ, $|L(r,0) - L_0| \leq A\epsilon, |H(r,0) - H_0| \leq A\epsilon, |F(r,0)| \leq A\epsilon$, *and* $R(0) = 1 - 2\epsilon$. *If* ϵ *is sufficiently small then* $\lim_{t\to\infty} R(t) = 1$. *i.e. the plaque will shrink.*

Theorem 2.4 *[112] If* $\frac{\lambda L_0}{\delta+H_0} - \mu_1 > 0$, *and* $R(0) < 1$, *then* $\lim_{t\to\infty} R(t) < 1$. *i.e the plaque will persist.*

It is to be noted that there have been recent works on infinite branches of symmetry-breaking stationary solutions that bifurcate from the stationary annular solution in the longitude-latitude direction, see [153,154,302,304,305].

2.2 MONOCYTES AND CELL MIGRATIONS AND FORMATION

Atherosclerosis emerges as a result of multiple dynamical cell processes [96,192,280]. Damage to the endothelial layer of the artery wall triggers an inflammatory response in which monocytes, T-lymphocytes and other immune cells are recruited to the region of damage. These cells penetrate the endothelial layer, reaching the "tunica intima", along with low density lipoprotein (LDL) and high-density lipoprotein (HDL)-particles. Stimulated by the presence of interferon gamma (IFN-γ) and macrophage colony stimulating factor (M-CSF), monocytes differentiate into macrophages once they have entered the artery wall. While embedded within the "tunica intima", both LDL and HDL become oxidized by free oxygen radicals. Macrophages will phagocytose oxidized LDL, but not oxidized HDL. Macrophages heavily loaded with oxidized LDL transform into foam cells that eventually undergo apoptosis. The resulting mass of debris embedded in the "tunica intima" is known as an atheroma. Foam cells, along with endothelial cells, secrete monocyte chemoattractant protein-1 (MCP-1) to recruit more monocytes to the site of inflammation. Naive T cells contained within the artery wall differentiate into individual T cell types that can secrete IFN-γ. Smooth muscle cells (SMCs) are also recruited into the 'tunica intima', where they undergo apoptosis and contribute to the formation of a plaque in the artery wall. This accumulation of cells and debris can cause a swelling of the artery wall that restricts blood flow, leading to stenosis. Although the simplified model in previous section captures some key variables (such as LDL and HDL), more variables should be involved to describe the plaque development process which involves oxidization of lipoprotein and monocytes and cell migrations and formations.

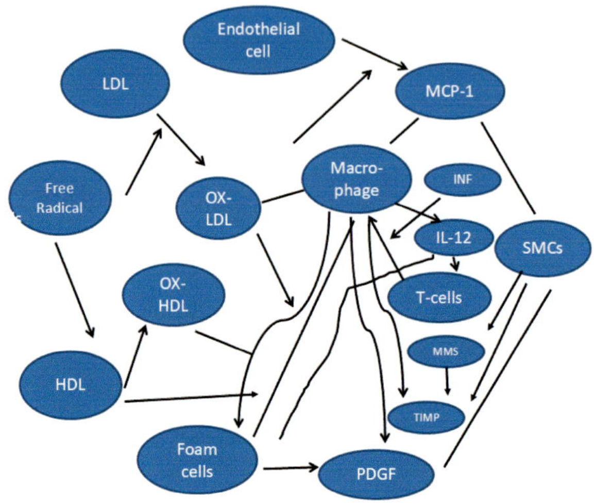

Figure 2.2 LDL and HDL are oxidized by free radicals, and become ox-LDL and ox-HDL respectively. Ox-LDL recruits macrophages to intima. By ingesting ox-LDL, macrophages are transformed to foam cells. SMCs are attracted into the intima by MCP-1 (secreted by endothelial cells) and PDGF (secreted by macrophages and foam cells). Macrophages, foam cells and SMCs secrete IL-12, which activates T cells. IFN-γ secreted by T cells enhance the activity of macrophages which contributes the plaque built-up.

2.2.1 A More Comprehensive Model

In this section, we discuss a more comprehensive model presented in [147]. The model consists of a system of partial differential equations. The mathematical model will be based on the network shown in Fig. 2.2. The variables included in the model are listed in Table 2.2.

We assume that all cells are moving with a common velocity $\mathbf{u}$; the velocity is the result of movement of macrophages, T-cells and SMCs into the

TABLE 2.2 The variables of the comprehensive model: concentrations and densities are in units of g/cm^3

L:	concentration of LDL	H:	concentration of HDL
L_{ox}:	concentration of ox-LDL	σ:	pressure (in gcm^2/day)
r:	concentration of free radicals	M:	density of macrophages
P:	concentration of MCP-1	G:	concentration of PDGF
S:	density of SMCs	ρ:	density of ECM
F:	density of foam cells	T:	density of T-cells
I_{12}:	concentration of IL-12	I_γ:	concentration of IFN-γ
Q:	concentration of MMPs	Q_r:	concentration of TIMP
$\mathbf{u}$:	fluid velocity (in cm/day)		

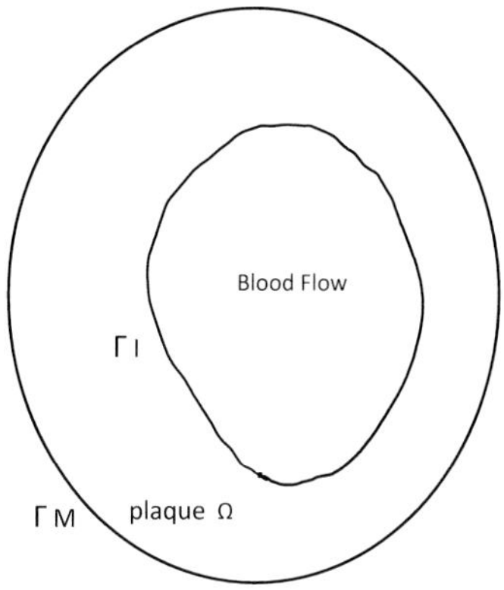

Figure 2.3 A 2D cross section of a plaque. Γ_M is the boundary of the intima in contact with the media, and Γ_I is the boundary of the intima in contact with the lumen.

intima. We also assume that all species are diffusing with appropriate diffusion coefficients. The equation for each species of cells X has the form

$$\frac{\partial X}{\partial t} + \nabla \cdot (\mathbf{u}X) - D_X \Delta X = F_X. \tag{2.21}$$

where the expression on the left side includes advection and diffusion, and F_X accounts for various growth factors, bio-chemical reactions, chemotaxis and haptotaxis. The equation for the chemical species are the same but without the advection term. In this work, we consider only two dimensional plaque for simplicity. Figure 2.3 shows a 2D cross section of a blood vessel with plaque Ω.

Equations for lipoproteins [LDL (L), HDL (H), ox-LDL (L_{ox}): The distribution of LDL, HDL and free radicals in the intima are described using reaction diffusion equations [7, 9, 10, 39]

$$\frac{\partial L}{\partial t} - D_L \Delta L = -k_L r L, \tag{2.22}$$

$$\frac{\partial H}{\partial t} - D_H \Delta H = -k_H r H, \tag{2.23}$$

$$\frac{\partial L_{ox}}{\partial t} - D_{L_{ox}} \Delta L_{ox} = k_L r L - \lambda_{M L_{ox}} M L_{ox}, \tag{2.24}$$

where k_L is reaction rates of oxidization, and $\lambda_{L_{ox}M}$ is the reduction rate of ox-LDL due to ingestion by macrophages. Equations (2.22) and (2.23) model the evolution of LDL and HDL concentrations. It is assumed that LDL and HDL are lost by reaction of oxidation with free radicals and LDL is ingested by macrophages. Equation (2.24) models the production of ox-LDL due to LDL oxidation by reaction with the radicals (first term on right-hand side) and a reduction of ox-LDL through ingestion by macrophages (second term on right-hand side).

Equation for free radicals (r): The equation for the concentration of free radicals is modeled by

$$\frac{\partial r}{\partial t} - D_r \Delta r = r_0 - r(k_L L + k_H H), \tag{2.25}$$

where r_0 is the base line growth.

Equation for SMCs (S): The equation of the SMCs density is given by

$$\frac{\partial S}{\partial t} + \nabla \cdot (\mathbf{u}S) - D_S \Delta S = -\nabla \cdot (S \chi_C \nabla P) - \nabla \cdot (S \chi_C \nabla G) - \nabla \cdot (S \chi_H \nabla \rho), \tag{2.26}$$

The first two terms on the right side account for chemostaxis by MCP-1 and PDGF (Platelet Driven Growth Factor) [148, 230, 231, 238],and the last term accounts for haptotaxis by ECM.

Equation for macrophages (M): The evolution of macrophage density is modeled by

$$\frac{\partial M}{\partial t} + \nabla \cdot (\mathbf{u}M) - D_M \Delta M = -\nabla \cdot (M \chi_C \nabla P) + \lambda_{MI_\gamma} \frac{M I_\gamma}{K_{I_\gamma} + I_\gamma} - d_M M, \tag{2.27}$$

Here the first term accounts for recruitment of macrophages by MCP-1 [148]; The second term accounts for activation of macrophages by I_γ [111, 147]. The third term accounts for the death of macrophages.

Equation for foam cells (F): The equation for foam cells is given by

$$\frac{\partial F}{\partial t} + \nabla \cdot (\mathbf{u}F) - D_F \Delta F = \lambda_{FM} \frac{M L_{ox}}{K_{L_{ox}} + L_{ox}} - d_F F, \tag{2.28}$$

where on the right side of the equation, a gain of foam cells from macrophages M ingesting L, and a loss of foam cells triggered by H. The death rate of foam cells is d_F.

Equation for MPC-1 (P): The MPC-1 is modeled by

$$\frac{\partial P}{\partial t} - D_P \Delta P = \lambda_{PE} \frac{L_{ox}}{K_{L_{ox}} + L_{ox}} - d_P P, \tag{2.29}$$

where the first term on the right-hand side is the production of MCP-1 by endothelial cells, whose density is assumed to be constant, under the influence of ox-LDL [111, 148].

Equation for T cells (T). The density of T cells satisfies

$$\frac{\partial T}{\partial t} + \nabla \cdot (\mathbf{u}T) - D_T \Delta T = \lambda_{TI_{12}} \frac{MI_{12}}{K_M + M} - d_T T. \tag{2.30}$$

In this equation, we assume that T cells are activated by IL-12 in conjunction with MHC-II (major histocompatibility complex, class II) [41,9.H-F].

Equation for PDGF (G), MMP(Q) and TIMP (Q_r: We have the following equation for PDFG

$$\frac{\partial G}{\partial t} - D_G \Delta G = \lambda_{GM} M + \lambda_{GF} F + \lambda_{GS} S - d_G G, \tag{2.31}$$

$$\frac{\partial Q}{\partial t} - D_Q \Delta Q = \lambda_{QS} S - d_{QQ_r} Q Q_r - d_Q Q, \tag{2.32}$$

$$\frac{\partial Q_r}{\partial t} - D_{Q_r} \Delta Q_r = \lambda_{Q_r S} S + \lambda_{Q_r M} M - d_{QQ_r} Q Q_r - d_{Q_r} Q_r, \tag{2.33}$$

where PDGF is produced by macrophages, foam cells, and SMCs [42,43,9]. In Eq. (2.32), MMP is secreted by SMCs and is lost by binding with TIMP [111, 147]. In Eq. (2.33), TIMP is produced by SMCs and macrophages [111, 147].

Equation for IFN-γ. The dynamics of IFN-γ is given by

$$\frac{\partial I_\gamma}{\partial t} - D_{I_\gamma} \Delta I_\gamma = \lambda_{TI_\gamma} T - d_{I_\gamma} I_\gamma. \tag{2.34}$$

where the first term on the right hand side is the production of I_γ by T cells [111, 147].

Equation for IL-12 (I_{12}): The equation for I_{12} is given by

$$\begin{aligned} \frac{\partial I_{12}}{\partial t} - D_{I_12} \Delta I_{12} = \lambda_{MI_{12}} \frac{M}{K_M + M} \left(1 + \frac{I_\gamma}{K_{I_{12}} H + I_\gamma}\right) \\ + \lambda_{I_{12}F} \frac{F}{K_F + F} - d_{I_12} I_{12}, \end{aligned} \tag{2.35}$$

The firs term of the right hand side is the production of I_{12} by macrophages enhanced by I_γ and resisted by HDL. The second term represents the production by the foam cells [111, 147].

Equation for pressure σ and ECM (ρ**:** We assume that the intima has the constituency of a porous medium. Then, by Darcy's law, the velocity $\mathbf{u}$ of the cells is given by

$$\mathbf{u} = -\nabla \sigma, \tag{2.36}$$

where σ is the pressure. We also assume that the total density of all the cells is constant. This constant should be smaller than the average density of a plaque, $1.22 \pm 0.03 g/cm^3$ [9], because plaques contain some debris, which are not included in our model. We take the constant to be 1 g/cm3, i.e.,

$$M + F + T + \rho + S = 1 \tag{2.37}$$

We assume that all cells are approximately of the same volume and surface area, so that the diffusion coefficients of the all cells have the same coefficient D. By adding Eqs. (2.26)–(2.28) and (2.30), and using (2.37), we get

$$-\frac{\partial \rho}{dt} - (1-\rho)\Delta\sigma + \nabla\sigma\dot{\nabla}\rho + D\Delta\rho = \phi, \tag{2.38}$$

where

$$\begin{aligned}\phi = &-\nabla\cdot(S\chi_C\nabla P) - \nabla\cdot(S\chi_C\nabla G) - \nabla\cdot(S\chi_H\nabla\rho)\\ &- \nabla\cdot(M\chi_C\nabla P) + \lambda_{TI_{12}}\frac{MI_{12}}{K_M+M} + \lambda_{MI_\gamma}\frac{MI_\gamma}{K_{I_\gamma}+I_\gamma}\\ &+ \lambda_{FM}\frac{ML_{ox}}{K_{L_{ox}}+L_{ox}} - d_T T - d_F F - d_M M. \end{aligned} \tag{2.39}$$

We next derive an equation for ρ. The ECM is degraded by MMP [27], and is remodeled by macrophages and SMCs [18, 27]. For simplicity, we take the remodeling rate to be a constant, λ_ρ, as in [28]. Then the equation of the density of ECM is given by

$$\frac{\partial \rho}{\partial t} + \nabla\cdot(\mathbf{u}\rho) = -\lambda_\rho\rho(1-\frac{\rho}{\rho_0}) - d_{\rho Q}Q. \tag{2.40}$$

Since $u = -\nabla\sigma$, this equation can be written in the form

$$\frac{\partial \rho}{\partial t} - \rho\Delta\sigma - \nabla\sigma\cdot\nabla\rho = \psi,$$

where

$$\psi = -\lambda_\rho\rho(1-\frac{\rho}{\rho_0}) - d_{\rho Q}Q. \tag{2.41}$$

Adding this equation and (2.38), we get our final equation for σ:

$$-\Delta\sigma + D\Delta\rho = \phi + \psi. \tag{2.42}$$

The equation for ρ can then be written as

$$\frac{\partial \rho}{\partial t} - D\rho\Delta\rho + (\phi+\psi) - \nabla\rho\cdot\nabla\sigma = \psi. \tag{2.43}$$

Boundary Conditions: For simplicity, we consider only 2-dimensional plaques as in Fig. 2.3. Then the boundary of the plaque consists of i) Γ_M, in contact with media; ii) a free boundary Γ_I, inside the lumen.

Boundary conditions on Γ_I: We assume flux boundary conditions of the form

$$\frac{\partial X}{\partial n} + \alpha_X(X - X_0) = 0, \tag{2.44}$$

for $X = L, H, M, T$, and α_X are constants.

Non-flux boundary conditions for all other variables

$$Y = r, S, F, L_o x, I_\gamma, I_{12}, G, Q, Q_r, P :$$
$$\frac{\partial Y}{\partial n} = 0. \tag{2.45}$$

The flux boundary condition for ρ is determined by $\rho = 1 - S - F - M$. The coefficient α_X is a constant except for M, and $\alpha_M(L_{ox}, H) = \tilde{\alpha}_M \frac{L_{ox}}{1+H}$ since ox-LDL attracts monocytes [H-F], while HDL limits the inflammation process. Note that L_0 and H_0 are the LDL and HDL concentrations in the blood, so we shall be interested to see how these concentrations determine whether a small plaque will grow or shrink.

As in [40, 41, 43], we assume that the free boundary Γ_I is held together by cell-to-cell adhesion forces so that

$$\sigma = \gamma\kappa \text{ on } \Gamma_I, \tag{2.46}$$

where κ is the mean curvature of the surface Γ_I. (If Γ_I is circular, then κ is the reciprocal of the radius) Furthermore, the continuity condition $u_n = V_n$, where n is the outward normal and V_n is the velocity of the free boundary Γ_I in the direction n, yields the relation

$$V_n = -\frac{\partial \sigma}{\partial n} \text{ on } \Gamma_I. \tag{2.47}$$

Boundary conditions on Γ_M: We assume non-flux boundary conditions for all variables except S and ρ on Γ_M: For S, we have

$$\frac{\partial S}{\partial n} + \tilde{\alpha}_S \frac{P+G}{P_0+G_0}(S - S_0) = 0 \text{ on } \Gamma_M, \tag{2.48}$$

where S_0 is SMCs density in the media and MCP-1 and PDGF attract SMCs from the media. The flux condition for ρ is determined by $\rho = 1-S-T-F-M$. **Parameter estimation**: Parameters on the right hand side of (2.22)–(2.48) can be found given in [111, 147] and are listed in Tables 2.3, 2.4, and 2.5.

2.2.2 Numerical Algorithm and Simulation Results of the More Comprehensive Model

In this section we discuss the numerical method and algorithm used in [147].

In order to illustrate the numerical method, we consider the following diffusion equation with Robin boundary conditions:

$$\begin{aligned} &\frac{dX}{dt} + \gamma\nabla \cdot (\mathbf{u}X) - D\Delta X = f(X), \\ &\frac{\partial X}{\partial n} + \alpha(X - X_I) = 0, on\Gamma_I, \\ &\frac{\partial X}{\partial n} + \beta(X - X_M) = 0, on\Gamma_M, \end{aligned} \tag{2.49}$$

TABLE 2.3 Parameters' description and value

Parameters	Description	Value
D_M	diffusion coefficient for macrophage	$8.64 \times 10^{-7}\, cm^2\ d^{-1}$ [147]
D_F	diffusion coefficient for foam cells	$8.64 \times 10^{-7}\, cm^2\ d^{-1}$ [147]
D_S	diffusion coefficient for SMC	$8.64 \times 10^{-1}\, cm^2\ d^{-1}$ [147]
D_G	diffusion coefficient for PDGF	$8.64 \times 10^{-1}\, cm^2\ d^{-1}$ [147]
$D_{I_{12}}$	diffusion coefficient for I_{12}	$1.08 \times 10^{2}\, cm^2\ d^{-1}$ [147]
D_{I_γ}	diffusion coefficient I_γ	$1.08 \times 10^{2}\, cm^2\ d^{-1}$ [147]
D_P	diffusion coefficient for MCP-1	$17.28\, cm^2\ d^{-1}$ [147]
D_r	diffusion coefficient for radicals	$2.05 \times 10^{-1}\, cm^2\ d^{-1}$ [147]
D_L	diffusion coefficient for LDL	$29.89\, cm^2\ d^{-1}$ [147]
D_H	diffusion coefficient for HDL	$3.93\, cm^2\ d^{-1}$ [147]
$D_{L_{ox}}$	diffusion coefficient for Oxidized LDL	$29.89\, cm^2\ d^{-1}$ [147]
D_T	diffusion coefficient for T cells	$8.64 \times 10^{-7}.89\, cm^2\ d^{-1}$ [147]
D_Q	diffusion coefficient for MMP	$4.32 \times 10^{-2}\, cm^2\ d^{-1}$ [147]
D_{Q_r}	diffusion coefficient for TIMPs	$4.32 \times 10^{-2}\, cm^2\ d^{-1}$ [147]
k_L	reaction rate of for LDL+ Radical	$2.35 \times 10^{-4}\, g^{-1}\, cm^3\ d^{-1}$ [147]
k_H	reaction rate of for HDL+ Radical	$5.29 \times 10^{-6}\, g^{-1}\, cm^3\ d^{-1}$ [147]
α_T	influx rate of T cells into intima	$0.05\, cm^{-1}$ [147]
$\tilde{\alpha}_S$	influx rate of SMCs into intima	$0.2\, cm^{-1}$ [147]
α_L	influx rate of LDL into intima	$1.0\, cm^{-1}$ [147]
α_H	influx rate of HDL into intima	$1.0\, cm^{-1}$ [147]
$\tilde{\alpha}_M$	influx rate of Macrophages into intima	$0.2\, cm^{-1}$ [147]
χ_C	Chemotactic sensitivity parameter	$8.64 \times 10^{-1} \sim 1.73 \times 10^{4}$ $cm^5\ g^{-1}\ day^{-1}$ [147]
χ_H	Haptotaxis parameter	$8.64 \times 10^{-2} \sim 8.64 \times 10^{4}$ $cm^5\ g^{-1}\ day^{-1}$ [147]

TABLE 2.4 Parameters' description and value

Parameters	Description	Value
λ_{GM}	production rate of PDGE by macrophages	$0.1\ d^{-1}$ [147]
λ_{GF}	production rate of PDGE by foam cells	$0.033\ d^{-1}$ [147]
λ_{GS}	production rate of PDGE by SMCs	$0.5\ d^{-1}$ [147]
λ_{QS}	production rate of MMP by SMCs	$3 \times 10^{-4}\ d^{-1}$ [147]
λ_{Q_rS}	production rate of TIMP by SMCs	$3 \times 10^{-5}\ d^{-1}$ [147]
λ_{Q_rM}	production rate of TIMP by macrophages	$6 \times 10^{-5}\ d^{-1}$ [147]
$\lambda_{ML_{ox}}$	rate of ox-LDL ingestion by macrophages	$10g\ cm^{-3}\ d^{-1}$ [147]
λ_{PE}	Production rate of MCP-1	$8.65 \times 10^{-10}g\ cm^{-3}\ d^{-1}$ [147]
$\lambda_{I_{12}M}$	production rate of I_{12} by macrophages	$3 \times 10^{-7}g\ cm^{-3}\ d^{-1}$ [147]
$\lambda_{I_{12}F}$	production rate of I_{12} by foam cells	$1 \times 10^{-7}g\ cm^{-3}\ d^{-1}$ [147]
$\lambda_{I_\gamma T}$	production rate of I_γ by T cells	$0.066g\ cm^{-3}\ d^{-1}$ [147]
λ_{MI_γ}	activation rate of macrophages by IFN_γ	$0.0005\ d^{-1}$ [147]
λ_{FM}	activation rate of by foam cells	$0.12\ d^{-1}$ [147]
$\lambda_{TI_{12}}$	activation rate of T cells by I_{12}	$1 \times 10^{6}\ d^{-1}$ [147]
λ_ρ	remodeling rate of ECM	$0.432\ d^{-1}$ [147]
d_M	death rate of macrophages	$0.015\ d^{-1}$ [147]
d_F	death rate of foam cells	$0.03\ d^{-1}$ [147]
d_P	degradation rate of MCP-1	$1.73\ d^{-1}$ [147]
d_T	death rate of T cells	$0.33\ d^{-1}$ [147]
d_S	death rate of SMCs	$0.86\ d^{-1}$ [147]
d_{I_γ}	degradation rate of I_γ	$0.69\ d^{-1}$ [147]
$d_{I_{12}}$	degradation rate of I_{12}	$1.188\ d^{-1}$ [147]
d_G	degradation rate of PDGF	$3.84\ d^{-1}$ [147]
d_Q	degradation rate of MMP	$4.32\ d^{-1}$ [147]
d_{Q_r}	degradation rate of TIMP	$21.6\ d^{-1}$ [147]
d_{QQ_r}	binding rate of MMP to TIMP	$4.98 \times 10^{8}\ g\ cm^{-3}\ d^{-1}$ [147]
d_{Q_rQ}	binding rate of TIMP to MMP	$1.04 \times 10^{8}\ g\ cm^{-3}\ d^{-1}$ [147]

TABLE 2.5 Parameters' description and value

Parameters	Description	Value
r_0	source/influx of radical into intima	$0.25\, g\, cm^{-3}\ d^{-1}$ [147]
M_0	source/influx of macrophage from blood	$5 \times 10^{-5}\, g\, cm^{-3}$ [147]
T_0	source/influx of T cells into intima	$1 \times 10^{-3}\, g\, cm^{-3}$ [147]
S_0	source/influx of SMCs into intima	$6 \times 10^{-3}\, g\, cm^{-3}$ [147]
L_0	source/influx of LDL in blood	$7 \times 10^{-4} - 1.9 \times 10^{-3}$ $g\, cm^{-3}$ [147]
H_0	source/influx of HDL in blood	$4 \times 10^{-4} - 6 \times 10^{-4}$ $g\, cm^{-3}$ [147]
ρ_0	ECM density	$1 \times 10^{-3}\, g\, cm^{-3}$ [147]
P_0	MCP-1 concentration	3×10^{-10} [147]
G_0	PDGF concentration	1.5×10^{-8} [147]
$K_{L_{ox}}$	ox-LDL saturation for production of MCP-1	$0.5\, g\, cm^{-3}$ [147]
K_M	macrophages saturation for production of I_{12}	$2.5 \times 10^{-5}\, g\, cm^{-3}$ [147]
K_F	foam cells saturation for production of I_{12}	$2.5 \times 10^{-5}\, g\, cm^{-3}$ [147]
$K_{I_{12}}$	I_{12} saturation for production of I_{12}	$7 \times 10^{-11}\, g\, cm^{-3}$ [147]
K_{I_γ}	I_γ saturation for activation of macrophage	$1 \times 10^{-11}\, g\, cm^{-3}$ [147]

where $\gamma\nabla \cdot (\mathbf{u}X)$ is an advection term, and either $\gamma = 1$ or $\gamma = 0$ (no advection), and $u = -\nabla\sigma$. Multiplying the differential equation by an arbitrary test function v, and performing integration by parts using the boundary conditions, we get

$$\begin{aligned}\int_\Omega \frac{dX}{dt} v dx + \gamma \int_\Omega X\nabla\sigma \cdot \nabla v dx + D\int_\Omega \nabla X \cdot \nabla v dx \\ = \int_\Omega f(X) v dx - \gamma \int_{\Gamma_I} Xv\frac{\partial\sigma}{\partial n} ds - \int_{\Gamma_M} v\beta(X - X_M) ds \\ + \int_{\Gamma_I} v\beta(X - X_I) ds \quad (2.50)\end{aligned}$$

This is an equivalent formulation of the system (2.49), which is better suited for simulation. Similarly, Eq. (2.42) for s has the equivalent form:

$$\int_\Omega \nabla\sigma \cdot \nabla v dx - D\int_\Omega \nabla\rho \cdot \nabla v dx = \int_\Omega (\phi + \psi) v dx - \gamma \int_{\Gamma_M} v\frac{\partial\rho}{\partial n} ds. \quad (2.51)$$

Galerkin discretization. The standard Galerkin discretization method uses finite dimensional subspaces V_h to approximate the solution X. Let $\{\omega_i\}_{i=1}^N$ be a basis of V_h, where N is the number of nodes within the triangulation K. Let $X_n \in V_h$ denote the numerical approximation of X at time $t = ndt$, where dt is the time step, X_h^n is written as a sum

$$X_h^n = \sum_{j=1}^{N} c_j^n \omega_j, \tag{2.52}$$

for coefficient c_j^n to be determined. If $\frac{X}{dt}$ is approximated by $\frac{X^{n+1}-X^n}{dt}$ then (2.50) is equivalent to

$$\int_\Omega X^{n+1}\omega_i dx + dt\left[\gamma\int_\Omega X^n\nabla\sigma\cdot\nabla\omega_i dx + D\int_\Omega \nabla X\cdot\nabla\omega_i dx\right]$$
$$= dt\Bigg(\int_\Omega f(X^n)\omega_i dx - \gamma\int_{\Gamma_I} X^n\omega_i\frac{\partial\sigma}{\partial n}ds - \int_{\Gamma_M}\omega_i\beta(X^n - X_M)ds$$
$$+\int_{\Gamma_I}\omega_i\beta(X^n - X_I)ds\Bigg) \tag{2.53}$$

Recalling (2.52), we can rewrite the system (2.53) as a linear system of equations

$$Ac^{n+1} = b, \tag{2.54}$$

where c^n is the vector of $((c_j^n)$, and the coefficient matrix $A = (A_{ij})$ and the right-hand side $b = (b_i)$ are defined by

$$A_{ij} = \int_\Omega \nabla\omega_i\cdot\nabla\omega_j dx + dt\int_\Omega \omega_i\omega_j dx,$$

and

$$b_i = \int_\Omega\sum_{j=1}^{N}(c_j^n\omega_j)\omega_i dx - dt\gamma\int_{Omega}\sum_{j=1}^{N}(c_j^n\omega_j)\nabla\sigma\cdot\nabla\omega_i dx$$
$$+ dt\Bigg(\int_\Omega f(\sum_{j=1}^{N}c_j^n\omega_j)\omega_i dx - \gamma\int_{\Gamma_I}\sum_{j=1}^{N}(c_j^n\omega_j)\omega_i\frac{\partial\sigma}{\partial n}ds$$
$$-\int_{\Gamma_M}\omega_i\beta(\sum_{j=1}^{N}c_j^n\omega_j - X_M)ds + \int_{\Gamma_I}\omega_i\alpha(\sum_{j=1}^{N}c_j^n\omega_j - X_I)ds\Bigg)$$

Similarly, setting $\sigma_h^n = \sum_j^N d_j^n\omega_j$, where σ_h^n is a numerical approximation of σ at time ndt, Eq. (2.51) can be written as follows

$$Bd^n = e, \tag{2.55}$$

where d^n is the vector (d_j^n), B is a matrix (B_{ij}), $B_{ij} = \int_\Omega \nabla\omega_i \cdot \nabla\omega_j dx$, and

$$e_j = D\int_\Omega \nabla\rho\cdot\nabla\omega_j dx + \int_\Omega(\phi+\psi)\omega_j dx - \int_{\Gamma_M}\omega_j\frac{\partial\rho}{\partial n}ds.$$

Outline of the procedure. A triangle mesh can be generated by MATLAB, and the algorithm is outlined in Algorithm for implementation. For the detailed implementations, such as: construct basis functions over the triangulation, assemble the stiffness matrix, etc, see references [187].

	Algorithm for implementation
Input:	The initial condition, time stepsize τ, the maximum time-steps N_T, step size for remeshing M. Generate a triangular mesh over the domain.
for $n = 0 : N_T$	**do**
	• Compute $L^{n+1}, H^{n+1}, r^{n+1}, L_{ox}^{n+1}, M^{n+1}, P^{n+1}$, $T^{n+1}, I_\gamma^{n+1}, S^{n+1}, I_{12}^{n+1}, G^{n+1}, Q^{n+1}, Q_r^{n+1}, \rho^{n+1}$, F^{n+1} by solving equation (2.54); • Compute the mean curvature of γ_I^n, κ^n; • Compute σ^{n+1} by solving equation (2.55); • Compute V_n in equation (2.47) and update Γ_I^{n+1}; • Remeshing every M steps.
end	

Results of simulation: Numerical simulation is initialized by a small formed plaque. Five combined levels of LDL and HDL (L_0 and H_0) are tested in [147] for 300 days:

(a) $(L_0, H_0) = (190, 40)$: a small plaque doubles in size at 300 days;

(b) $(L_0, H_0) = (150, 45)$: a small plaque increases approximately 50% at 300 days;

(c) $(L_0, H_0) = (130, 50)$: a small plaque remains small at 300 days;

(d) $(L_0, H_0) = (110, 52)$: a small plaque decreases approximately 30% at 300 days;

(e) (L_0, H_0) $(70, 60)$: a small plaque almost disappear at 300 days.

A risk-map of plaque development has been created in [147] by computing the weight of the plaque, the summation of total cells, namely, $\int_\Omega(M + F + S + T)d\Omega$, and form the risk matrix.

2.3 MODELING OF DIABETIC ATHEROSCLEROSIS

Diabetes and atherosclerosis are chronic inflammatory conditions. Diabetic patients have an increased risk of cardiovascular disease (CVD), and have a more than twofold increase in the risk of dying from CVD [17]. Myeloid cells (neutrophils, monocytes, and macrophages) are involved in both atherosclerosis and diabetes. The migration of circulating monocytes into the vessel wall is critical for the development of diabetic atherosclerosis. Moreover, intercellular cell adhesion molecule-1 (ICAM-1), chemoattractant protein-1 (MCP-1), and macrophage migration inhibitory factor (MIF), which regulate the adhesion of monocytes, are dysregulated in hyperglycemia-induced atherosclerosis. Increased foam cells derived from macrophages promote the acceleration of atherosclerotic lesions in diabetic mice [164,252]. A more inflammatory monocyte/macrophage phenotype with secretion of higher levels of proinflammatory cytokines was detected in both animal models and patients with diabetes mellitus [166]. In addition, T-cell function is closely related to atherosclerosis in the diabetic environment, and inflammatory monocytes have been shown to activate Th17 cells under diabetic conditions [36].

Diabetes cause endothelial cell dysfunction: Endothelial dysfunction due to inflammation and oxidative stress is a crucial characteristic in diabetes mellitus-linked atherosclerosis. Endothelial dysfunction is associated with decreased nitric oxide (NO) availability, either through loss of NO production or NO biological activity [228,270]. The excess generation of free oxygen radicals leads to apoptosis in endothelial cells [20]. In hyperglycemia, chronic inflammation increases vascular permeability, promotes the generation of adhesion molecules and chemokines, and stimulates accumulation of monocytes in the artery wall.

Diabetes cause vascular smooth muscle cell dysfunction. Proliferation and accumulation of smooth muscle cells are detected in both type 1 and type 2 diabetes mellitus. The changes in smooth muscle cells are a result of the diabetic environment directly [64, 196, 210]. Diabetes stimulates atherogenic activities of SMCs. SMCs cultured from patients with type 2 diabetes demonstrate enhanced migration [17]. Advanced atherosclerotic lesions in diabetic patients have fewer SMCs compared with those of controls [17].

Diabetes impair platelet function. Platelets from patients with diabetes have been shown to have decreased sensitivity to antiaggregation agents, such as prostacyclin (PGI2) and NO [204]. Glycated low-density lipoprotein (GlyLDL-) and hyperinsulinemia-induced impairment of calcium homeostasis, activation of protein kinase C (PKC), increased generation of reactive oxygen species (ROS), and decreased NO bioactivity result in hyperactivation of platelets [100].

Animal studies of diabetic atherosclerosis exist for mouse, rabbit and pig [133, 164]. As atherosclerosis is a cardiovascular condition that affects critical circulatory systems, studying human atheroma poses logistical and ethical problems, as access to live atherosclerotic tissue is limited and disturbances risk triggering plaque rupture. As a result, it is compelling to study diabetic atherosclerosis by mathematical model which is biologically relevant and can be used to simulate pathway dynamics of the disease.

2.3.1 Risk of Hyperglycaemia: A Simplified Model

The metabolic milieu of T2DM, including insulin resistance, hyperglycemia and release of excess free fatty acids, along with other metabolic abnormalities affects vascular wall by a series of events including endothelial dysfunction, oxidative stress and low-grade inflammation [17, 150, 161, 163, 168, 282]. Activation of these events further enhances vasoconstriction and promotes thrombus formation, ultimately resulting in the development of atherosclerosis. Hyperglycemia is thought to trigger vascular damage by creating imbalance between NO bioavailability and accumulation of ROS as well as reactive nitrogen species (RNS), resulting in endothelial dysfunction [235, 246].

In this section, we discuss a model proposed in [288,290]. The model establishes governing equations for the mechanism whereby excess glucose metabolites inhibits production of NO by blocking eNOS synthase activation and increase the production of ROS, governing equations for the mechanism that insulin resistance decrease endothelium-derived NO and increase the production of ROS, governing equations for the mechanism where diabetes stimulates atherogenic activity of vascular smooth muscle cells.

We will use a system of partial differential equations to develop a mathematical model of plaque formation in diabetic atherosclerosis. The mathematical model will be based on the network shown in Fig. 2.4. The variables included in the model are listed in Table 2.6. We assume that all cells are moving with a common velocity $\mathbf{u}$ [9, 10]; the velocity is the result of movement of macrophages, T-cells and SMCs into the intima. We also assume that all species are diffusing with appropriate diffusion coefficients. The equation for each species of cells X has the form

$$\frac{dX}{dt} + \nabla \cdot (\mathbf{u}X) - D_X \Delta X = F_X. \tag{2.56}$$

where the expression on the left side includes advection and diffusion, and F_X accounts for various growth factors, bio-chemical reactions, chemotaxis and haptotaxis. The equation for the chemical species are the same but without the advection term.

Equations for glucose, insulin, and β-cells: The distribution of G and I and β density are modeled by

$$\frac{\partial G}{\partial t} - D_G \Delta G = \tilde{G}_0 - (E_{G0} + S_I I)G - \lambda_{GH}(G - G_s)H, \tag{2.57}$$

$$\frac{d\beta}{dt} + \nabla \cdot (\mathbf{u}\beta) - D_\beta \Delta\beta = (-d_0 + r_1 G - r_2 G^2)\beta, \tag{2.58}$$

$$\frac{dI}{dt} - D_I \Delta I = \frac{\tilde{\sigma} G^2 \beta}{\alpha + G^2} - k_I I - \lambda_{RI} RI; \tag{2.59}$$

Equation (2.57) describes the dynamics of glucose and insulin,the third term on the right side of (2.57) represents that HDL helps lower glucose. G_s is the steady glucose concentration. Equation (2.58) describes the formation and loss

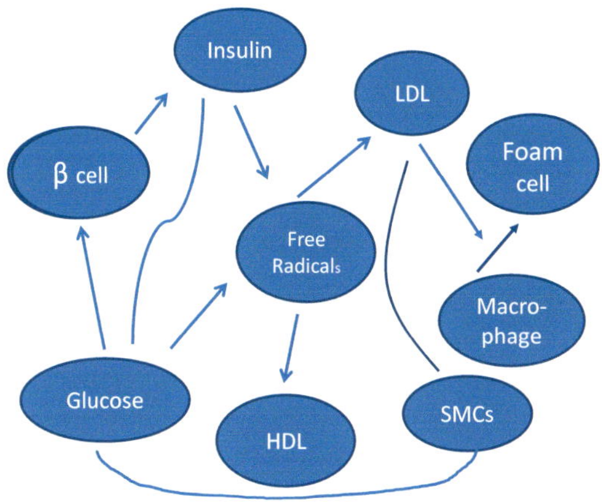

Figure 2.4 Glucose production and uptake depend on blood glucose and insulin levels. Insulin is secreted by pancreatic β cells, cleared by the liver, kidneys, and insulin receptors. β cells replication and death vary nonlinearly with glucose. Glucose metabolites inhibits production of NO and increase the production of ROS. Insulin resistance decrease endothelium-derived NO and increase the production of ROS. Diabetes stimulates atherogenic activity of vascular smooth muscle cells. LDL and HDL are oxidized by free radicals, Ox- LDL recruits macrophages to intima. By ingesting ox-LDL, macrophages are transformed to foam cells. In this figure, LDL and oxidized LDL are merged.

of β-cells [265]. The first term on the right hand side of (2.59) is secretion of insulin [35], the second term is clearance of insulin. The third term on the right side of (2.59) models that ROS, in excess and over time, cause chronic oxidation stress, which in turn result in reduction of insulin secretion as well as increased apoptosis [235, 246], where λ_{RI} is the reduction rate of insulin due to ROS.

Equations for lipoproteins [LDL (L), HDL (H)]: The distribution of LDL, HDL and free radicals in the intima are described using reaction diffusion equations [7, 9, 10, 39]

$$\frac{\partial L}{\partial t} - D_L \Delta L = -k_L R L + \lambda_{GL}(G - G_s)L - \lambda_{ML}\frac{ML}{K_{ML} + L}, \tag{2.60}$$

$$\frac{\partial H}{\partial t} - D_H \Delta H = -k_H R H - \lambda_{HF}\frac{HF}{(K_{HF} + H)}, \tag{2.61}$$

TABLE 2.6 The variables of the model: concentrations and densities are in units of g/cm^3

L:	concentration of LDL	H:	concentration of HDL
G:	concentration of Glucose	I:	concentration of Insulin
R:	concentration of free radicals	M:	density of macrophages
S:	density of SMCs	β:	density of β-cells
F:	density of foam cells		
u:	fluid velocity (in cm/day)	σ:	pressure (in gcm^2/day)

where k_L and k_H are reaction rates of oxidization. Equations (2.60) and (2.61) model the evolution of LDL and HDL concentrations. It is assumed that LDL and HDL are lost by reaction of oxidation with free radicals. LDL is ingested by macrophages and its production is enhanced by AGEs which is assumed to be proportional to the glucose. A reduction of ox-HDL through ingestion by foam cells is represented by the second term on right-hand side of (2.61). λ_{FH} is the reduction rate of ox-HDL due to ingestion by the foam cells. We merge LDL and HDL with oxidized LDL and oxidized HDL in these equations.

Equation for free radicals (R): The equation for the concentration of free radicals is modeled by

$$\frac{dR}{dt} - D_R \Delta R = R_0 - R(k_L L + k_H H) + \lambda_{GR}(G - G_s) + \lambda_{IR} IR, \qquad (2.62)$$

where R_0 is the base line growth, the third term on the right hand of the equation models the mechanism whereby excess glucose metabolites inhibits production of NO by blocking eNOS synthase activation and increase the production of ROS [163, 282]; where λ_{GR} is the growth rate of ROS due to excess glucose. The fourth term on the right hand of the equation models the mechanism that insulin resistance decrease endothelium-derived NO and increase the production of ROS [33, 34]; where λ_{IR} is the growth rate of ROS due to insulin resistance.

Equation for SMCs (S): The equation of the SMCs density is given by

$$\frac{dS}{dt} + \nabla \cdot (\mathbf{u}S) - D_S \Delta S = -\nabla \cdot (S\chi_C \nabla G) - \lambda_{GL}(G - G_s)L, \qquad (2.63)$$

Diabetes stimulates atherogenic activities of SMCs. SMCs cultured from patients with type 2 diabetes demonstrate enhanced migration [17]. Advanced atherosclerotic lesions in diabetic patients have fewer SMCs compared with those of controls [17]. The first term in the right hand side models haptotaxis by glucose. The second term models that oxidized glycated LDL can induce apoptosis of SMCs [17].

Equation for macrophages (M): The evolution of macrophage density is modeled by

$$\frac{\partial M}{\partial t} + \nabla \cdot (\mathbf{u}M) - D_M \Delta M = -\lambda_{ML} \frac{ML}{K_{ML} + L} + \lambda_{HF} \frac{HF}{(K_{HF} + H)} + \lambda \frac{ML}{K_{MH} + H} - d_M M, \quad (2.64)$$

Here the first and the second term on right-hand side accounts for the transition between M and L: when L molecules are ingested by a macrophage, the macrophage becomes a foam cell; when H combines with membrane protein on a foam cell in a process that clears it from the bad cholesterol, the foam cell turns into a macrophage. The third term is phenomenological [111]: the factor ML accounts for a sequence of reactions, stemming from oxidized LDL, which results in the activation of inflammatory macrophages, while the inhibition factor $\frac{1}{K_{MH}+H}$ is introduced to account for the fact that by oxidizing with radicals, HDL removes some of the radicals available to oxidize LDL. The fourth term accounts for the death of macrophages.

Equation for foam cells (F): The equation for foam cells is given by

$$\frac{dF}{dt} + \nabla \cdot (\mathbf{u}F) - D_F \Delta F = \lambda_{ML} \frac{ML}{K_{ML} + L} - \lambda_{HF} \frac{HF}{K_{HF} + H} - d_F F, \quad (2.65)$$

where on the right side of the equation, a gain of foam cells from macrophages M ingesting L, and a loss of foam cells triggered by H. The death rate of foam cells is d_F.

Equations pressure (σ): We assume that the intima has the constituency of a porous medium. Then, by Darcy's law, the velocity $\mathbf{u}$ of the cells is given by

$$\mathbf{u} = -\nabla \sigma, \quad (2.66)$$

where σ is the pressure. We also assume that the total density of all the cells is constant. This constant should be smaller than the average density of a plaque, $1.22 \pm 0.03 g/cm^3$ [9], because plaques contain some debris, which are not included in our model. We take the constant to be 1 g/cm3, i.e.,

$$M + F + \beta + S = 1 \quad (2.67)$$

We assume that all cells are approximately of the same volume and surface area, so that the diffusion coefficients of the all cells have the same coefficient. By adding Eqs. (2.58)–(2.64), and (2.65), and using (2.67), we get

$$-\Delta \sigma = (-d_0 + r_1 G - r_2 G^2)\beta - \nabla \cdot (S \chi_G \nabla G) - \lambda_{GL} GL + \lambda \frac{(M_0 - F - \beta)L}{K_{MH} + H} - d_F F - d_M M. \quad (2.68)$$

Boundary Conditions: For simplicity, we consider only 2-dimensional plaques as in Fig. 2.3. Then the boundary of the plaque consists of i) Γ_M, in contact with media; ii) a free boundary Γ_I, inside the lumen.

Boundary conditions on Γ_I: We assume flux boundary conditions of the form

$$\frac{\partial X}{\partial n} + \alpha_X(X - X_0) = 0, \quad \frac{\partial Y}{\partial n} = 0 \tag{2.69}$$

for $X = G, I, L, H, \beta$, and non-flux boundary conditions for all other variables $Y = R, S, F$. The flux boundary condition for M is determined by $M = 1 - S - \beta - F$. Note that G_0, I_0, L_0 and H_0 are the glucose, insulin, LDL, and HDL concentrations in the blood, so we shall be interested to see how these concentrations determine whether a small plaque will grow or shrink.

As in [40, 41, 43], we assume that the free boundary Γ_I is held together by cell-to-cell adhesion forces so that

$$\sigma = \gamma\kappa \text{ on } \Gamma_I, \tag{2.70}$$

where κ is the mean curvature of the surface Γ_I. (If Γ_I is circular, then κ is the reciprocal of the radius) Furthermore, the continuity condition $u_n = V_n$, where n is the outward normal and V_n is the velocity of the free boundary Γ_I in the direction n, yields the relation

$$V_n = -\frac{\partial \sigma}{\partial n} \text{ on } \Gamma_I. \tag{2.71}$$

Boundary conditions on Γ_M: We assume non-flux boundary conditions for all variables except S and M on Γ_M: For S, we have

$$\frac{\partial S}{\partial n} + \alpha_S(S - S_0) = 0 \text{ on } \Gamma_M, \tag{2.72}$$

where S_0 is SMCs density in the media. The flux condition for M is determined by $M = 1 - S - \beta - F$.

Parameter estimation: Most parameters on the right hand side of (2.57)–(2.59) are given in [265] and most estimates of parameters on the right hand side of (2.60)-(2.72) can be found given in [111, 147]. See Table 2.8 and Table 2.9.

To estimate some of the parameters in the equations for proteins, we shall use the concept of accessible surface area [65, 162] of a protein p, or briefly A_p, which is roughly the minimum surface area of the smooth shapes containing the protein.

$$A_p = 11.1 M_p^{2/3}, \tag{2.73}$$

where M_p is the molecular weight of the protein. The molecular weights of insulin, glucose and radical are:

$$M_I = 5734\ g/mol\ (daltons), M_G = 180\ daltons, M_R = 500\ daltons.$$

TABLE 2.7 Steady concentrations of proteins and densities of cells are in units of g/cm^3

Proteins and cells	Concentrations (gcm^{-3})	Explaination
L: LDL	$7 \times 10^{-4} - 1.9 \times 10^{-3}$	Range is $70 - 190$ mg/dl [147]
H: HDL	$4 \times 10^{-4} - 1.6 \times 10^{-4}$	Range is $40 - 60$ mg/dl [147]
G: Glucose	10^{-3}	100 mg/dl [265]
I: Insulin	10^{-4}	10 mg/dl [265]
β: β-cells	10^{-3}	100 mg/dl [265]

From (2.73), we obtain

$$A_I = 3555.9974 \times 10^{-16} cm^2, A_G = 353.8653 \times 10^{-16} cm^2, \\ A_R = 699.2562 \times 10^{-16} cm^2. \tag{2.74}$$

Diffusion coefficients. We assume that the diffusion coefficients of all the cells are the same, and take them to be $8.64 \times 10^{-7} cm^2\ d^{-1}$ [111, 147]. In order to estimate the diffusion coefficients of the various proteins, we assume that the diffusion coefficient of protein p, D_p, is proportional to its area A_p, i.e., $D_p \sim KA_p$, where we take $K = 2.93 \times 10^{12}\ d^{-1}$ to be the same for all small molecules. Using (2.74), we have $D_I = 1.04\ cm^2\ d^{-1}$, $D_G = 0.104\ cm^2\ d^{-1}$.
Production rates: production rates in (2.62) will be estimated from the steady state and the data in the existing literature.
First from (2.73), we have

$$\lambda_{IR} = \frac{A_I}{A_G} \lambda_{GR} = 10.049\, \lambda_{GR}. \tag{2.75}$$

From (2.62) we have

$$R_0 = \lambda_{IR}\, I_{steady} + \lambda_{GR}\, G_{steady}, \tag{2.76}$$

where $I_{steady} = 10^{-4}\, g\, cm^{-3}$, $G_{steady} = 10^{-3} g\, cm^{-3}$ from Table 2.7 and $R_0 = 0.25$ from Table 2.9.

Solving (2.75) and (2.76), we obtain

$$\lambda_{GR} = 124.69\, d^{-1},\ \lambda_{IR} = 1253.055\, d^{-1}. \tag{2.77}$$

Since the death rate of SMC is $0.86\, d^{-1}$ [147], we estimate that $\lambda_{GL} = 0.86 \times 10^3\, d^{-1}\, cm^3 g^{-1}$ in the Eq. (2.63).

We take the flux rates $\alpha_G = \alpha_I = \alpha_L = \alpha_H = 1.0\, cm^{-1}$ and $\alpha_\beta = \alpha_M = 0.2\, cm^{-1}$ [147].

TABLE 2.8 Parameters' description and value

Parameters	Description	Value
$\tilde{G}_0$	net rate of production at zero glucose	$864\ mg\, dl^{-1}\, d^{-1}$ [265]
E_{G0}	total glucose effectiveness at zero insulin	$1.44\ d^{-1}$ [265]
S_I	total insulin sensitivity	$0.72\ ml\, \mu U^{-1}\, d^{-1}$ [265]
d_0	death rate at zero glucose for β cell	$0.06\ d^{-1}$ [265]
r_1	rate constant	$0.84 \times 10^{-3}\ mg^{-1}\, dl\, d^{-1}$ [265]
r_2	rate constant	$0.24 \times 10^{-3}\ mg^{-1}\, dl^2\, d^{-1}$ [265]
$\tilde{\sigma}$	max secretion rate for insulin	$43.2\ \mu U\, ml^{-1}\, d^{-1}$ [265]
α	constant in hill function with coefficient 2	$20000\, mg^2\ dl^{-2}$ [265]
k_I	clearance rate for insulin	$432\ d^{-1}$ [265]
D_G	diffusion coefficient for glucose	$1.04 \times 10^{-1}\ cm^2\ d^{-1}$ [147]
D_I	diffusion coefficient for Insulin	$1.042\, cm^2\ d^{-1}$ estimated
D_β	diffusion coefficient for β cell	$8.64 \times 10^{-7}\ cm^2\ d^{-1}$ [147]
D_R	diffusion coefficient for radicals	$2.05 \times 10^{-1}\ cm^2\ d^{-1}$ [147]
D_L	diffusion coefficient for LDL	$29.89\, cm^2\ d^{-1}$ [147]
D_H	diffusion coefficient for HDL	$3.93\, cm^2\ d^{-1}$ [147]
D_S	diffusion coefficient for SMC	$8.64 \times 10^{-7}\ cm^2\ d^{-1}$ [147]
χ_C	Chemotactic sensitivity parameter	$8.64 \times 10^{-1} \sim 1.73 \times 10^4$ $cm^5\ g^{-1}\ day^{-1}$ [147]
S_0	source/influx of SMCs into intima	$6 \times 10^{-3}\, g\, cm^{-3}$ [147]

2.3.2 Mathematical Analysis of the Simplified Model

In this section we are going to study the well-posedness of the simplified model [288] and the existence and stability of steady radially symmetric solution of the simplified model [290].

2.3.2.1 *Well Posedness*

Models for the glucose-insulin control system, typically span the short time (minutes) along which perturbation experiments (IVGTT, OGTT, or clamps) are performed and blood concentration of metabolites are obtained. Long time

TABLE 2.9 Parameters' description and value

Parameters	Description	Value
D_M	diffusion coefficient for macrophage	$8.64 \times 10^{-7}\, cm^2\, d^{-1}$ [147]
D_F	diffusion coefficient for foam cells	$8.64 \times 10^{-7}\, cm^2\, d^{-1}$ [147]
k_L	reaction rate of for LDL+ Radical	$2.35 \times 10^{-4}\, g^{-1}\, cm^3\, d^{-1}$ [147]
k_H	reaction rate of for HDL+ Radical	$5.29 \times 10^{-6}\, g^{-1}\, cm^3\, d^{-1}$ [147]
λ_{GR}	growth rate of radical due to excess glucose	$124.69\, d^{-1}$ estimated
λ_{IR}	growth rate of radical due to excess insulin	$1253.055\, d^{-1}$ estimated
λ_{GH}	rate of reduction due to HDL	$860\, cm^3\, g^{-1}\, d^{-1}$ estimated
λ_{GL}	rate of production due to excess glucose	$860\, cm^3\, g^{-1}\, d^{-1}$ estimated
λ	parameter in Eq. (2.63) for M	$2.573 \times 10^{-3} d^{-1}$ [147]
λ_{ML}	rate of LDL ingestion by macrophages	$144.5\, d^{-1}$ [147]
λ_{HF}	rate of HDL ingestion by foam cells	$10\, d^{-1}$ [147]
d_M	death rate of macrophages	$0.015\, d^{-1}$ [147]
d_F	death rate of foam cells	$0.03\, d^{-1}$ [147]
K_{ML}	LDL saturation for production of macrophages	$10^{-2}\, g\, cm^{-3}$ [147]
K_{FH}	HDL saturation for production of foam cells	$0.5\, g\, cm^{-3}$ [147]
K_{MH}	parameter in Equation (2.64)	$-2.541 \times 10^{-3}\, g\, cm^{-3}$ [111]
R_0	source/influx of radical into intima	$0.25\, g\, cm^{-3}\, d^{-1}$ [147]
α_G	influx rate of glucose into intima	$1.0\, cm^{-1}$ estimated
α_I	influx rate of insulin into intima	$1.0\, cm^{-1}$ estimated
α_L	influx rate of LDL into intima	$1.0\, cm^{-1}$ [147]
α_H	influx rate of HDL into intima	$1.0\, cm^{-1}$ [147]
α_β	influx rate of β cell into intima	$0.2\, cm^{-1}$ [147]
α_M	influx rate of Macrophages into intima	$0.2\, cm^{-1}$ [147]
α_S	influx rate of SMCs into intima	$0.2\, cm^{-1}$ [147]

spans (months, years) are used when assessing the response to antidiabetic therapy during clinical trials. As in [93, 211], we may substitute the fast-scale time t with a slow scale time τ in the glucose-insulin system (2.57) and (2.59) by setting $\tau = \epsilon t$ where ϵ is a very small parameter. Letting $\epsilon \to 0$, then we can replace the glucose-insulin system (2.57) and (2.59) by the following slow equations for the glucose and insulin:

$$-D_G \Delta G = \tilde{G}_0 - (E_{G0} + S_I I)G, \tag{2.78}$$

$$-D_I \Delta I = \frac{\sigma G^2 \beta}{\alpha + G^2} - kI - \lambda_{RI} R; \tag{2.79}$$

Using (2.78), we can write (2.68) as

$$-\Delta\sigma + \nabla S \cdot (\chi_G \nabla G) = F_1(G, S, \beta, I, L, F), \tag{2.80}$$

where

$$\begin{aligned} F_1(G, S, \beta, I, L, F) &= (-d_0 + r_1 G - r_2 G^2)\beta - \lambda_{GL} GL \\ &- \chi_G D_G^{-1}[\tilde{G}_0 - (E_{G0} + S_I I)G] - d_F F - d_M(1 - \beta - S - F). \end{aligned} \tag{2.81}$$

Using (2.78) and (2.66), we can write (2.58) as

$$\frac{d\beta}{dt} - \nabla\sigma \cdot \nabla\beta + \beta \nabla S \cdot (\chi_G \nabla G) - D_\beta \Delta\beta = F_2(G, S, \beta, I, L, F); \tag{2.82}$$

where

$$F_2(G, S, \beta, I, L, F) = (-d_0 + r_1 G - r_2 G^2)\beta - \beta F_1(G, S, \beta, I, L, F). \tag{2.83}$$

(2.62) can be written as

$$\frac{dR}{dt} - D_R \Delta R = F_3(G, I, L, H, R), \tag{2.84}$$

where

$$F_3(G, I, L, H, R) = R_0 - R(k_L L + k_H H) + \lambda_{GR} G + \lambda_{IR} I. \tag{2.85}$$

Using (2.79) and (2.66), we can write (2.63) as

$$\frac{dS}{dt} + [(\chi_G + S)\nabla G - \nabla\sigma] \cdot \nabla S - D_S \Delta S = F_4(G, S, \beta, I, L, F), \tag{2.86}$$

where

$$\begin{aligned} F_4(G, S, \beta, I, L, F) &= -S F_1(G, S, \beta, I, L, F) \\ &+ \chi_G S D_G^{-1}[\tilde{G}_0 - (E_{G0} + S_I I)G] - \lambda_{GL} GL. \end{aligned} \tag{2.87}$$

Using (2.80) and (2.66), we can write (2.65) as

$$\frac{dF}{dt} - \nabla\sigma \cdot \nabla F + F\nabla S \cdot (\chi_G \nabla G) - D_F \Delta F = F_5(G, S, \beta, I, L, F); \quad (2.88)$$

where

$$F_5(G, S, \beta, I, L, F) = \lambda_{ML}\frac{ML}{K_{ML} + L} - \lambda_{HF}\frac{HF}{K_{HF} + H} - d_F F - FF_1(G, S, \beta, I, L, F). \quad (2.89)$$

Now the slow model consists of functions $\{L, H, G, I, \beta, R, S, F, \sigma\}$ which satisfy Eqs. (2.60), (2.61), (2.78)–(2.89) in the region $\Omega(t)$ bounded by a free boundary $\Gamma_I(t)$ an a fixed boundary Γ_M and the following boundary conditions:

On the free boundary $\Gamma_I(t)$,

$$\begin{aligned}
&\frac{\partial L}{\partial n} + \alpha_L(L - L_0) = 0, \quad \frac{\partial H}{\partial n} + \alpha_H(H - H_0) = 0,\\
&\frac{\partial G}{\partial n} + \alpha_G(G - G_0) = 0, \quad \frac{\partial I}{\partial n} + \alpha_I(I - I_0) = 0,\\
&\frac{\partial \beta}{\partial n} + \alpha_\beta(\beta - \beta_0) = 0, \quad \frac{\partial R}{\partial n} = \frac{\partial S}{\partial n} = \frac{\partial F}{\partial n} = 0,\\
&\sigma = \gamma\kappa, \quad V_n = -\frac{\partial \sigma}{\partial n}
\end{aligned} \quad (2.90)$$

and on the fixed boundary Γ_M:

$$\begin{aligned}
&\frac{\partial L}{\partial n} = \frac{\partial H}{\partial n} = \frac{\partial G}{\partial n} = 0\\
&\frac{\partial R}{\partial n} = \frac{\partial \beta}{\partial n} = \frac{\partial I}{\partial n} = \frac{\partial F}{\partial n} = 0\\
&\frac{\partial S}{\partial n} + \alpha_S(S - L_0) = 0\\
&\sigma = 0.
\end{aligned} \quad (2.91)$$

We impose the following initial conditions: for $x \in \Omega_0$,

$$\begin{aligned}
&L(0, x) = L_0(x), \ H(0, x) = H_0(x), \ \beta(0, x) = \beta_0(x),\\
&R(0, x) = R_0(x), \ S(0, x) = S_0(x), \ F(0, x) = F_0(x), \ \Gamma_I|_{t=0} = \Gamma_0,
\end{aligned} \quad (2.92)$$

where the initial free boundary Γ_0 is assumed to not intersect the fixed boundary Γ_M and Ω_0 is the region between Γ_0 and Γ_M.

We are interested in the question of well-posedness of the free boundary problem for the system(2.78)-(2.92). To answer the question, we will first use the Hanzawa transformation [146] to reduce the domain $\Omega(t)$ to a fixed domain Ω_0, the free boundary $\Gamma_I(t)$ is described by a function $\rho(\omega, t)$ which is defined on the fixed boundary Γ_0. The free boundary problem will be changed into a system of PDEs in a fixed domain domain Ω_0 with boundary conditions on the fixed boundaries Γ_0 and Γ_M. Then we will further reduce the fixed boundary problem to an abstract evolution equation in Banach spaces, and we will obtain existence uniqueness of solution employing the analytic semigroup theory [76, 191].

We assume that $\Gamma_0 \in C^{m,\alpha}$, where $C^{m,\alpha}$ is the classical Hölder space with norm $\|\cdot\|_{m,\alpha}$; $m \geq 4$ is an integer, and $0 < \alpha < 1$.

Let ω be a variable point of Γ_0 and $n(\omega)$ the unit exterior normal to Γ_0 at ω.

Let γ_0 be a given sufficiently small positive number such that the mapping

$$x : \Gamma_0 \times [-\gamma_0, \gamma_0] \to N_0 \subset R^2, x(\omega, \lambda) = \omega + \lambda n(\omega)$$

is a $C^{m-1,\alpha}$ diffeomorphism.

We define $\Gamma_{0,T} = \Gamma_0 \times [0, T]$ and $\Omega_{0,T} = \Omega_0 \times [0, T]$. For $\rho(\omega, t) \in C([0, T], C^{m,\alpha}(\Gamma_0))$ with $\|\rho\|_{m,\alpha} \leq \gamma_0$. Let

$$\Gamma_{\rho,T} = \{\omega + \rho(\omega, t)n(\omega); (\omega, t) \in \Gamma_{0,T}\}$$

and $\Omega_{\rho,T}$ be the domain bounded by $\Gamma_{\rho,T}$ and Γ_M.

Let δ_0 be sufficiently small so that $4\delta_0 < \gamma_0$. Choose a function $\chi(\lambda) \in C^\infty(R)$ so that

(1) $\chi(\lambda) = 1,$ for $|\lambda| \leq \delta_0$.

(2) $\chi(\lambda) = 0,$ for $\lambda > 3\delta_0$.

(3) $|\chi'(\lambda)| \leq \frac{3}{4\delta_0}$ for $\lambda \in R$.

For $\rho(\omega, t) \in C([0, T], C^{m,\alpha}(\Gamma_0)) \cap C^1([0, T], C^{m-1,\alpha}(\Gamma_0))$, with $|\rho|_{m+\alpha} \leq \delta_0$, we define Hanzawa diffeomorphism:

$$\begin{aligned} &e_\rho : R_y^2 \times [0, T] \to R_x^2 \times [0, T] \\ &e_\rho(y, t) = (x(\omega, \lambda + \chi(\lambda)\rho(\omega, t)), t) \\ &\qquad \text{for } (y, t) = (x(\omega, \lambda), t) \in N_0 \times [0, T] \\ &e_\rho(y, t) = (y, t) \text{ for } (y, t) \in (R^2 - N_0) \times [0, T] \end{aligned} \tag{2.93}$$

Note that $e_\rho(\Omega_{0,T}) = \Omega_{\rho,T}, e_\rho(\Gamma_{0,T}) = \Gamma_{\rho,T}$.

Define a function $\eta : R \times [-\delta_0, \delta_0] \to R$ by $\eta(\lambda, \mu) + \chi_0(\eta(\lambda, \mu))\mu = \lambda$ for $(\lambda, \mu) \in R \times [-\delta_0, \delta_0]$. Since $|\chi'(\lambda)| \leq \frac{3}{4\delta_0}$, the function η is well defined and C^∞. And we have

$$\begin{aligned} &e_\rho^{-1} : R_x^2 \times [0, T] \to R_y^2 \times [0, T] \\ &e_\rho^{-1}(x(\omega, \lambda), t) = (x(\omega, \eta(\lambda, \rho(\omega, t)), t) \\ &\qquad \text{for } (x, t) = (x(\omega, \lambda), t) \in N_0 \times [0, T] \\ &e_\rho^{-1}(x, t) = (x, t) \text{ for } (x, t) \in (R^2 - N_0) \times [0, T] \end{aligned} \tag{2.94}$$

We define the following operators: for $v \in C^2(\overline{\Omega_{0T}})$

$$\mathcal{L}_\rho v \equiv \Delta(v \circ e_\rho^{-1}) \circ e_\rho = \sum_{k,j=1}^{2} A_{\rho,kj}(y,t)\partial^2_{y_k y_j} v + \sum_{k=1}^{2} A_{\rho,k}\partial_{y_k} v,$$

$$\begin{aligned} &A_{\rho,kj}(y,t) = A_{kj}(y, \rho(\omega(y),t); \partial_\omega \rho(\omega(y),t)), \\ &\quad \text{for } k,j = 1,2, \text{ and } (y,t) \in N_0 \times [0,T], \\ &A_{\rho,kj}(y,t) = \delta_{kj} \text{ for } k,j = 1,2, (y,t) \in (R^n - N_0) \times [0,T]. \end{aligned} \tag{2.95}$$

$$A_{\rho,k}(y,t) = A_k(y, \rho(\omega(y),t), \partial_\omega \rho(\omega(y),t), \partial^2_\omega \rho(\omega(y),t)) \quad k = 1,2; \tag{2.96}$$

$$S_\rho = 1 + |\partial_\omega \rho \nabla_x \omega(x(\omega, \rho(\omega,t)))|^2 . \tag{2.97}$$

For $v \in C^1(\overline{\Omega_{0T}})$ we define the operator

$$\nabla_\rho v = \nabla(v \circ e_\rho^{-1}) \circ e_\rho. \tag{2.98}$$

For given $\rho(\omega,t) \in C^1([0,T] \times \Gamma_0)$, we define the function

$$\psi_\rho : N_0 \to R, \qquad \psi_\rho(x) = \lambda(x) - \rho(\omega(x),t), \text{ for } x \in N_0. \tag{2.99}$$

So $\Gamma_\rho = \{x \in N_0 : \psi_\rho(x) = 0\}$, the unit outward normal vector on Γ_ρ is given by

$$\mathbf{n}_\rho(x) = \frac{\nabla \psi_\rho(x)}{|\nabla \psi_\rho(x)|} \text{ for } x \in \Gamma_\rho. \tag{2.100}$$

The normal velocity V_n is given by

$$V_n = \frac{\partial_t \rho(\omega(x),t)}{|\nabla \psi_\rho(x)|} \text{ for } x \in \Gamma_\rho. \tag{2.101}$$

For $v \in C^1(\overline{\Omega_{0T}})$ we define the operator

$$\mathcal{D}_\rho v = \left(\nabla(v \circ e_\rho^{-1})|_{\Gamma_\rho} \cdot \nabla \psi_\rho|_{\Gamma_\rho}\right) \circ e_\rho. \tag{2.102}$$

We define

$$\mathcal{M}_\rho(y) = \begin{cases} \chi(\lambda)\partial_\lambda x(\omega(y), \lambda + \chi(\lambda)\rho(\omega(y),t)), \\ \qquad \text{for } (y,t) = (x(\omega,\lambda),t) \in N_0 \times [0,T], \\ 0, \qquad \text{for } (y,t) = (x(\omega,\lambda),t) \in \Omega_{0T}/N_0 \times [0,T]. \end{cases} \tag{2.103}$$

Set

$$\tilde{G} = G \circ e_\rho, \; \tilde{I} = I \circ e_\rho, \; \tilde{\sigma} = \sigma \circ e_\rho, \; \tilde{\beta} = \beta \circ e_\rho, \; \tilde{R} = R \circ e_\rho,$$

$$\tilde{S} = S \circ e_\rho, \; \tilde{L} = I \circ e_\rho, \; \tilde{H} = H \circ e_\rho, \; \tilde{F} = F \circ e_\rho.$$

Then the system (2.60)–(2.61) and (2.72)-(2.89) become

$$-D_G \mathcal{L}_\rho \tilde{G} = \tilde{G}_0 - (E_{G0} + S_I \tilde{I})\tilde{G}, \tag{2.104}$$

$$-D_I\mathcal{L}_\rho\tilde{I} = \frac{\sigma_0\tilde{G}^2\tilde{\beta}}{\alpha+\tilde{G}^2} - k\tilde{I} - \lambda_{RI}\tilde{R}; \tag{2.105}$$

$$-\mathcal{L}_\rho\tilde{\sigma} + \nabla_\rho\tilde{S}\cdot(\chi_G\nabla_\rho\tilde{G}) = \tilde{F}_1(\tilde{G},\tilde{S},\tilde{\beta},\tilde{I},\tilde{L},\tilde{F}), \tag{2.106}$$

where

$$\begin{aligned}\tilde{F}_1(\tilde{G},\tilde{S},\tilde{\beta},\tilde{I},\tilde{L},\tilde{F}) &= (-d_0 + r_1\tilde{G} - r_2\tilde{G}^2)\tilde{\beta} - \lambda_{GL}\tilde{G}\tilde{L}\\ &- \chi_G D_G^{-1}[\tilde{G}_0 - (E_{G0} + S_I\tilde{I})\tilde{G}] - d_F\tilde{F} - d_M(1-\tilde{\beta}-\tilde{S}-\tilde{F}).\end{aligned} \tag{2.107}$$

$$\begin{aligned}&\frac{d\tilde{\beta}}{dt} - (\nabla_\rho\tilde{\sigma} + (\mathcal{D}_\rho\tilde{\sigma})\mathcal{M}(y))\cdot\nabla_\rho\tilde{\beta} + \beta\nabla_\rho\tilde{S}\cdot(\chi_G\nabla_\rho\tilde{G}) - D_\beta\mathcal{L}_\rho\tilde{\beta}\\ &\qquad = \tilde{F}_2(\tilde{G},\tilde{S},\tilde{\beta},\tilde{I},\tilde{L},\tilde{F});\end{aligned} \tag{2.108}$$

where

$$\tilde{F}_2(\tilde{G},\tilde{S},\tilde{\beta},\tilde{I},\tilde{L},\tilde{F}) = (-d_0 + r_1\tilde{G} - r_2\tilde{G}^2)\tilde{\beta} - \tilde{\beta}\tilde{F}_1(\tilde{G},\tilde{S},\tilde{\beta},\tilde{I},\tilde{L},\tilde{F}). \tag{2.109}$$

$$\frac{d\tilde{L}}{dt} - D_L\mathcal{L}_\rho\tilde{L} - (\mathcal{D}_\rho\tilde{\sigma})\mathcal{M}_\rho(y)\cdot\nabla_\rho\tilde{L} = -k_L\tilde{R}\tilde{L}, \tag{2.110}$$

$$\frac{d\tilde{H}}{dt} - D_H\mathcal{L}_\rho\tilde{H} - (\mathcal{D}_\rho\tilde{\sigma})\mathcal{M}_\rho(y)\cdot\nabla_\rho\tilde{H} = -k_L\tilde{R}\tilde{H}, \tag{2.111}$$

$$\frac{d\tilde{R}}{dt} - D_R\mathcal{L}_\rho\tilde{R} - (\mathcal{D}_\rho\tilde{\sigma})\mathcal{M}_\rho(y)\cdot\nabla_\rho\tilde{R} = \tilde{F}_3(\tilde{G},\tilde{I},\tilde{L},\tilde{H},\tilde{R}), \tag{2.112}$$

where

$$\tilde{F}_3(\tilde{G},\tilde{I},\tilde{L},\tilde{H},\tilde{R}) = R_0 - \tilde{R}(k_L\tilde{L} + k_H\tilde{H}) + \lambda_{GR}\tilde{G} + \lambda_{IR}\tilde{I}. \tag{2.113}$$

$$\frac{d\tilde{S}}{dt} + [(\chi_G+\tilde{S})\nabla_\rho\tilde{G} - \nabla_\rho\tilde{\sigma} - (\mathcal{D}_\rho\tilde{\sigma})\mathcal{M}_\rho(y)]\cdot\nabla_\rho\tilde{S} - D_S\mathcal{L}_\rho\tilde{S} = \tilde{F}_4(\tilde{G},\tilde{S},\tilde{\beta},\tilde{I},\tilde{L},\tilde{F}), \tag{2.114}$$

where

$$\begin{aligned}\tilde{F}_4(\tilde{G},\tilde{S},\tilde{\beta},\tilde{I},\tilde{L},\tilde{F}) &= -\tilde{S}\tilde{F}_1(\tilde{G},\tilde{S},\tilde{\beta},\tilde{I},\tilde{L},\tilde{F})\\ &+ \chi_G\tilde{S}D_G^{-1}[\tilde{G}_0 - (E_{G0} + S_I\tilde{I})\tilde{G}] - \lambda_{GL}\tilde{G}\tilde{L}.\end{aligned} \tag{2.115}$$

$$\begin{aligned}&\frac{d\tilde{F}}{dt} - (\nabla_\rho\tilde{\sigma} + (\mathcal{D}_\rho\tilde{\sigma})\mathcal{M}_\rho(y))\cdot\nabla_\rho\tilde{F} + \tilde{F}\nabla_\rho\tilde{S}\cdot(\chi_G\nabla_\rho\tilde{G}) - D_F\mathcal{L}_\rho\tilde{F}\\ &\qquad = \tilde{F}_5(\tilde{G},\tilde{S},\tilde{\beta},\tilde{I},\tilde{L},\tilde{H},\tilde{F});\end{aligned} \tag{2.116}$$

where

$$\begin{aligned}\tilde{F}_5(\tilde{G},\tilde{S},\tilde{\beta},\tilde{I},\tilde{L},\tilde{H},\tilde{F}) &= \lambda_{ML}\frac{\tilde{M}\tilde{L}}{K_{ML}+\tilde{L}} - \lambda_{HF}\frac{\tilde{H}\tilde{F}}{K_{HF}+\tilde{H}}\\ &- d_F\tilde{F} - \tilde{F}\tilde{F}_1(\tilde{G},\tilde{S},\tilde{\beta},\tilde{I},\tilde{L},\tilde{F}).\end{aligned} \tag{2.117}$$

The boundary conditions (2.90) and (2.91) becomes the following conditions on $\Gamma \times [0, T]$:

$$\partial_t \rho + \mathcal{D}_\rho \tilde{\sigma} = 0; \tag{2.118}$$

$$\tilde{\sigma} = \gamma \kappa_\rho(\omega, t) \text{ on } \Gamma_{0T}; \tag{2.119}$$

where

$$\kappa_\rho(\omega, t) = \nabla(|\nabla \psi_\rho|^{-1} \nabla \psi_\rho)(\omega, t). \tag{2.120}$$

$$\begin{aligned}
&\mathcal{D}_\rho \tilde{L} + S_\rho \alpha_L(\tilde{L} - L_0) = 0, \ \mathcal{D}_\rho \tilde{H} + S_\rho \alpha_H(\tilde{H} - H_0) = 0,\\
&\mathcal{D}_\rho \tilde{G} + S_\rho \alpha_G(\tilde{G} - G_0) = 0, \ \mathcal{D}_\rho \tilde{I} + S_\rho \alpha_I(\tilde{I} - I_0) = 0,\\
&\mathcal{D}_\rho \tilde{\beta} + S_\rho \alpha_\beta(\tilde{\beta} - \beta_0) = 0, \ \mathcal{D}_\rho \tilde{R} = \mathcal{D}_\rho \tilde{S} = \mathcal{D}_\rho \tilde{F} = 0.
\end{aligned} \tag{2.121}$$

and on the fixed boundary Γ_M:

$$\begin{aligned}
&\frac{\partial \tilde{L}}{\partial n} = \frac{\partial \tilde{H}}{\partial n} = \frac{\partial \tilde{G}}{\partial n} = 0\\
&\frac{\partial \tilde{R}}{\partial n} = \frac{\partial \tilde{\beta}}{\partial n} = \frac{\partial \tilde{I}}{\partial n} = \frac{\partial \tilde{F}}{\partial n} = 0\\
&\frac{\partial \tilde{S}}{\partial n} + \alpha_S(\tilde{S} - S_0) = 0\\
&\tilde{\sigma} = 0.
\end{aligned} \tag{2.122}$$

The initial conditions are: for $x \in \Omega_0$,

$$\begin{aligned}
&\tilde{L}(0, x) = L_0(x), \ \tilde{H}(0, x) = H_0(x), \ \tilde{\beta}(0, x) = \beta_0(x),\\
&\tilde{R}(0, x) = R_0(x), \ \tilde{S}(0, x) = S_0(x), \ \tilde{F}(0, x) = F_0(x), \ \rho(\omega, t)|_{t=0} = 0.
\end{aligned} \tag{2.123}$$

We denote by $h^{m,\alpha}$ the closure of $C^\infty(\Omega_0)$ in the usual Hölder space $C^{m,\alpha}(\Omega_0)$ with norm $\|\cdot\|_{m,\alpha}$. Similarly we define $h^{m,\alpha}(\Gamma_0)$ and $h^{m,\alpha}_{\delta_0}(\Gamma_0) = \{\rho \in h^{m,\alpha}(\Gamma_0) \mid \|\rho\|_{m,\alpha} < \delta_0\}$. We are going to prove the following main theorem:

Theorem 2.5 *Assume that $m \geq 4, 0 < \alpha < 1$, Ω_0 is of class $C^{m,\alpha}$. Given that all initial data in (2.123) are in $h^{m,\alpha}(\Omega_0)$ and satisfy the corresponding boundary conditions (2.121) and (2.122). Then there exist $T > 0$ such that the system (2.104)-(2.123) has a unique solution $\rho \in L^\infty([0, T]), h^{m,\alpha}(\Gamma_0)) \cap C([0, T]), h^{m-3,\alpha}(\Gamma_0)) \cap C((0, T], h^{m,\alpha}(\Gamma_0)) \cap C^1((0, T]), h^{m-3,\alpha}(\Gamma_0))$,$\tilde{G}, \tilde{I}, \tilde{L}, \tilde{H}, \tilde{S}, \tilde{\beta}, \tilde{\sigma}, \tilde{R}$, and $\tilde{F}$ all belong to $L^\infty([0, T]), h^{m-1,\alpha}(\Omega_0)) \cap C([0, T]), h^{m-3,\alpha}(\Omega_0)) \cap C((0, T], h^{m-1,\alpha}(\Omega_0))$ $\cap C^1((0, T]), h^{m-3,\alpha}(\Omega_0))$.*

To prove the main theorem, we are going to use similar steps to that in [76]. We first rewrite the system (2.104)-(2.123) as a quasi-linear abstract evolution equation in Banach spaces and then apply the analytic semigroup theory [191].

Lemma 2.6 *If* $\rho \in h^{m,\alpha}(\Gamma_0), \tilde{R}, \tilde{\beta} \in h^{k-2,\alpha}(\Omega_0)$*, then the problem*

$$\begin{cases} -D_G\mathcal{L}_\rho\tilde{G} = \tilde{G}_0 - (E_{G0} + S_I\tilde{I})\tilde{G} \ in\ \Omega_0, \\ -D_I\mathcal{L}_\rho\tilde{I} = \frac{\sigma_0\tilde{G}^2\tilde{\beta}}{\alpha+\tilde{G}^2} - k\tilde{I} - \lambda_{RI}\tilde{R} \ in\ \Omega_0; \\ \mathcal{D}_\rho\tilde{G} + S_\rho\alpha_G(\tilde{G} - G_0) = 0,\ \mathcal{D}_\rho\tilde{I} + S_\rho\alpha_I(\tilde{I} - I_0) = 0 \ on\ \Gamma_0, \\ \frac{\partial\tilde{G}}{\partial n} = \frac{\partial\tilde{I}}{\partial n} = 0 \ on\ \Gamma_M \end{cases} \tag{2.124}$$

has a unique solution $\tilde{G}, \tilde{I} \in h^{k,\alpha}(\Omega_0)$*. Moreover there are operators* $\mathcal{U}_j(\rho), \mathcal{V}_j(\rho), j = 1, 2$ *such that*

$$\mathcal{U}_j(\rho) \in \bigcap_{2\le k\le m} L(h^{k-2,\alpha}(\Omega_0), h^{k,\alpha}(\Omega_0)),\ \mathcal{V}_j(\rho) \in \bigcap L(h^{k-2,\alpha}(\Omega_0), h^{k,\alpha}(\Omega_0))$$

and

$$\tilde{G} = \mathcal{U}_1(\rho)\tilde{R} + \mathcal{V}_1(\rho)\tilde{\beta}, \quad \tilde{I} = \mathcal{U}_2(\rho)\tilde{R} + \mathcal{V}_2(\rho)\tilde{\beta}. \tag{2.125}$$

Furthermore we have

$$\mathcal{U}_j \in C^\infty(h^{m,\alpha}(\Gamma_0), L(h^{k-2,\alpha}(\Omega_0), h^{k,\alpha}(\Omega_0))),$$

$$\mathcal{V}_j \in C^\infty(h^{m,\alpha}(\Gamma_0), L(h^{k-2,\alpha}(\Omega_0), h^{k,\alpha}(\Omega_0))).$$

Proof. The proof follows from Theorem 5.1 of chapter 8 in [176]. ■

Lemma 2.7 *If* $\rho \in h^{m,\alpha}(\Gamma_0), \tilde{h} \in h^{k-2,\alpha}(\Omega_0), \phi \in h^{m,\alpha}(\Gamma_0)$*, then the problem*

$$\begin{cases} \mathcal{L}_\rho\tilde{\sigma} = \tilde{h} & in\ \Omega_0 \\ \tilde{\sigma} = \tilde{\phi} & on\ \Gamma_0 \\ \tilde{\sigma} = 0 & on\ \Gamma_M \end{cases} \tag{2.126}$$

has a unique solution $\tilde{\sigma} \in h^{k,\alpha}(\Omega_0)$*. Moreover there are operators* $\mathcal{U}(\rho), \mathcal{V}(\rho), j = 1, 2$ *such that*

$$\mathcal{U}(\rho) \in \bigcap_{2\le k\le m} L(h^{k-2,\alpha}(\Omega_0), h^{k,\alpha}(\Omega_0)),\ \mathcal{V}(\rho) \in \bigcap L(h^{k,\alpha}(\Gamma_0), h^{k,\alpha}(\Omega_0))$$

and

$$\tilde{\sigma} = \mathcal{U}(\rho)\tilde{h} + \mathcal{V}(\rho)\tilde{\phi}. \tag{2.127}$$

Furthermore we have

$$\mathcal{U} \in C^\infty(h^{m,\alpha}(\Gamma_0), L(h^{k-2,\alpha}(\Omega_0), h^{k,\alpha}(\Omega_0))),$$

$$\mathcal{V} \in C^\infty(h^{m,\alpha}(\Gamma_0), L(h^{k,\alpha}(\Gamma_0), h^{k,\alpha}(\Omega_0))).$$

Lemma 2.8 *The curvature κ_ρ can be written as*

$$\kappa_\rho(\omega) = \mathcal{L}(\rho)\rho + \mathcal{K}(\rho)\rho, \tag{2.128}$$

where $\mathcal{L}(\rho)$ is a second order elliptic operator with coefficients being functions of ρ and its first order derivative and $\mathcal{K}(\rho)$ is a first order nonlinear operator. Moreover

$$\mathcal{L} \in C^\infty(h^{m,\alpha}(\Gamma_0), L(h^{k,\alpha}(\Gamma_0), h^{k-2,\alpha}(\Gamma_0))),$$
$$\mathcal{K} \in C^\infty(h^{m,\alpha}(\Gamma_0), L(h^{k,\alpha}(\Gamma_0), h^{m-1,\alpha}(\Gamma_0))).$$

Proof. The proof follows from (2.120) and (2.99). ■ Using (2.106), (2.119), (2.125), (2.127), and (2.128), we have

$$\tilde{\sigma} = \gamma\mathcal{V}(\rho)\mathcal{L}(\rho)\rho + \mathcal{A}_{1,\rho}(\tilde{R}, \tilde{\beta}, \tilde{L}, \tilde{S}, \tilde{F}); \tag{2.129}$$

where

$$\begin{aligned}\mathcal{A}_{1,\rho}(\tilde{R}, \tilde{\beta}, \tilde{L}, \tilde{S}, \tilde{F}) = {} & \gamma\mathcal{V}(\rho)\mathcal{K}(\rho)\rho - \mathcal{U}(\rho)\left(\nabla_\rho\tilde{S}\cdot(\chi_G\nabla_\rho(\mathcal{U}_1(\rho)\tilde{R} + \mathcal{V}_1(\rho)\tilde{\beta}))\right) \\ & + \mathcal{U}(\rho)\tilde{F}_1((\mathcal{U}_1(\rho)\tilde{R} + \mathcal{V}_1(\rho)\tilde{\beta}), \tilde{S}, \tilde{\beta}, (\mathcal{U}_2(\rho)\tilde{R} + \mathcal{V}_2(\rho)\tilde{\beta}), \tilde{L}, \tilde{F}). \end{aligned} \tag{2.130}$$

We define the following operators:

$$\mathcal{B}(\rho)v = \gamma\mathcal{D}_\rho\mathcal{V}(\rho)\mathcal{L}(\rho)v \quad \text{for } v \in h^{m,\alpha}(\Gamma_0); \tag{2.131}$$

$$\mathcal{C}(\rho, u)v = (\mathcal{B}(\rho)v)M_\rho(y)\cdot\nabla_\rho u \quad \text{for } u \in h^{k,\alpha}(\Omega_0),\ v \in h^{m,\alpha}(\Gamma_0); \tag{2.132}$$

$$\begin{aligned}\mathcal{E}(\rho, u)v = {} & (\mathcal{B}(\rho)v + \gamma\nabla_\rho\mathcal{V}(\rho)\mathcal{L}(\rho)v)\, M_\rho(y)\cdot\nabla_\rho u \quad \text{for } u \in h^{k,\alpha}(\Omega_0), \\ & v \in h^{m,\alpha}(\Gamma_0). \end{aligned} \tag{2.133}$$

Equations (2.108)-(2.117) can be written as

$$\frac{d\tilde{L}}{dt} - D_L\mathcal{L}_\rho\tilde{L} - \mathcal{C}(\rho, \tilde{L})\rho = \mathcal{G}_1(\tilde{R}, \tilde{\beta}, \tilde{L}, \tilde{S}, \tilde{F}); \tag{2.134}$$

where

$$\mathcal{G}_1(\tilde{R}, \tilde{\beta}, \tilde{L}, \tilde{S}, \tilde{F}) = (\mathcal{D}_\rho\mathcal{A}_{1,\rho}(\tilde{R}, \tilde{\beta}, \tilde{L}, \tilde{S}, \tilde{F}))\mathcal{M}_\rho(y)\cdot\nabla_\rho\tilde{L} - k_L\tilde{R}\tilde{L}; \tag{2.135}$$

$$\frac{d\tilde{H}}{dt} - D_H\mathcal{L}_\rho\tilde{H} - \mathcal{C}(\rho, \tilde{H})\rho = \mathcal{G}_2(\tilde{R}, \tilde{\beta}, \tilde{L}, \tilde{H}, \tilde{S}, \tilde{F}); \tag{2.136}$$

where

$$\mathcal{G}_2(\tilde{R}, \tilde{\beta}, \tilde{L}, \tilde{H}, \tilde{S}, \tilde{F}) = (\mathcal{D}_\rho\mathcal{A}_{1,\rho}(\tilde{R}, \tilde{\beta}, \tilde{L}, \tilde{S}, \tilde{F}))\mathcal{M}_\rho(y)\cdot\nabla_\rho\tilde{H} - k_L\tilde{R}\tilde{H}; \tag{2.137}$$

$$\frac{d\tilde{R}}{dt} - D_R\mathcal{L}_\rho\tilde{R} - \mathcal{C}(\rho, \tilde{R})\rho = \mathcal{G}_3(\tilde{R}, \tilde{\beta}, \tilde{L}, \tilde{H}, \tilde{S}, \tilde{F}); \tag{2.138}$$

Obviously, we have $\mathcal{X}_0 \hookrightarrow \mathcal{X}$.We denote by $\boldsymbol{H}(\mathcal{X}_0, \mathcal{X})$ the set of all linear operators $\mathcal{A}$ such that $\mathrm{dom}(\mathcal{A}) = \mathcal{X}_0$ and $-\mathcal{A}$ generates an analytic semigroup.

Lemma 2.9 *Let $U \in \mathcal{O}_{\delta_0}$, then $\mathcal{A}(U) \in \boldsymbol{H}(\mathcal{X}_0, \mathcal{X})$. Moreover*

$$\mathcal{A} \in C^\infty(\mathcal{O}_{\delta_0}, \boldsymbol{H}(\mathcal{X}_0, \mathcal{X})).$$

Proof. By adapting the proofs of Lemmas 4.1 and 4.2 in [76], we have the proof of the lemma. ∎

Applying Theorems 8.1.1 and 8.3.4 in [191], we obtain the following theorem

Theorem 2.10 *Let $m \geq 4$, $0 < \alpha < 1$, given that $U_0 \in \mathcal{O}_{\delta_0}$,then there exists $T > 0$ such that the problem (2.149) has a unique solution $U \in L^\infty([0,T], \mathcal{X}_0) \cap C([0,T], \mathcal{X}) \cap C((0,T], \mathcal{X}_0) \cap C^1((0,T], \mathcal{X})$.*

The main Theorem 2.5 follows easily from the above theorem.

2.3.2.2 Steady Solution and its Stability

We assume $S = constant = 0$ in the model and instead of $M + F + \beta = 1$ we assume that

$$M + F + \beta = M_0. \tag{2.150}$$

We get an equation for $\mathbf{u} = u(r)\vec{e}_r$:

$$\begin{aligned} M_0 \frac{1}{r} \partial_r(ru) &= (-d_0 + r_1 G - r_2 G^2)\beta \\ &\quad + \lambda \frac{(M_0 - F - \beta)L}{K_{MH} + H} - d_F F - d_M(M_0 - F - \beta). \end{aligned} \tag{2.151}$$

For simplicity, we consider radially symmetric plaques. Then the boundary of the plaque consists of i) $\Gamma_M = \{r = 1\}$, in contact with media; ii) a free boundary $\Gamma_I = \{r = B(t)\}$, inside the lumen.
We assume flux boundary conditions of the form on the free boundary $r = B(t)$:

$$-\frac{\partial L}{\partial n} + \alpha_L(L - L_0) = 0, \quad -\frac{\partial H}{\partial n} + \alpha_H(H - H_0) = 0, \tag{2.152}$$

$$-\frac{\partial G}{\partial n} + \alpha_G(G - G_0) = 0, \quad -\frac{\partial I}{\partial n} + \alpha_I(I - I_0) = 0, -\frac{\partial R}{\partial n} + \alpha_R(R - R_0) = 0, \tag{2.153}$$

$$-\frac{\partial M}{\partial n} + \alpha_M(M - \bar{M}_0) = 0, \quad -\frac{\partial \beta}{\partial n} + \alpha_M(\beta - \beta_0) = 0, \quad -\frac{\partial F}{\partial n} + \alpha_M F = 0, \tag{2.154}$$

where we assume $\bar{M}_0 + \beta_0 = M_0$. Note that G_0, I_0, L_0 and H_0 are the glucose, insulin, LDL and HDL concentrations in the blood, so we shall be interested to see how these concentrations determine whether a small plaque will grow

or shrink.
The equation for the free boundary is

$$\frac{dB(t)}{dt} = u(B(t)). \tag{2.155}$$

We assume no flux condition on the fixed boundary $r = 1$:

$$\frac{\partial L}{\partial n} = \frac{\partial H}{\partial n} = \frac{\partial G}{\partial n} = \frac{\partial I}{\partial n} = \frac{\partial R}{\partial n} = \frac{\partial M}{\partial n} = \frac{\partial \beta}{\partial n} = \frac{\partial F}{\partial n} = 0. \tag{2.156}$$

and

$$u(1) = 0. \tag{2.157}$$

In this section, we are going to prove that there exist stationary small plaque solutions $B(t) = 1 - \epsilon$ for any sufficiently small ϵ. Dropping the time derivatives, the stationary solution satisfies

$$-D_G \Delta G = \tilde{G}_0 - (E_{G0} + S_I I)G - \lambda_{GH}(G - G_s)H, \tag{2.158}$$

$$\nabla \cdot (\mathbf{u}\beta) - D_\beta \Delta \beta = (-d_0 + r_1 G - r_2 G^2)\beta, \tag{2.159}$$

$$-D_I \Delta I = \frac{\sigma G^2 \beta}{\alpha + G^2} - k_I I - \lambda_{RI} RI; \tag{2.160}$$

$$-D_L \Delta L = -k_L RL + \lambda_{GL}(G - G_s)L - \lambda_{ML}\frac{ML}{K_{ML} + L}, \tag{2.161}$$

$$-D_H \Delta H = -k_H RH - \lambda_{HF}\frac{HF}{(K_{HF} + H)}, \tag{2.162}$$

$$-D_R \Delta R = R_0 - R(k_L L + k_H H) + \lambda_{GR}(G - G_s)R + \lambda_{IR} IR, \tag{2.163}$$

$$\nabla \cdot (\mathbf{u}F) - D_F \Delta F = \lambda_{ML}\frac{(M_0 - F - \beta)L}{K_{ML} + L} - \lambda_{HF}\frac{HF}{(K_{HF} + H)} - d_F F, \tag{2.164}$$

$$\begin{aligned} M_0 \frac{1}{r}\partial_r(ru) &= (-d_0 + r_1 G - r_2 G^2)\beta \\ &\quad + \lambda\frac{(M_0 - F - \beta)L}{K_{MH} + H} - d_F F - d_M(M_0 - F - \beta). \end{aligned} \tag{2.165}$$

No flux condition on the boundary $r = 1$:

$$\frac{\partial L}{\partial n} = \frac{\partial H}{\partial n} = \frac{\partial G}{\partial n} = \frac{\partial I}{\partial n} = \frac{\partial R}{\partial n} = \frac{\partial \beta}{\partial n} = \frac{\partial F}{\partial n} = u(1) = 0. \tag{2.166}$$

The boundary conditions on $r = 1 - \epsilon$ are

$$-\frac{\partial L}{\partial n} + \alpha(L - L_0) = 0, \quad -\frac{\partial H}{\partial n} + \alpha(H - H_0) = 0, \tag{2.167}$$

$$-\frac{\partial G}{\partial n} + \alpha_G(G - G_0) = 0, \quad -\frac{\partial I}{\partial n} + \alpha_I(I - I_0) = 0, -\frac{\partial R}{\partial n} + \alpha_R(R - R_0) = 0, \tag{2.168}$$

$$-\frac{\partial \beta}{\partial n} + \alpha_M(\beta - \beta_0) = 0, \quad -\frac{\partial F}{\partial n} + \alpha_M F = 0, \tag{2.169}$$

$$u(1 - \epsilon) = 0. \tag{2.170}$$

Lemma 2.11 *For sufficiently small $\epsilon > 0$, there exists a unique solution $(G, I, \beta, R, L, H, F, u)$ to the problem (2.158)-(2.169).*

Proof. We define a Banach space

$$\mathcal{B} = \{(G, I, \beta, R, L, H, F, u) \in (C[1-\epsilon, 1])^8, G_s \le G \le G_0, 0 \le I \le I_0, \\ 0 \le R \le R_0, 0 \le L \le L_0, 0 \le H \le H_0, 0 \le \beta \le \beta_0, 0 \le F \le M_0\}$$

where $C[1-\epsilon, 1]$ is the space of continuous functions on $[1-\epsilon, 1]$.
We define a map $\mathcal{M}$ from $\mathcal{B} \to \mathcal{B}$: $(G, I, \beta, R, L, H, F, u) \to (\bar{G}, \bar{I}, \bar{\beta}, \bar{R}, \bar{L}, \bar{H}, \bar{F}, \bar{u})$, where $(\bar{G}, \bar{I}, \bar{\beta}, \bar{R}, \bar{L}, \bar{H}, \bar{F}, \bar{u})$ is given by

$$-D_G \Delta \bar{G} = \tilde{G}_0 - (E_{G0} + S_I I)\bar{G} - \lambda_{GH}(\bar{G} - G_s)H, \tag{2.171}$$

$$\nabla \cdot (\mathbf{u}\bar{\beta}) - D_\beta \Delta \bar{\beta} = (-d_0 + r_1 G - r_2 G^2)\bar{\beta}, \tag{2.172}$$

$$-D_I \Delta \bar{I} = \frac{\sigma G^2 \beta}{\alpha + G^2} - k_I \bar{I} - \lambda_{RI} R \bar{I}; \tag{2.173}$$

$$-D_L \Delta \bar{L} = -k_L R \bar{L} + \lambda_{GL}(G - G_s)\bar{L} - \lambda_{ML} \frac{(M_0 - F - \beta)\bar{L}}{K_{ML} + L}, \tag{2.174}$$

$$-D_H \Delta \bar{H} = -k_H R \bar{H} - \lambda_{HF} \frac{\bar{H} F}{(K_{HF} + H)}, \tag{2.175}$$

$$-D_R \Delta \bar{R} = \tilde{R}_0 - \bar{R}(k_L L + k_H H) + \lambda_{GR}(G - G_s)\bar{R} + \lambda_{IR} I \bar{R}, \tag{2.176}$$

$$\nabla \cdot (\mathbf{u}\bar{F}) - D_F \Delta \bar{F} = \lambda_{ML} \frac{(M_0 - \bar{F} - \beta)L}{K_{ML} + L} - \lambda_{HF} \frac{H\bar{F}}{(K_{HF} + H)} - d_F \bar{F}, \tag{2.177}$$

$$M_0 \frac{1}{r} \partial_r (r\bar{u}) = (-d_0 + r_1 G - r_2 G^2)\beta \\ + \lambda \frac{(M_0 - F - \beta)L}{K_{MH} + H} - d_F F - d_M(M_0 - F - \beta). \tag{2.178}$$

No flux condition on the boundary $r = 1$:

$$\frac{\partial \bar{L}}{\partial n} = \frac{\partial \bar{H}}{\partial n} = \frac{\partial \bar{G}}{\partial n} = \frac{\partial \bar{I}}{\partial n} = \frac{\partial \bar{R}}{\partial n} = \frac{\partial \bar{\beta}}{\partial n} = \frac{\partial \bar{F}}{\partial n} = \bar{u}(1) = 0. \tag{2.179}$$

The boundary conditions on $r = 1 - \epsilon$ are

$$-\frac{\partial \bar{L}}{\partial n} + \alpha(\bar{L} - L_0) = 0, \quad -\frac{\partial \bar{H}}{\partial n} + \alpha(\bar{H} - H_0) = 0, \tag{2.180}$$

$$-\frac{\partial \bar{G}}{\partial n}+\alpha_G(\bar{G}-G_0)=0, \quad -\frac{\partial \bar{I}}{\partial n}+\alpha_I(\bar{I}-I_0)=0, -\frac{\partial \bar{R}}{\partial n}+\alpha_R(\bar{R}-R_0)=0, \tag{2.181}$$

$$-\frac{\partial \bar{\beta}}{\partial n}+\alpha_M(\bar{\beta}-\beta_0)=0, \quad -\frac{\partial \bar{F}}{\partial n}+\alpha_M\bar{F}=0, \tag{2.182}$$

From Comparison Theorem, we can see that $G_s \leq \bar{G} \leq G_0, 0 \leq \bar{I} \leq I_0$, $0 \leq \bar{R} \leq R_0, 0 \leq \bar{L} \leq L_0, 0 \leq \bar{H} \leq H_0, 0 \leq \bar{\beta} \leq \beta_0, 0 \leq \bar{F} \leq M_0$, hence $(\bar{G}, \bar{I}, \bar{\beta}, \bar{R}, \bar{L}, \bar{H}, \bar{F}, \bar{u}) \in \mathcal{B}$. To prove that $\mathcal{M}$ is a contraction, we introduce function:

$$\eta(r)=\frac{1-r^2}{4}+\frac{1}{2}\log r; \tag{2.183}$$

then

$$\eta(1)=\eta_r(1)=0, \eta<0; \Delta\eta=-1, \eta=O(\epsilon^2), \eta_r=O(\epsilon) \text{ as } \epsilon \to 0. \tag{2.184}$$

Let $C(\gamma, \epsilon)$ be a number satisfying

$$-\frac{\partial(\eta+C(\gamma,\epsilon)}{\partial n}+\gamma(\eta+C(\gamma,\epsilon))=0, \text{ on } r=1-\epsilon; \tag{2.185}$$

then

$$\eta+C(\gamma,\epsilon)>0, \quad C(\gamma,\epsilon)=\frac{\epsilon}{\gamma}+O(\epsilon^2). \tag{2.186}$$

Let

$$(\bar{G}_j, \bar{I}_j, \bar{\beta}_j, \bar{R}_j, \bar{L}_j, \bar{H}_j, \bar{F}_j, \bar{u}_j)=\mathcal{M}(G_j, I_j, \beta_j, R_j, L_j, H_j, F_j, u_j),$$

$$A=|G_1-G_2|+|I_1-I_2|+|\beta_1-\beta_2|+|R_1-R_2|+|L_1-L_2|+|H_1-H_2|+|F_1-F_2|;$$

$$B=|\bar{G}_1-\bar{G}_2|+|\bar{I}_1-\bar{I}_2|+|\bar{\beta}_1-\bar{\beta}_2|+|\bar{R}_1-\bar{R}_2|+|\bar{L}_1-\bar{L}_2|+|\bar{H}_1-\bar{H}_2|+|\bar{F}_1-\bar{F}_2|;$$

then for some constant C,

$$|\Delta(\bar{G}_1-\bar{G}_2)| \leq C(A+B);$$

$$|\Delta(\bar{I}_1-\bar{I}_2)| \leq C(A+B);$$

$$|\Delta(\bar{\beta}_1-\bar{\beta}_2)-\nabla\cdot(\mathbf{u}(\bar{\beta}_1-\bar{\beta}_2))| \leq C(A+B);$$

$$|\Delta(\bar{R}_1-\bar{R}_2)| \leq C(A+B);$$

$$|\Delta(\bar{L}_1-\bar{L}_2)| \leq C(A+B);$$

$$|\Delta(\bar{H}_1-\bar{H}_2)| \leq C(A+B);$$

$$|\Delta(\bar{F}_1-\bar{F}_2)-\nabla\cdot(\mathbf{u}(\bar{F}_1-\bar{F}_2))| \leq C(A+B);$$

and use the maximum principle to get

$$|(\bar{G}_1-\bar{G}_2)| \leq C(A+B)(\eta+C(\alpha_G,\epsilon));$$

$$|(\bar{I}_1-\bar{I}_2)| \leq C(A+B)(\eta+C(\alpha_I,\epsilon));$$

$$|(\bar{\beta}_1 - \bar{\beta}_2)| \le C(A+B)(\eta + C(\alpha_M, \epsilon));$$
$$|(\bar{R}_1 - \bar{R}_2)| \le C(A+B)(\eta + C(\alpha_R, \epsilon));$$
$$|(\bar{L}_1 - \bar{L}_2)| \le C(A+B)(\eta + C(\alpha_L, \epsilon));$$
$$|(\bar{H}_1 - \bar{H}_2)| \le C(A+B)(\eta + C(\alpha_H, \epsilon));$$
$$|(\bar{F}_1 - \bar{F}_2) - \nabla \cdot (\mathbf{u}(\bar{F}_1 - \bar{F}_2))| \le C(A+B)(\eta + C(\alpha_M, \epsilon).$$

Using the above, we have

$$B \le C(A+B)(C(\alpha_G, \epsilon) + C(\alpha_I, \epsilon) + 2C(\alpha_M, \epsilon) + C(\alpha_R, \epsilon) + C(\alpha_L, \epsilon) + C(\alpha_H, \epsilon))$$

From (2.186) and above, we can see $B < C^*A$ for some constant $C^* < 1$, hence the mapping $\mathcal{M}$ is a contraction and the lemma holds.

■

As in [112], we assume that

$$\frac{\lambda L_0}{K_{MH} + H_0} - d_M = O(\epsilon). \tag{2.187}$$

We assume that $\tilde{G}_s$ is the root of $-d_0 + r_1 G^2 - r_2 G^2 = 0$ such that $\tilde{G}_s > G_s$.

Theorem 2.12 *For ϵ small, given $M_0 > \beta_0 > 0$, L_0 and H_0 satisfy (2.187). Then there exist G_0 satisfying $G_0 = \tilde{G}_s + O(\epsilon)$ such that the solution in Lemma 2.11 satisfies $u(1-\epsilon) = 0$.*

Proof. Since

$$|\Delta(G - G_0)| \le C;$$
$$|\Delta(I - I_0)| \le C;$$
$$|\Delta(\beta_1 - \beta_0) - \nabla \cdot (\mathbf{u}(\beta - \beta_0))| \le C;$$
$$|\Delta(R - R_0)| \le C;$$
$$|\Delta(L - L_0)| \le C;$$
$$|\Delta(H - H_0)| \le C;$$
$$|\Delta F - \nabla \cdot (\mathbf{u}F)| \le C;$$

and use the maximum principle to get

$$\begin{aligned}
&|(G - G_0)| \le C(\eta + C(\alpha_G, \epsilon));\\
&|(I - I_0)| \le C(\eta + C(\alpha_I, \epsilon));\\
&|(\beta_1 - \beta_0)| \le C(\eta + C(\alpha_M, \epsilon));\\
&|(R - R_0)| \le C(\eta + C(\alpha_R, \epsilon));\\
&|(L - L_0)| \le C; (\eta + C(\alpha_L, \epsilon));\\
&|(H - H_0)| \le C(\eta + C(\alpha_H, \epsilon));\\
&|F| \le C(\eta + C(\alpha_M, \epsilon)).
\end{aligned} \tag{2.188}$$

We obtain from (2.178)

$$\frac{M_0}{r}\partial_r(ru) = (M_0-\beta_0)\left(\frac{\lambda L_0}{K_{MH}+H_0} - d_M\right) + \beta_0(-d_0+r_1G_0^2-r_2G_0^2)+O(\epsilon). \tag{2.189}$$

Using (2.187) we have

$$\frac{M_0}{r}\partial_r(ru) = \beta_0(-d_0+r_1G_0^2-r_2G_0^2)+O(\epsilon) \tag{2.190}$$

which implies that

$$M_0(1-\epsilon)u(1-\epsilon) = -\int_{1-\epsilon}^{1} r\beta_0(-d_0+r_1G_0^2-r_2G_0^2)dr + O(\epsilon^2). \tag{2.191}$$

The above implies that $u(1-\epsilon) > 0$ for $G_0 > \tilde{G}_s$ while $u(1-\epsilon) < 0$ for $G_0 < \tilde{G}_s$. So there is $G_0 = \tilde{G}_s + O(\epsilon)$ such that $u(1-\epsilon) = 0$. ■

We now proceed to prove some sharper estimates for the steady solution, these estimates are useful in the future sections. From (2.158) to (2.164), we have

$$\begin{aligned}
&|\Delta\left(G - [G_0 + (\tilde{G}_0 - (E_{G0}+S_I I_0)G_0 - \lambda_{GH}(G_0-G_s)H_0)\eta(r)]\right)| \le O(\epsilon);\\
&\left|\Delta\left(I - \left[I_0 + \left(\frac{\sigma G_0^2\beta_0}{\alpha+G_0^2} - k_I I_0 - \lambda_{RI}R_0 I_0\right)\eta(r)\right]\right)\right| \le O(\epsilon);\\
&|\Delta\left(\beta_1 - [\beta_0 + (-d_0 + r_1G_0 - r_2G_0^2)\beta_0\eta(r)]\right)| \le O(\epsilon));\\
&\left|\Delta\bigg(R - \bigg[R_0 + \bigg(\tilde{R}_0 - R_0(k_L L_0 + k_H H_0) + \lambda_{GR}(G_0-G_s)R_0\right.\\
&\qquad\left. + \lambda_{IR}I_0R_0\bigg)\eta(r)\bigg]\bigg)\right| \le O(\epsilon);\\
&\left|\Delta\bigg(L - \bigg[L_0 + \bigg(- k_L R_0 L_0 + \lambda_{GL}(G_0-G_s)L_0\right.\\
&\qquad\left. - \lambda_{ML}\frac{(M_0-\beta_0)L_0}{K_{ML}+L_0}\bigg)\eta(r)\bigg]\bigg)\right| \le O(\epsilon);\\
&\left|\Delta\left(H - \left[H_0 + \left(-k_H R_0 H_0 - \lambda_{HF}\frac{H_0F_0}{(K_{HF}+H_0)}\right)\eta(r)\right]\right)\right| \le O(\epsilon);\\
&\left|\Delta\left(F - \left(\lambda_{ML}\frac{(M_0-\beta_0)L_0}{K_{ML}+L_0}\right)\eta(r)\right)\right| \le O(\epsilon).
\end{aligned} \tag{2.192}$$

Integrating above to obtain

$$
\begin{aligned}
&|\partial_r\left(G-[G_0+(\tilde{G}_0-(E_{G0}+S_I I_0)G_0-\lambda_{GH}(G_0-G_s)H_0)\eta(r)]\right)| \leq O(\epsilon^2);\\
&\left|\Delta\left(I-\left[I_0+\left(\frac{\sigma G_0^2\beta_0}{\alpha+G_0^2}-k_I I_0-\lambda_{RI}R_0 I_0\right)\eta(r)\right]\right)\right| \leq O(\epsilon^2);\\
&|\partial_r\left(\beta_1-\left[\beta_0+(-d_0+r_1G_0-r_2G_0^2)\beta_0\eta(r)\right]\right)| \leq O(\epsilon^2));\\
&\left|\partial_r\left(R-\left[R_0+\left(\tilde{R}_0-R_0(k_L L_0+k_H H_0)+\lambda_{GR}(G_0-G_s)R_0\right.\right.\right.\right.\\
&\qquad\left.\left.\left.\left.+\lambda_{IR}I_0R_0\right)\eta(r)\right]\right)\right| \leq O(\epsilon^2);\\
&\left|\partial_r\left(L-\left[L_0+\left(-k_L R_0 L_0+\lambda_{GL}(G_0-G_s)L_0\right.\right.\right.\right.\\
&\qquad\left.\left.\left.\left.-\lambda_{ML}\frac{(M_0-\beta_0)L_0}{K_{ML}+L_0}\right)\eta(r)\right]\right)\right| \leq O(\epsilon^2);\\
&\left|\partial_r\left(H-\left[H_0+\left(-k_H R_0 H_0-\lambda_{HF}\frac{H_0F_0}{(K_{HF}+H_0)}\right)\eta(r)\right]\right)\right| \leq O(\epsilon^2);\\
&\left|\partial_r\left(F-\left(\lambda_{ML}\frac{(M_0-\beta_0)L_0}{K_{ML}+L_0}\right)\eta(r)\right)\right| \leq O(\epsilon^2).
\end{aligned}
\tag{2.193}
$$

Integrating the above and using (2.185) and (2.186), we can write

$$
\begin{aligned}
G&=[G_0+(\tilde{G}_0-(E_{G0}+S_I I_0)G_0-\lambda_{GH}(G_0-G_s)H_0)(\eta(r)+\frac{\epsilon}{\alpha_G})]\\
&\quad+G^*\epsilon^2+O(\epsilon^3=:G_0+G_1\epsilon+G_2\epsilon^2+O(\epsilon^3),\\
I&=\left[I_0+\left(\frac{\sigma G_0^2\beta_0}{\alpha+G_0^2}-k_I I_0-\lambda_{RI}R_0I_0\right)(\eta(r)+\frac{\epsilon}{\alpha_I})\right]+I^*\epsilon^2+O(\epsilon^3)\\
&\quad=:I_0+I_1\epsilon+L_2\epsilon^2+O(\epsilon^3),\\
\beta&=\left[\beta_0+(-d_0+r_1G_0-r_2G_0^2)\beta_0(\eta(r)+\frac{\epsilon}{\alpha_M})\right]+\beta^*\epsilon^2+O(\epsilon^3));\\
R&=\left[R_0+\left(\tilde{R}_0-R_0(k_L L_0+k_H H_0)+\lambda_{GR}(G_0-G_s)R_0\right.\right.\\
&\quad\left.\left.+\lambda_{IR}I_0R_0\right)(\eta(r)+\frac{\epsilon}{\alpha_R})\right]\\
&\qquad+R^*\epsilon^2+O(\epsilon^3)\\
&\quad=:R_0+R_1\epsilon+R_2\epsilon^2+O(\epsilon^3)
\end{aligned}
$$

$$
\begin{aligned}
L = & \left[L_0 + \left(-k_L R_0 L_0 + \lambda_{GL}(G_0 - G_s)L_0 - \lambda_{ML}\frac{(M_0-\beta_0)L_0}{K_{ML}+L_0} \right) \right. \\
& \left. \times (\eta(r) + \frac{\epsilon}{\alpha_L}) \right] + L^* \epsilon^2 + O(\epsilon^3) \\
=: & \; L_0 + L_1\epsilon + L_2\epsilon^2 + O(\epsilon^3) \\
H = & \left[H_0 + \left(-k_H R_0 H_0 - \lambda_{HF}\frac{H_0 F_0}{(K_{HF}+H_0)} \right) (\eta(r) + \frac{\epsilon}{\alpha_H}) \right] \\
& + H^*\epsilon^2 + O(\epsilon^3) \\
=: & \; H_0 + H_1\epsilon + H_2\epsilon^2 + O(\epsilon^3), \\
F = & \left(\lambda_{ML}\frac{(M_0-\beta_0)L_0}{K_{ML}+L_0} \right)(\eta(r) + \frac{\epsilon}{\alpha_M}) + F^*\epsilon^2 + O(\epsilon^3) \\
=: & \; F_1\epsilon + F_2\epsilon^2 + O(\epsilon^3),
\end{aligned} \tag{2.194}
$$

where the constants $G^*, I^*, \beta^*, L^*, H^*$, and F^* are of order $O(1)$. Plugging (2.194) into (2.165), we have

$$
\begin{aligned}
\frac{M_0}{r}\partial_r(ru) = (M_0-\beta_0)\left(\frac{\lambda L_0}{K_{MH}+H_0} - d_M \right) + \beta_0(-d_0 + r_1 G_0^2 - r_2 G_0^2) \\
+ K_1\epsilon + K_2\epsilon^2 + O(\epsilon^3),
\end{aligned} \tag{2.195}
$$

where

$$
\begin{aligned}
K_1 = & \lambda_{HF}\frac{(M_0-\beta_0)L_1}{(K_{HF}+H_0)} - \frac{L_0(\beta_1+F_1)}{(K_{HF}+H_0)} - \frac{(M_0-\beta_0)L_0}{(K_{HF}+H_0)}\frac{H_1}{(K_{HF}+H_0)} \\
& - d_M(F_1+\beta_1) - d_F F_1 + \beta_0(r_1 G_1 - 2r_2 G_0 G_1) + \beta_1(-d_0 + r_1 G_0^2 - r_2 G_0^2),
\end{aligned} \tag{2.196}
$$

and $G_1,\ I_1,\ L_1,\ H_1, \beta_1$ and F_1 are defined in (2.194).
Using the fact

$$
\int_{1-\epsilon}^{1} u_r(s)ds = 0 \tag{2.197}
$$

and (2.195) we conclude that

$$
(M_0-\beta_0)\left(\frac{\lambda L_0}{K_{MH}+H_0} - d_M \right) + \beta_0(-d_0 + r_1 G_0^2 - r_2 G_0^2) + K_1\epsilon = O(\epsilon^2). \tag{2.198}
$$

Now using (2.165), (2.194), and (2.198), we can write

$$
\frac{M_0}{r}\partial_r(ru) = S_0\eta(r) + K_2^*\epsilon^2 + O(\epsilon^3), \tag{2.199}
$$

where K_2^* is a constant and S_0 is given by

$$\begin{aligned}
S_0 &= (M_0 - \beta_0)\frac{\lambda}{K_{MH} + H_0}[(E_{G0} + S_I I_0)G_0 - \lambda_{GL}(G_0 - G_s)L_0] \\
&\quad + \frac{\lambda L_0}{K_{MH} + H_0}\left[(-d_0 + r_1 G_0 - r_2 G_0^2)\beta_0 - \lambda_{ML}\frac{(M_0 - \beta_0)L_0}{K_{ML} + L_0}\right] \\
&\quad + \lambda_{HF}\frac{(M_0 - \beta_0)L_0}{(K_{HF} + H_0)^2}[\lambda_{HR}H_0 R_0] + (d_M - d_F)\lambda_{ML}\frac{(M_0 - \beta_0)L_0}{K_{ML} + L_0} \\
&\quad + d_M\left[(-d_0 + r_1 G_0 - r_2 G_0^2)\beta_0\right] + \left[(-d_0 + r_1 G_0 - r_2 G_0^2)\beta_0\right]^2 \\
&\quad + (r_1 - 2r_2)[(E_{G0} + S_I I_0)G_0 - \lambda_{GL}(G_0 - G_s)L_0]. \qquad (2.200)
\end{aligned}$$

Now using (2.197) and (2.199), we can write

$$\frac{M_0}{r}\partial_r(ru) = S_0[\eta(r) - \eta^*] + O(\epsilon^3), \qquad (2.201)$$

where

$$\eta^* = \frac{1}{\epsilon}\int_{1-\epsilon}^{1}\eta(s)ds = -\frac{1}{6}\epsilon^2 + O(\epsilon^3).$$

Taking $r = 1 - \epsilon$ in (2.201), we get

$$\frac{M_0}{r}\partial_r(ru)(1 - \epsilon) = -\frac{1}{3}S_0\epsilon^2 + O(\epsilon^3), \qquad (2.202)$$

Now we look into the linear stability of the steady solutions. Let $(\tilde{G}, \tilde{I}, \tilde{\beta}, \tilde{R}, \tilde{L}, \tilde{H}, \tilde{F}, \tilde{u})$ be the steady solution as in Theorem 1, we are going to study its linear stability. Let

$$\begin{aligned}
G(r,t) &= \tilde{G}(r) + \tau G^1(r,t) + O(\tau^2), \\
I(r,t) &= \tilde{I}(r) + \tau I^1(r,t) + O(\tau^2), \\
L(r,t) &= \tilde{L}(r) + \tau L^1(r,t) + O(\tau^2), \\
H(r,t) &= \tilde{H}(r) + \tau H^1(r,t) + O(\tau^2), \\
R(r,t) &= \tilde{R}(r) + \tau R^1(r,t) + O(\tau^2), \qquad (2.203) \\
\beta(r,t) &= \tilde{\beta}(r) + \tau \beta^1(r,t) + O(\tau^2), \\
F(r,t) &= \tilde{F}(r) + \tau F^1(r,t) + O(\tau^2), \\
B(t) &= 1 - \epsilon + \tau B^1(t) + O(\tau^2), \\
u(r,t) &= \tilde{u}(r) + \tau u^1(r,t) + O(\tau^2).
\end{aligned}$$

The linearized equations are

$$\frac{\partial G^1}{\partial t} - D_G \Delta G^1 = S_I \tilde{I} G^1 - \lambda_{GH}[(\tilde{G} - G_s)H^1 + G^1 \tilde{L}], \tag{2.204}$$

$$\frac{\partial \beta^1}{\partial t} + \nabla \cdot (\mathbf{u}\beta^1) - D_\beta \Delta \beta^1 = (-d_0 + r_1 \tilde{G} - r_2 \tilde{G}^2)\beta^1 + \tilde{\beta}(r_1 - 2r_2 \tilde{G})G^1, \tag{2.205}$$

$$\frac{\partial I^1}{\partial t} - D_I \Delta I^1 = \frac{\sigma \tilde{G}^2 \beta^1}{\alpha + \tilde{G}^2} - k_I I^1 - \lambda_{RI}(\tilde{R} I^1 + \tilde{I} R^1) + \frac{2\sigma G^1 \tilde{\beta}}{\alpha + \tilde{G}^2} - \frac{2\sigma \tilde{G}^3 \tilde{\beta} G^1}{(\alpha + \tilde{G}^2)^2}; \tag{2.206}$$

$$\begin{aligned} \frac{\partial L^1}{\partial t} - D_L \Delta L^1 &= -k_L(\tilde{R} L^1 + \tilde{L} R^1) + \lambda_{GL}[(\tilde{G} - G_s)L^1 + \tilde{L} G^1] \\ &- \lambda_{ML} \frac{(M_0 - \tilde{\beta} - \tilde{F})L^1}{K_{ML} + \tilde{L}} + \lambda_{ML} \frac{(\beta^1 + F^1)\tilde{L}}{K_{ML} + \tilde{L}} + \lambda_{ML} \frac{(M_0 - \tilde{\beta} - \tilde{F})\tilde{L} L^1}{(K_{ML} + \tilde{L})^2}, \end{aligned} \tag{2.207}$$

$$\begin{aligned} \frac{\partial H^1}{\partial t} - D_H \Delta H^1 &= -k_H(\tilde{R} H^1 + \tilde{H} R^1) - \lambda_{HF} \frac{\tilde{H} F^1 + \tilde{F} H^1}{(K_{HF} + \tilde{H})} \\ &+ \lambda_{HF} \frac{\tilde{H} F^1 \tilde{F}}{(K_{HF} + \tilde{H})^2}, \end{aligned} \tag{2.208}$$

$$\begin{aligned} \frac{\partial R^1}{\partial t} - D_R \Delta R^1 &= -\tilde{R}(k_L L^1 + k_H H^1) - R^1(k_L \tilde{L} + k_H \tilde{H}) \\ &+ \lambda_{GR}[(\tilde{G} - G_s)R^1 + \tilde{R} G^1] + \lambda_{IR}(\tilde{I} R^1 + \tilde{R} I^1), \end{aligned} \tag{2.209}$$

$$\begin{aligned} \frac{\partial F^1}{\partial t} + \nabla \cdot (\mathbf{u} F^1) - D_F \Delta F^1 &= \lambda_{ML} \frac{(M_0 - \tilde{\beta} - \tilde{F})L^1}{K_{ML} + \tilde{L}} - \lambda_{ML} \frac{(\beta^1 + F^1)\tilde{L}}{K_{ML} + \tilde{L}} \\ - \lambda_{ML} \frac{(M_0 - \tilde{\beta} - \tilde{F})\tilde{L} L^1}{(K_{ML} + \tilde{L})^2} &- \lambda_{HF} \frac{\tilde{H} F^1 + \tilde{F} H^1}{(K_{HF} + \tilde{H})} + \lambda_{HF} \frac{\tilde{H} \tilde{F} H^1}{(K_{HF} + \tilde{H})^2} - d_F F^1. \end{aligned} \tag{2.210}$$

The equation for u^1 is as follows from (2.151):

$$\begin{aligned} M_0 \frac{1}{r} \partial_r (r u^1) &= (-d_0 + r_1 \tilde{G} - r_2 \tilde{G}^2)\beta^1 + ((r_1 - 2r_2 G^1)\tilde{\beta} - d_F F^1 - d_M(-F^1 - \beta^1) \\ &+ \lambda \frac{(M_0 - \tilde{F} - \tilde{\beta})L^1}{K_{MH} + \tilde{H}} - \lambda \frac{(M_0 - \tilde{F} - \tilde{\beta})\tilde{L} H^1}{(K_{MH} + H)^2} - \lambda \frac{(F^1 + \beta^1)\tilde{L}}{K_{MH} + \tilde{H}}. \end{aligned} \tag{2.211}$$

No flux condition on the fixed boundary $r = 1$:

$$\frac{\partial L^1}{\partial n} = \frac{\partial H^1}{\partial n} = \frac{\partial G^1}{\partial n} = \frac{\partial I^1}{\partial n} = \frac{\partial R^1}{\partial n} = \frac{\partial M^1}{\partial n} = \frac{\partial \beta^1}{\partial n} = \frac{\partial F^1}{\partial n} = u^1(1) = 0. \tag{2.212}$$

Flux boundary conditions on the free boundary $r = 1 - \epsilon$:

$$-\frac{\partial L^1}{\partial n} + \alpha_L L^1 = \frac{\partial}{\partial r}\left[\frac{\partial \tilde{L}}{\partial n} - \alpha_L \tilde{L}\right] B^1, \tag{2.213}$$

$$-\frac{\partial H^1}{\partial n} + \alpha_H H^1 = \frac{\partial}{\partial r}\left[\frac{\partial \tilde{H}}{\partial n} - \alpha_H \tilde{H}\right] B^1, \tag{2.214}$$

$$-\frac{\partial G^1}{\partial n} + \alpha_G G^1 = \frac{\partial}{\partial r}\left[\frac{\partial \tilde{G}}{\partial n} - \alpha_G \tilde{G}\right] B^1, \tag{2.215}$$

$$-\frac{\partial I^1}{\partial n} + \alpha_I I^1 = \frac{\partial}{\partial r}\left[\frac{\partial \tilde{I}}{\partial n} - \alpha_I \tilde{I}\right] B^1, \tag{2.216}$$

$$-\frac{\partial R^1}{\partial n} + \alpha_R R^1 = \frac{\partial}{\partial r}\left[\frac{\partial \tilde{R}}{\partial n} - \alpha_R \tilde{R}\right] B^1, \tag{2.217}$$

$$-\frac{\partial \beta^1}{\partial n} + \alpha_M \beta^1 = \frac{\partial}{\partial r}\left[\frac{\partial \tilde{\beta}}{\partial n} - \alpha_M \tilde{\beta}\right] B^1, \tag{2.218}$$

$$-\frac{\partial F^1}{\partial n} + \alpha_M F^1 = \frac{\partial}{\partial r}\left[\frac{\partial \tilde{F}}{\partial n} - \alpha_M \tilde{F}\right] B^1, \tag{2.219}$$

The equation for the free boundary leads

$$\frac{dB^1(t)}{dt} = u^1(1-\epsilon, t) + \tilde{u}_r(1-\epsilon). \tag{2.220}$$

Using (2.194) and (2.213)-(2.219), we have

$$-\frac{\partial L^1}{\partial n} + \alpha_L L^1 = \left[k_L R_0 L_0 - \lambda_{GL}(G_0 - G_s)L_0 + \lambda_{ML}\frac{(M_0 - \beta_0)L_0}{K_{ML} + L_0} + O(\epsilon)\right] B^1 =: \eta_L B^1, \tag{2.221}$$

$$-\frac{\partial H^1}{\partial n} + \alpha_H H^1 = \left[k_H R_0 H_0 + \lambda_{HF}\frac{H_0 F_0}{(K_{HF} + H_0)} + O(\epsilon)\right] B^1 =: \eta_H B^1, \tag{2.222}$$

$$-\frac{\partial G^1}{\partial n} + \alpha_G G^1 =$$
$$-\left[\tilde{G}_0 - (E_{G0} + S_I I_0)G_0 - \lambda_{GH}(G_0 - G_s)H_0 + O(\epsilon)\right] B^1 =: \eta_G B^1, \quad (2.223)$$

$$-\frac{\partial I^1}{\partial n} + \alpha_I I^1 = \left[\frac{\sigma G_0^2 \beta_0}{\alpha + G_0^2} - k_I I_0 - \lambda_{RI} R_0 I_0 + O(\epsilon)\right] =: \eta_I B^1 B^1, \quad (2.224)$$

$$-\frac{\partial R^1}{\partial n} + \alpha_R R^1 = -\Big[\tilde{R}_0 - R_0(k_L L_0 + k_H H_0) + \lambda_{GR}(G_0 - G_s)R_0$$
$$+ \lambda_{IR} I_0 R_0 + O(\epsilon)\Big] B^1 =: \eta_R B^1, \quad (2.225)$$

$$-\frac{\partial \beta^1}{\partial n} + \alpha_M \beta^1 = -\left[(-d_0 + r_1 G_0 - r_2 G_0^2)\beta_0 + O(\epsilon)\right] B^1 =: \eta_\beta B^1, \quad (2.226)$$

$$-\frac{\partial F^1}{\partial n} + \alpha_M F^1 = -\left[\lambda_{ML}\frac{(M_0 - \beta_0)L_0}{K_{ML} + L_0} + O(\epsilon)\right] B^1 =: \eta_F B^1. \quad (2.227)$$

Now using (2.211) and (2.220)-(2.227), we can write

$$M_0 \partial_r u^1 = J_1 + J_2 B^1, \quad (2.228)$$

where

$$J_1 = (M_0 - \tilde{\beta} - \tilde{F})\frac{\lambda}{K_{MH} + \tilde{H}}\left(L^1 - \frac{\eta_L}{\alpha_L}B^1\right)$$
$$- (M_0 - \tilde{F} - \tilde{\beta})\frac{\lambda \tilde{L}}{K_{MH} + \tilde{H}}\left[\beta^1 - \left(\frac{\eta_\beta}{\alpha_M}B^1 + F^1 - \frac{\eta_F}{\alpha_M}B^1\right)\right]$$
$$- (M_0 - \tilde{\beta} - \tilde{F})\frac{\lambda}{(K_{MH} + \tilde{H})^2}\left(H^1 - \frac{\eta_H}{\alpha_H}B^1\right)$$
$$+ d_M\left(\beta^1 - \frac{\eta_\beta}{\alpha_M}B^1 + F^1 - \frac{\eta_F}{\alpha_M}B^1\right)$$
$$- d_F\left(F^1 - \frac{\eta_F}{\alpha_M}B^1\right) + \beta_0\left(r_1\left(G^1 - \frac{\eta_G}{\alpha_G}B^1\right) - 2r_2\tilde{G}\left(G^1 - \frac{\eta_G}{\alpha_G}\right)\right)$$
$$+ (-d_0 + r_1\tilde{G} - r_2\tilde{G}^2)\left(\beta^1 - \frac{\eta_\beta}{\alpha_M}B^1\right); \quad (2.229)$$

$$J_2 = (M_0 - \beta_0)\frac{\lambda}{K_{MH} + H_0}\frac{\eta_L}{\alpha_L} - (M_0 - \beta_0)\frac{\lambda L_0}{K_{MH} + H_0}\left(\frac{\eta_\beta}{\alpha_M} + \frac{\eta_F}{\alpha_M}\right)$$
$$- (M_0 - \beta_0)\frac{\lambda}{(K_{MH} + H_0)^2}\frac{\eta_H}{\alpha_H} + d_M\left(\frac{\eta_\beta}{\alpha_M} + \frac{\eta_F}{\alpha_M}\right)$$
$$- d_F\frac{\eta_F}{\alpha_M} + \beta_0\left(r_1\frac{\eta_G}{\alpha_G} - 2r_2 G_0\frac{\eta_G}{\alpha_G}\right) + (-d_0 + r_1 G_0 - r_2 G_0^2)\frac{\eta_\beta}{\alpha_M}. \quad (2.230)$$

Integrating (2.228) we obtain:

$$u^1(1-\epsilon,t) = -\frac{1}{M_0}\int_{1-\epsilon}^{1} J_1 dr - \frac{B^1}{M_0}\int_{1-\epsilon}^{1} J_2 dr \tag{2.231}$$

Set

$$\begin{aligned}
S_1 = &-\frac{(M_0-\beta_0)}{M_0}\frac{\lambda}{K_{MH}+H_0} \\
&\times \frac{\left[k_L R_0 L_0 - \lambda_{GL}(G_0-G_s)L_0 + \lambda_{ML}\frac{(M_0-\beta_0)L_0}{K_{ML}+L_0}\right]}{\alpha_L} \\
&-\frac{(M_0-\beta_0)}{M_0}\frac{\lambda L_0}{K_{MH}+H_0}\left(\frac{\left[(-d_0+r_1G_0-r_2G_0^2)\beta_0\right]}{\alpha_M} + \frac{\left[\lambda_{ML}\frac{(M_0-\beta_0)L_0}{K_{ML}+L_0}\right]}{\alpha_M}\right) \\
&+\frac{(M_0-\beta_0)}{M_0}\frac{\lambda}{(K_{MH}+H_0)^2}\frac{\left[k_H R_0 H_0 + \lambda_{HF}\frac{H_0F_0}{(K_{HF}+H_0)}\right]}{\alpha_H} \\
&+\frac{d_M}{M_0}\left(\frac{\left[(-d_0+r_1G_0-r_2G_0^2)\beta_0\right]}{\alpha_M} + \frac{\left[\lambda_{ML}\frac{(M_0-\beta_0)L_0}{K_{ML}+L_0}\right]}{\alpha_M}\right) \\
&-\frac{d_F}{M_0}\frac{\left[\lambda_{ML}\frac{(M_0-\beta_0)L_0}{K_{ML}+L_0}\right]}{\alpha_M} \\
&+\frac{\beta_0}{M_0}\left(r_1\frac{\left[\tilde{G}_0-(E_{G0}+S_I I_0)G_0-\lambda_{GH}(G_0-G_s)H_0\right]}{\alpha_G}\right) \\
&-\frac{\beta_0}{M_0}\left(\frac{2r_2G_0}{M_0}\frac{\left[\tilde{G}_0-(E_{G0}+S_I I_0)G_0-\lambda_{GL}(G_0-G_s)L_0\right]}{\alpha_G}\right) \\
&+\frac{(-d_0+r_1G_0-r_2G_0^2)}{M_0}\frac{\left[(-d_0+r_1G_0-r_2G_0^2)\beta_0\right]}{\alpha_M}.
\end{aligned} \tag{2.232}$$

Then from (2.220), (2.231), and (2.202), we have

$$\frac{dB^1(t)}{dt} = (S_1\epsilon + O(\epsilon^2))B^1 + a_1. \tag{2.233}$$

where

$$a_1 = -\frac{1}{M_0}\int_{1-\epsilon}^{1} J_1 dr. \tag{2.234}$$

Using (2.229) and (2.204)-(2.210), we can show that

$$|a_1| \le C\epsilon^{3/2}\Bigg(\int_{1-\epsilon}^{1} [|G^1_{rr}|^2 + |I^1_{rr}|^2 + |R^1_{rr}|^2 + |L^1_{rr}|^2 + |H^1_{rr}|^2 + |\beta^1_{rr}|^2 + |F^1_{rr}|^2]\Bigg)^{1/2}. \quad (2.235)$$

We conclude from (2.233), (2.234), and (2.235) that

Theorem 2.13 *For fixed ϵ, the steady solution in Theorem 2.12 is linearly asymptotically stable if $S_1 < 0$, and linearly unstable if $S_1 > 0$.*

For patients without diabetes, i.e. $G_0 = G_s$, it is shown in [112] that an ϵ initial plague shrinks to zero if

$$\frac{\lambda L_0}{K_{MH} + H_0} - d_M < 0 \quad (2.236)$$

Here, we are going to show that for patients with hyperglycemia, where the following inequality (2.237) holds, an initial plaque will persist even if (2.236) holds.

$$(M_0 - \beta_0)\left(\frac{\lambda L_0}{K_{MH} + H_0} - d_M\right) + \beta_0(-d_0 + r_1 G_0^2 - r_2 G_0^2) > 0. \quad (2.237)$$

Theorem 2.14 *If (2.237) holds, assume that*

$$\begin{aligned} 0 < L(r,0) \le L_0 + A\epsilon, H(r,0) < H_0 + A\epsilon, F(r,0) \le A\epsilon, \\ G_s < G(r,0) < G_0 + A\epsilon, \beta < \beta_0 + A\epsilon, B(0) = 1 - \epsilon/2 \end{aligned} \quad (2.238)$$

for some constant $A \ge 0$, then

$$\limsup_{t\to\infty} B(t) < 1. \quad (2.239)$$

Proof. Using strong maximum principle, we can show that

$$L_0 - k^*\epsilon \le L(r,t) \le L_0 + A^*\epsilon + \max |L(r,0)|e^{-c_1 t}, \quad (2.240)$$

$$H_0 - k_1\epsilon \le H(r,t) \le H_0 + A_1\epsilon + \max |H(r,0)|e^{-c_1 t}, \quad (2.241)$$

$$0 < F(r,t) < A^*\epsilon, \quad (2.242)$$

$$G_0 - k_2\epsilon \le G(r,t) \le G_0 + A_2\epsilon + \max |H(r,0)|e^{-c_2 t}, \quad (2.243)$$

$$\beta_0 - k_3\epsilon \le \beta(r,t) < \beta_0 + A_3\epsilon; \quad (2.244)$$

where k^*, k_1, k_2, k_3 and A_1, A_2, A_3, A^* are positive constants.
Using (2.151) and the above inequalities, we have for sufficiently large t

$$M_0\partial_r u(r,t) = (M_0 - \beta_0)\left(\frac{\lambda L_0}{K_{MH} + H_0} - d_M\right) + \beta_0(-d_0 + r_1 G_0^2 - r_2 G_0^2) + O(\epsilon). \quad (2.245)$$

Integrating above to obtain

$$u(r,t) = -\frac{1}{M_0}\int_r^1 \left[(M_0-\beta_0)\left(\frac{\lambda L_0}{K_{MH}+H_0}-d_M\right) + \beta_0(-d_0+r_1G_0^2-r_2G_0^2)+O(\epsilon)\right] < 0. \quad (2.246)$$

Now (2.155) and (2.246) imply that $B(t)$ is decreasing, so (2.239) holds.
■

2.3.3 A More Comprehensive Model for Diabetic Atherosclerosis

Hyperglycemia damage the vascular bed by several cellular mechanisms, comprising of enhanced production of intracellular advanced glycation end products (AGEs), increased expression of AGE receptors (RAGE) and ligands, augmented polyol and hexosamine flux, activation of protein kinase C (PKC) and over activation of hexosamine pathway [60, 239, 279]. AGEs formation further lead to alteration of structural, functional and receptor recognition properties of matrix components. Sequentially, AGEs binding to its receptor (RAGE) increases superoxide production that promotes macrophage induced vascular inflammation [60, 239, 279]. Furthermore, AGEs also induces decreased endothelial NO synthase (eNOS) expression as well as NO synthesis and increased ET-1 expression, leading to endothelial dysfunction [55, 229, 294].

Although some key variables such as LDL, HDL, Glucose, Insulin, free radicals, SMC and foam cells are included in the simplified model discussed in the previous sections, some important variables such as AGEs are missing in the model. The risk of diabetic cardiovascular complications after exposure to high glucose levels for a certain period of time is called "metabolic memory" or "legacy effect". One of the possible mechanisms of this effect is the formation of advanced glycation end-products (AGEs), which occurs when the blood glucose level is high. These compounds are not easily metabolized, accumulating in patients with a long history of inadequate blood glucose control. Such accumulation may accelerate the progression of vascular disease in diabetic patients [145, 249]. In this section we present a more comprehensive model in [289].

We will use a system of partial differential equations to develop a mathematical model of plaque formation in diabetic atherosclerosis. The mathematical model will be based on the network shown in Fig. 2.5. The variables included in the model are listed in Table 2.10.

Equations for glucose, insulin, and β-cells: The distribution of G and I and β density are modeled by

$$\frac{\partial G}{\partial t} - D_G\Delta G = \tilde{G}_0 - (E_{G0}+S_I I)G - k_{GL}(G-G_s)L, \quad (2.247)$$

$$\frac{\partial \beta}{\partial t} + \nabla\cdot(\mathbf{u}\beta) - D_\beta\Delta\beta = (-d_0+r_1G-r_2G^2)\beta, \quad (2.248)$$

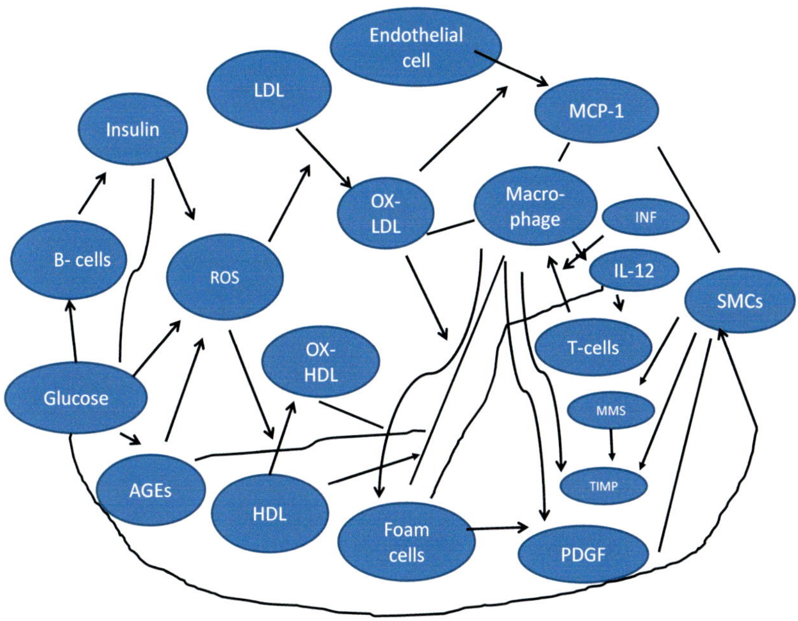

Figure 2.5 Glucose production and uptake depend on blood glucose and insulin levels. Insulin is secreted by pancreatic β cells, cleared by the liver, kidneys, and insulin receptors. β cells replication and death vary nonlinearly with glucose. Glucose metabolites inhibits production of NO and increase the production of ROS. High glucose level leads to formation of AGEs. AGEs increases ROS production and induces decreased NO production; AGE may inhibit reverse cholesterol transport by reducing ABCA1 and ABCG1. Insulin resistance decrease endothelium-derived NO and increase the production of ROS. Diabetes stimulates atherogenic activity of vascular smooth muscle cells. LDL and HDL are oxidized by free radicals, and become ox-LDL and ox-HDL respectively. Ox- LDL recruits macrophages to intima. By ingesting ox-LDL, macrophages are transformed to foam cells. SMCs are attracted into the intima by MCP-1 (secreted by endothelial cells) and PDGF (secreted by macrophages and foam cells). Macrophages, foam cells and SMCs secrete IL-12, which activates T cells. IFN-c secreted by T cells enhance the activity of macrophages which contributes the plaque built-up.

$$\frac{\partial I}{\partial t} - D_I \Delta I = \frac{\sigma G^2 \beta}{\alpha + G^2} - kI - \lambda_{RI} RI; \tag{2.249}$$

Equation (2.247) describes the dynamics of glucose and insulin,the third term on the right side of (2.247) represents glycation of LDL; and Eq. (2.248) describes the formation and loss of β-cells [265]. The first term on the right hand side of (2.249) is secretion of insulin [265], the second term is clearance

TABLE 2.10 The variables of the model: concentrations and densities are in units of g/cm^3

L:	concentration of LDL	H:	concentration of HDL
L_{ox}:	concentration of ox-LDL	H_{ox}:	concentration of ox-HDL
G:	concentration of Glucose	I:	concentration of Insulin
R:	concentration of ROS	M:	density of macrophages
N:	concentration of NO	A:	concentration of AGEs
P:	concentration of MCP-1	D:	concentration of PDGF
S:	density of SMCs	β:	density of β-cells
F:	density of foam cells	T:	density of T-cells
I_{12}:	concentration of IL-12	I_γ:	concentration of IFN-γ
Q:	concentration of MMPs	Q_r:	concentration of TIMP
u:	fluid velocity (in cm/day)	σ:	pressure (in gcm^2/day)

of insulin. The third term on the right side of (2.249) models that ROS, in excess and over time, cause chronic oxidation stress, which in turn result in reduction of insulin secretion as well as increased apoptosis [235, 246], where λ_{RI} is the reduction rate of insulin due to ROS.

Equations for lipoproteins [LDL (L), HDL (H), ox-LDL (L_{ox}) and ox-HDL (H_{ox})]: The distribution of LDL, HDL and free radicals in the intima are described using reaction diffusion equations [68, 111, 147, 200]

$$\frac{\partial L}{\partial t} - D_L \Delta L = -k_L RL - \lambda_{AL} AL - k_{ML} \frac{ML}{K_{ML} + L}, \tag{2.250}$$

$$\frac{\partial H}{\partial t} - D_H \Delta H = -k_H RH - \lambda_{HF} \frac{HF}{(K_{HF} + H)(K_{MA} + A)}, \tag{2.251}$$

$$\frac{\partial L_{ox}}{\partial t} - D_{L_{ox}} \Delta L_{ox} = k_L RL - \lambda_{ML_{ox}} ML_{ox}, \tag{2.252}$$

$$\frac{\partial H_{ox}}{\partial t} - D_{H_{ox}} \Delta H_{ox} = k_H RH - k_{FH_{ox}} \frac{F}{K_F + F} H_{ox}, \tag{2.253}$$

where k_L and k_H are reaction rates of oxidization, and $\lambda_{L_{ox}M}$ is the reduction rate of ox-LDL due to ingestion by macrophages. Equations (2.250) and (2.251) model the evolution of LDL and HDL concentrations. It is assumed that LDL and HDL are lost by reaction of oxidation with free radicals and LDL is ingested by macrophages and glycated by AGEs. Equation (2.252) models the production of ox-LDL due to LDL oxidation by reaction with the radicals (first term on right-hand side) and a reduction of ox-LDL through ingestion by macrophages (second term on right-hand side). Equation (2.253) models the production of ox-HDL due to HDL oxidation by reaction with the radicals (first term on right-hand side) and a reduction of ox-HDL through ingestion by foam cells (second term on right-hand side). $k_{FH_{ox}}$ is the reduction rate of ox-HDL due to ingestion by the foam cells.

Equation for ROS (R): The equation for the concentration of free radicals is modeled by

$$\frac{\partial R}{\partial t} - D_R \Delta R = R_0 - R(k_L L + k_H H) + \lambda_{GR} G + \lambda_{IR} I + \lambda_{AR} A, \quad (2.254)$$

where R_0 is the base line growth, the third term on the right hand of the equation models the mechanism whereby excess glucose metabolites inhibits production of NO by blocking eNOS synthase activation and increase the production of ROS [163, 282]; where λ_{GR} is the growth rate of ROS due to excess glucose. The fourth term on the right hand of the equation models the mechanism that insulin resistance decrease endothelium-derived NO and increase the production of ROS [150,161]; where λ_{IR} is the growth rate of ROS due to insulin resistance. The fifth term accounts for that AGEs also induces increased ROS and decreased endothelial NO synthase (eNOS) expression as well as NO synthesis and increased ET-1 expression, leading to endothelial dysfunction [55, 229, 294]; where λ_{AR} is the growth rate of ROS due to the formation of AGEs.

Equation for AGEs (A): The equation for the concentration of AGEs is modeled by

$$\frac{\partial A}{\partial t} - D_A \Delta A = \lambda_{GA} G + k_{GL} GL + \lambda_{AL} LA - d_A A, \quad (2.255)$$

where the first two terms are the production due to high glucose concentration and glycation of LDL , the third term represents that AGEs enhance glycation of LDC [10, 168], the fourth term represents the natural death of AGEs.

Equation for SMCs (S): The equation of the SMCs density is given by

$$\frac{\partial S}{\partial t} + \nabla \cdot (\mathbf{u} S) - D_S \Delta S = -\nabla \cdot (S \chi_C \nabla P) - \nabla \cdot (S \chi_C \nabla D) - \nabla \cdot (S \chi_G \nabla G) - \lambda_{GL} GL, \quad (2.256)$$

The first two terms on the right side account for chemostaxis by MCP-1 and PDGF [111, 147]. Diabetes stimulates atherogenic activities of SMCs. SMCs cultured from patients with type 2 diabetes demonstrate enhanced migration [17]. Advanced atherosclerotic lesions in diabetic patients have fewer SMCs compared with those of controls [17]. The third term in the right hand side models haptotaxis by glucose. The fourth term models that oxidized glycated LDL can induce apoptosis of SMCs [17].

Equation for macrophages (M): The evolution of macrophage density is modeled by

$$\frac{\partial M}{\partial t} + \nabla \cdot (\mathbf{u} M) - D_M \Delta M = -\nabla \cdot (M \chi_C \nabla P) - \lambda_{ML_{ox}} \frac{M L_{ox}}{K_{ML_{ox}} + L_{ox}} + \lambda_{HF} \frac{HF}{(K_{MA} + A)(K_{HF} + H)} + \lambda_{MI_\gamma} \frac{M I_\gamma}{K_{I_\gamma} + I_\gamma} - d_M M, \quad (2.257)$$

Here the first term accounts for recruitment of macrophages by MCP-1 [111, 147]; the second and third term on right-hand side accounts for the transition between M and L: when L molecules are ingested by a macrophage, the macrophage becomes a foam cell; when H combines with membrane protein on a foam cell in a process that clears it from the bad cholesterol, the foam cell turns into a macrophage. The factor $(K_{MA}+A)$ on the denominator of the third term represents that AGEs inhibit reverse cholesterol transportation [10, 168]. The fourth term accounts for activation of macrophages by I_γ [111, 147]. The fifth term accounts for the death of macrophages.

Equation for foam cells (F): The equation for foam cells is given by

$$\frac{\partial F}{\partial t} + \nabla \cdot (\mathbf{u}F) - D_F \Delta F = \lambda_{ML_{ox}} \frac{ML_{ox}}{K_{ML} + L_{ox}} - \lambda_{HF} \frac{HF}{(K_{MA}+A)(K_{HF}+H)} - d_F F, \quad (2.258)$$

where on the right side of the equation, a gain of foam cells from macrophages M ingesting L, and a loss of foam cells triggered by H. The death rate of foam cells is d_F.

Equation for MPC-1 (P): The MPC-1 is modeled by

$$\frac{\partial P}{\partial t} - D_P \Delta P = \lambda_{PL_{ox}} \frac{L_{ox}}{K_{L_{ox}} + L_{ox}} - d_P P, \quad (2.259)$$

where the first term on the right-hand side is the production of MCP-1 by endothelial cells, whose density is assumed to be constant, under the influence of ox-LDL [111, 148].

Equation for T cells (T). The density of T cells satisfies

$$\frac{\partial T}{\partial t} + \nabla \cdot (\mathbf{u}T) - D_T \Delta T = \lambda_{TM} \frac{M}{K_{TM} + M} - d_T T. \quad (2.260)$$

In this equation, we assume that T cells are activated by macrophages [111, 231].

Equation for PDGF (D), MMP(Q), and TIMP (Q_r): We have the following equation for PDFG

$$\frac{\partial D}{\partial t} - D_D \Delta D = \lambda_{DM} M + \lambda_{DF} F + \lambda_{DS} S - d_D D, \quad (2.261)$$

$$\frac{\partial Q}{\partial t} - D_Q \Delta Q = \lambda_{QS} S - d_{QQ_r} Q Q_r - d_Q Q, \quad (2.262)$$

$$\frac{\partial Q_r}{\partial t} - D_{Q_r} \Delta Q_r = \lambda_{Q_r S} S + \lambda_{Q_r M} M - d_{QQ_r} Q Q_r - d_{Q_r} Q_r, \quad (2.263)$$

where PDGF is produced by macrophages, foam cells, and SMCs [111, 230, 238]. In Eq. (2.262), MMP is secreted by SMCs and is lost by binding with

TIMP [111,147]. In Eq. (2.263), TIMP is produced by SMCs and macrophages [111, 147].

Equation for IFN-γ. The dynamics of IFN-γ is given by

$$\frac{\partial I_\gamma}{\partial t} - D_{I_\gamma}\Delta I_\gamma = \lambda_{TI_\gamma}T - d_{I_\gamma}I_\gamma. \tag{2.264}$$

where the first term on the right hand side is the production of I_γ by T cells [111, 147].

Equation for IL-12 (I_{12}): The equation for I_{12} is given by

$$\frac{\partial I_{12}}{\partial t} - D_{I_12}\Delta I_{12} = \lambda_{MI_{12}}\frac{M}{K_M + M}\left(1 + \frac{I_\gamma}{K_{I_{12}}H + I_\gamma}\right) + \lambda_{I_{12}F}\frac{F}{K_F + F} - d_{I_12}I_{12}, \tag{2.265}$$

The firs term of the right hand side is the production of I_{12} by macrophages enhanced by I_γ and resisted by HDL. The second term represents the production by the foam cells [111, 147].

Equation for pressure σ: We assume that the intima has the constituency of a porous medium. Then, by Darcy's law, the velocity $\mathbf{u}$ of the cells is given by

$$\mathbf{u} = -\nabla\sigma, \tag{2.266}$$

where σ is the pressure. We also assume that the total density of all the cells is constant. This constant should be smaller than the average density of a plaque, $1.22 \pm 0.03g/cm^3$[9], because plaques contain some debris, which are not included in our model. We take the constant to be 1 g/cm3, i.e.,

$$M + F + T + \beta + S = 1 \tag{2.267}$$

We assume that all cells are approximately of the same volume and surface area, so that the diffusion coefficients of the all cells have the same coefficient. By adding Eqs. (2.248), (2.253), (2.254), and (2.255), and using (2.257), we get

$$-\Delta\sigma = (-d_0 + r_1G - r_2G^2)\beta - \nabla\cdot(S\chi_G\nabla G) - \nabla\cdot(S\chi_C\nabla P) - \nabla\cdot(S\chi_C\nabla D) - \nabla\cdot(M\chi_C\nabla P) + \lambda_{TM}\frac{M}{K_{TM} + M} + \lambda_{MI_\gamma}\frac{MI_\gamma}{K_{MI_\gamma} + I_\gamma} - d_TT - \lambda_{GL}GL - d_FF - d_MM. \tag{2.268}$$

Boundary Conditions: For simplicity, we consider only 2-dimensional plaques as in Fig. 2.3. Then the boundary of the plaque consists of i) Γ_M, in contact with media; ii) a free boundary Γ_I, inside the lumen.

Boundary conditions on Γ_I: We assume flux boundary conditions of the form

$$\frac{\partial X}{\partial n} + \alpha_X(X - X_0) = 0, \tag{2.269}$$

for $X = G, I, L, H, \beta$, and α_X are constants. M satisfies

$$\frac{\partial M}{\partial n} + \alpha_M \frac{L_{ox} A}{1 + H}(M - M_0) = 0, \tag{2.270}$$

since ox-LDL attracts monocytes and AGEs promotes the entrance of monocytes and macrophages into the subendothelial space. Non-flux boundary conditions for all other variables $Y = R, A, S, F, L_o x, I_\gamma, I_{12}, D, Q, Q_r, P$:

$$\frac{\partial Y}{\partial n} = 0. \tag{2.271}$$

The flux boundary condition for T is determined by $T = 1 - S - \beta - F - M$. Note that G_0, I_0, L_0, and H_0 are the glucose, insulin, LDL, and HDL concentrations in the blood, so we shall be interested to see how these concentrations determine whether a small plaque will grow or shrink.

As in [40,41,43], we assume that the free boundary Γ_I is held together by cell-to-cell adhesion forces so that

$$\sigma = \gamma\kappa \text{ on } \Gamma_I, \tag{2.272}$$

where κ is the mean curvature of the surface Γ_I. (If Γ_I is circular, then κ is the reciprocal of the radius) Furthermore, the continuity condition $u_n = V_n$, where n is the outward normal and V_n is the velocity of the free boundary Γ_I in the direction n, yields the relation

$$V_n = -\frac{\partial \sigma}{\partial n} \text{ on } \Gamma_I. \tag{2.273}$$

Boundary conditions on Γ_M: We assume non-flux boundary conditions for all variables except S and T on Γ_M: For S, we have

$$\frac{\partial S}{\partial n} + \alpha_S \frac{P + D}{P_0 + D_0}(S - S_0) = 0 \text{ on } \Gamma_M, \tag{2.274}$$

where S_0 is SMCs density in the media and MCP-1 and PDGF attract SMCs from the media. The flux condition for T is determined by $T = 1 - S - \beta - F - M$.

Parameter estimation: Most parameters in (2.247)–(2.274) can be found in Tables 2.3–2.5 and Tables 2.8–2.9. The remaining parameters are in the following table.

2.4 A MULTI-LAYER MODEL

The typical anatomical structure of an arterial wall is shown schematically in Fig. 2.6. Going from the lumen to the most external layer, a large artery is

TABLE 2.11 Parameters' description and value

Parameters	Description	Value
D_A	diffusion coefficient for AGEs	$1.04 \times 10^{-1}\,cm^2\,d^{-1}$ [147]
λ_{AL}	reaction rate of for LDL+ AGEs	$2.35 \times 10^{-4}\,g^{-1}\,cm^3\,d^{-1}$ [147]
λ_{AR}	growth rate of radical due to AGEs	$124.69\,d^{-1}$ estimated
λ_{AR}	growth rate of AGEs due to radicals	$124.69\,d^{-1}$ estimated
d_A	death rate of AGEs	$0.015\,d^{-1}$ [147]
d_F	death rate of foam cells	$0.03\,d^{-1}$ [147]
K_{MA}	AGEs saturation for production of macrophage	$0.5\,g\,cm^{-3}$ [147]

comprised of the following five layers: glycocalyx, endothelium, intima, media, and adventitia. The luminal glycocalyx is a thin layer of macromolecules which is believed to cover the plasma membrane of a single layer of endothelial cells, and the entrance of the intercellular junctions. The thickness of the glycocalyx is usually less than 100 nm (average thickness 60 nm). Immediately in contact with the glycocalyx is endothelium, a single layer of endothelial cells, which are elongated in the direction of blood flow. Endothelial cells are interconnected through intercellular junctions. Internal elastic lamina (IEL), an impermeable elastic tissue with fenestral pores, is lying between intima and media. In contrast to the media, which contains alternating layers of smooth muscle cells and elastic connective tissue, the intima is mainly comprised of proteoglycan and collagen fibers. The media layer is surrounded by loose connective tissue, the adventitia, in which there are some capillaries (lymphatic and vasa vasorum). Except via transport from luminal blood supplies, proteins can be transported from the adventitia to the media through the vasa vasorum.

The main focus of the present section is to present a four-layer model developed in [169, 297, 298] for the description of the mass transport in the arterial wall coupled with the mass transport in the arterial lumen. The endothelium, intima, IEL and media layers are all treated as macroscopically homogeneous porous media and mathematically modeled using proper types of the volume averaged porous media equations, with the Staverman filtration and osmotic reflection coefficients employed to account for selective permeability of each porous layer to certain solutes. In particular, the effects of hypertension on the LDL transport within the arterial wall are studied based on our new mathematical model, to identify possible factors that might be responsible for enhanced arterial wall uptake of LDL under hypertensive conditions.

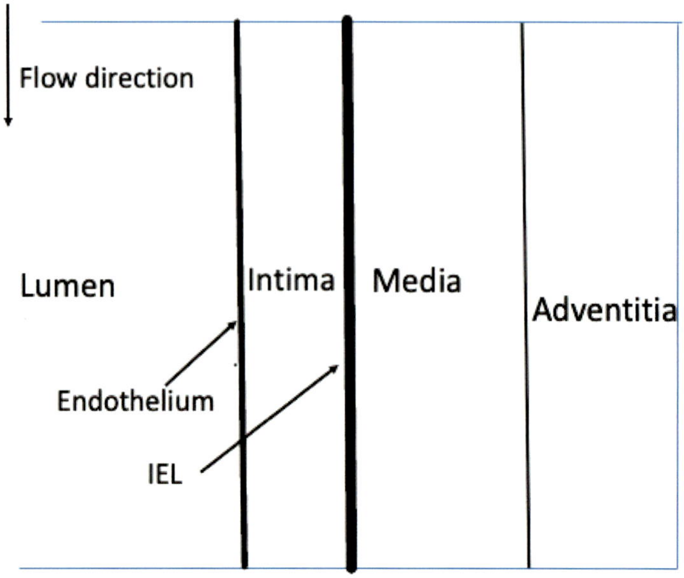

Figure 2.6 Transverse section of a large artery.

2.4.1 Mathematical Formulation

In the lumen layer, the blood flow can be modeled by the Navier-Stokes equations:

$$\rho\left(\frac{\partial u}{\partial t}+u\cdot\nabla u\right)=-\nabla p+\mu\nabla^2 u, \tag{2.275}$$

$$\nabla\cdot u=0; \tag{2.276}$$

$$\frac{\partial X}{\partial t}+\nabla\cdot(uX)=D_L\nabla^2 X, \tag{2.277}$$

where u is the blood velocity vector, p is the blood pressure, ρ is the blood density and μ is the viscosity of blood, X is a protein such as LDL.

In endothelium and internal elastic lamina (IEL) are treated as biological porous membranes. The Staverman filtration and osmotic reflection coefficients are employed to account for selective rejection of species by the membranes and for the effects of osmotic pressure. Let V_e be the velocity, p_e be the pressure and X_e be a protein such as LDL, the following equations may be employed:

$$\frac{\partial V_e}{\partial t}+K_eV_e=-\nabla p_e+R_e\nabla X_e+\mu_e\nabla^2 V_e, \tag{2.278}$$

$$\frac{\partial X_e}{\partial t}+\sigma_eV_e\cdot\nabla X_e=D_e\nabla^2 X_e, \tag{2.279}$$

where the coefficients K_e, R_e, and μ_e are related to porosity, permeability and viscosity, σ_e is the filtration reflection coefficient.

The intima and media layer are modeled as macroscopically homogeneous porous media. Since the porous media are selectively permeable to certain species such as LDL, the Staverman filtration reflection coefficient has to be introduced to account for this effect. The osmotic effect in the transport modeling is not included in this part since the maximum osmotic pressure gradient in the medial layer is far below the hydraulic pressure gradient [10]. Therefore, the volume averaged governing equations of the intima and media layers are

$$\frac{\partial V_I}{\partial t} + K_I V_I = -\nabla p_I + \mu_I \nabla^2 V_I, \tag{2.280}$$

$$\frac{\partial X_I}{\partial t} + \sigma_I V_I \cdot \nabla X_I = D_I \nabla^2 X_I + F(X_I), \tag{2.281}$$

where $F(X_I)$ ia a function of X_I representing the interaction of proteins, and the other coefficients (2.280) and (2.281) are parallel to that in (2.278) and (2.279).

On the free boundary of the plaque, we impose the pressure condition:

$$p_e - p = \gamma\kappa. \tag{2.282}$$

The boundary conditions for the flow are as follows: a fully developed (parabolic) velocity profile at the inlet of the arterial lumen is taken and it is assumed that $u = 0$, both at the inlet and outlet sections of the arterial wall. In addition we employ the zero cross flow condition which exists on the axis of symmetry, and constant pressure at the outlet of the arterial lumen and the media adventitia interface. At the interfaces between the lumen, endothelium, intima, IEL, and media continuity of velocity and shear stress is applied.

The concentration boundary conditions are: $X/X_0 = 1$ at the lumen inlet, zero normal diffusive mass flux at the axis of symmetry, at the lumen outlet, and the inlet and outlet of the arterial wall. Three types of boundary conditions are employed at the media adventitia interface: $X/X_0 = 0, X/X_0 = 0.01$, and $\frac{\partial X}{\partial n} = 0$. Note that X_0 is the reference concentration at the lumen inlet for LDL. These boundary conditions are reflective of the physiological conditions that exist within an artery.

Parameters in equations (2.275)–(2.282) are discussed in [297].

2.4.2 Risk of Hypertension

The effects of hypertension on the LDL transport in the arterial wall are studied in [297] based on the multi-layer model in an attempt to explain how the hypertension increases the uptake of LDL by the arterial wall. The effects of transmural pressure on the LDL "concentration polarization", i.e. the accumulation of LDL at the lumen endothelium interface due to the higher resistance offered by the endothelium were studied. As it can be seen, transmural pressure has a significant impact on the species accumulation at the lumen endothelium interface. As the transmural pressure increases, the species accumulation is found to increase substantially. This might be explained by an increase in the convective rejection fluxes as the transmural pressure increases. As the endothelial diffusivity increases, the LDL concentration at the interface drops very slightly.

The impact of the "concentration polarization" on the LDL transport across the endothelium was examined. It can be seen that the uptake of LDL into the intima is slightly dependent of axial location, while this dependence diminishes significantly in the IEL and media layers. This interesting result suggests the elevated species accumulation at the lumen endothelium interface leads to a higher species concentration in the intima layer. However, this higher species accumulation produces only minor effects on the species profiles in the IEL and media layers. The influence of transmural pressure and endothelial diffusivity on the species concentration within the different layers was studied. It was found that the LDL uptake within different layers is largely affected by the transmural pressure and endothelial diffusivity. More specifically, increasing the transmural pressure to 160 mmHg while maintaining the normal value of endothelial LDL diffusivity results in an almost 50% increase in the average species concentration as compared to the normal condition. On the other hand, when there is four-folder increase in the endothelial LDL diffusivity at 160 mmHg, the mean LDL concentration in the wall increases by a factor of 2.3 compared to normal case. This result is close to the experimental measurements. The results suggest that a pressure-induced increase in the endothelial diffusivity, combined with pressure-driven convection, most probably is a major determinant of the LDL transport across the arterial wall, which might explain increased atherosclerosis susceptibility in the presence of hypertension. In contrast, concentration polarization only plays a minor role in the enhanced LDL uptake within the arterial wall at higher transmural pressure. This contention is consistent with the conclusions in previous studies except that the present study demonstrates pressure-driven convection also plays an essential role in hypertension.

2.5 STOCHASTIC MODELS

The aforementioned studies in the previous sections focused on a deterministic model without discussing variability in the model parameters due to uncertainty. Given the large number of inputs to the diabetic atherosclerosis simulation, several sources of uncertainty exist. For example, uncertainty may come from clinical measurements, image based geometries, biological properties, boundary conditions, choice of models, etc. In this section, we study a stochastic model for diabetic atherosclerosis, which account for the situation where some parameters in the deterministic model are perturbed by white noise; the model is given by a system of stochastic partial differential equations with a free boundary.

2.5.1 A Simplified SPDE Model

Deterministic model in section 2.3.1 can be used to study the diabetic atherosclerosis if the parameters in the model can be obtained accurately. However, estimation of parameters are not easy due to the uncertainty of the data collection on individual patients. For example, the parameter E_{G0} in Eq. (2.57) may not be estimated accurately, instead we may add to it an error which can be given by $\delta_G \dot{W}_G(t)$, where $\dot{W}_G(t)$ is a white noise. Some parameters in the equations for other variables may have the same situations, and it leads us to consider the following system of stochastic PDEs:

$$\frac{\partial G}{\partial t} - D_G \Delta G = \tilde{G}_0 - (E_{G0} + S_I I)G - \lambda_{GL}(G - G_s)L + \delta_G G \dot{W}_G(t), \quad (2.283)$$

$$\frac{\partial I}{\partial t} - D_I \Delta I = \frac{\sigma G^2 \beta}{\alpha + G^2} - k_I I - \lambda_{RI} RI + \delta_I I \dot{W}_I(t); \quad (2.284)$$

$$\frac{\partial L}{\partial t} - D_L \Delta L = -k_L RL - \lambda_{GL}(G - G_s)L - \lambda_{ML} \frac{ML}{K_{ML} + L} + \delta_L L \dot{W}_L(t), \quad (2.285)$$

$$\frac{\partial H}{\partial t} - D_H \Delta H = -k_H RH - \lambda_{HF} \frac{HF}{(K_{HF} + H)} + \delta_H H \dot{W}_H(t), \quad (2.286)$$

$$\frac{\partial R}{\partial t} - D_R \Delta R = R_0 - R(k_L L + k_H H) + \lambda_{GR}(G - G_s)R + \lambda_{IR} IR + \delta_R R \dot{W}_R(t), \quad (2.287)$$

$$\frac{\partial \beta}{\partial t} + \nabla \cdot (\mathbf{u}\beta) - D_\beta \Delta \beta = (-d_0 + r_1 G - r_2 G^2)\beta + \delta_\beta \dot{W}_\beta(t), \quad (2.288)$$

$$\begin{aligned}\frac{\partial M}{\partial t} + \nabla \cdot (\mathbf{u}M) - D_M \Delta M &= -\lambda_{ML} \frac{ML}{K_{ML} + L} \\ &+ \lambda_{HF} \frac{HF}{(K_{HF} + H)} + \lambda \frac{ML}{K_{MH} + H} - d_M M + \delta_M \dot{W}_M(t), \end{aligned} \quad (2.289)$$

$$\frac{\partial F}{\partial t} + \nabla \cdot (\mathbf{u}F) - D_F \Delta F = \lambda_{ML} \frac{ML}{K_{ML} + L} - \lambda_{HF} \frac{HF}{(K_{HF} + H)} - d_F F + \delta_F \dot{W}_F(t), \quad (2.290)$$

where $W_X(t), X = G, \beta \cdots, M$ are independent real valued Wiener processes on a probability space $(\mathbf{\Omega}, \mathcal{F}, \mathbf{P})$ with filtration $\mathcal{F}_t$.

By adding Eqs. (2.288), (2.289), and (2.290) and using (2.67), we get an equation for $\mathbf{u} = u(r)\vec{e}_r$:

$$M_0\nabla\mathbf{u} = (-d_0+r_1G-r_2G^2)\beta+\lambda\frac{(M_0-F-\beta)L}{K_{MH}+H}-d_FF-d_M(M_0-F-\beta)$$
$$+\delta_\beta\dot{W}_\beta(t)+\delta_F\dot{W}_F(t)+\delta_M\dot{W}_M(t). \quad (2.291)$$

By Eqs. (2.291) and (2.66), we get

$$-\Delta\sigma = F_1(G,\beta,L,H,F)+M_0^{-1}\delta_\beta\dot{W}_\beta(t)+M_0^{-1}\delta_F\dot{W}_F(t)+M_0^{-1}\delta_M\dot{W}_M(t), \quad (2.292)$$

where

$$F_1(G,\beta,L,H,F) = M_0^{-1}(-d_0+r_1G-r_2G^2)\beta$$
$$+M_0^{-1}\left(\lambda\frac{(M_0-F-\beta)L}{K_{MH}+H}-d_FF-d_M(M_0-F-\beta)\right). \quad (2.293)$$

Using (2.292) and (2.66), we can write (2.288) as

$$\frac{d\beta}{dt}-\nabla\sigma\cdot\nabla\beta-D_\beta\Delta\beta = F_2(G,\beta,L,H,F)$$
$$+\delta_\beta\dot{W}_\beta(t)-\beta[M_0^{-1}\delta_\beta\dot{W}_\beta(t)+M_0^{-1}\delta_F\dot{W}_F(t)+M_0^{-1}\delta_M\dot{W}_M(t)]; \quad (2.294)$$

where

$$F_2(G,\beta,L,H,F) = (-d_0+r_1G-r_2G^2)\beta-\beta F_1(G,\beta,L,H,F). \quad (2.295)$$

Using (2.292) and (2.66), we can write (2.290) as

$$\frac{dF}{dt}-\nabla\sigma\cdot\nabla F-D_F\Delta F = F_3(G,\beta,L,H,F)$$
$$+\delta_F\dot{W}_F-F[M_0^{-1}\delta_\beta\dot{W}_\beta(t)+M_0^{-1}\delta_F\dot{W}_F(t)+M_0^{-1}\delta_M\dot{W}_M(t)]; \quad (2.296)$$

where

$$F_3(G,\beta,L,H,F) = \lambda_{ML}\frac{(M_0-F-\beta)L}{K_{ML}+L}$$
$$-\lambda_{HF}\frac{HF}{K_{HF}+H}-d_FF-FF_1(G,\beta,I,L,F). \quad (2.297)$$

Now the stochastic model consists of functions $\{L,H,G,I,\beta,R,F,\sigma\}$ which satisfy Eqs. (2.283)–(2.287), (2.294)–(2.297) in the region $\Omega(t)$ bounded by a free boundary $\Gamma_I(t)$ an a fixed boundary Γ_M and the following boundary

conditions:
On the free boundary $\Gamma_I(t)$,

$$\begin{aligned}
&\frac{\partial L}{\partial n} + \alpha_L(L - L_0) = 0, \ \frac{\partial H}{\partial n} + \alpha_H(H - H_0) = 0, \\
&\frac{\partial G}{\partial n} + \alpha_G(G - G_0) = 0, \ \frac{\partial I}{\partial n} + \alpha_I(I - I_0) = 0, \\
&\frac{\partial \beta}{\partial n} + \alpha_M(\beta - \beta_0) = 0, \ \frac{\partial R}{\partial n} + \alpha_R(R - R_0) = 0, \frac{\partial F}{\partial n} + \alpha_M F = 0, \\
&\sigma = \gamma\kappa, \ \ V_n = -\frac{\partial \sigma}{\partial n}
\end{aligned} \tag{2.298}$$

and on the fixed boundary Γ_M:

$$\begin{aligned}
&\frac{\partial L}{\partial n} = \frac{\partial H}{\partial n} = \frac{\partial G}{\partial n} = 0 \\
&\frac{\partial R}{\partial n} = \frac{\partial \beta}{\partial n} = \frac{\partial I}{\partial n} = \frac{\partial F}{\partial n} = 0 \\
&\sigma = 0.
\end{aligned} \tag{2.299}$$

We impose the following initial conditions: for $x \in \Omega_0$,

$$\begin{aligned}
&L(0, x) = L_0(x), \ H(0, x) = H_0(x), \ \beta(0, x) = \beta_0(x), \\
&G(0, x) = G_0(x), \ I(0, x) = I_0(x) \\
&R(0, x) = R_0(x), \ F(0, x) = F_0(x), \ \Gamma_I|_{t=0} = \Gamma_0,
\end{aligned} \tag{2.300}$$

where the initial free boundary Γ_0 is assumed to not intersect the fixed boundary Γ_M and Ω_0 is the region between Γ_0 and Γ_M.

2.5.2 Mathematical Analysis of the SPDE Model

In this section we are interested in the question of well-posedness of the free boundary problem for the stochastic model proposed in the previous section. To answer the question, we will first use the Hanzawa transformation [146] to reduce the domain $\Omega(t)$ to a fixed domain Ω_0, the free boundary $\Gamma_I(t)$ is described by a function $\rho(\omega, t)$ which is defined on the fixed boundary Γ_0. The free boundary problem will be changed into a system of stochastic PDEs in a fixed domain domain Ω_0 with boundary conditions on the fixed boundaries Γ_0 and Γ_M. Then we will further reduce the fixed boundary problem to an abstract evolution stochastic equation in Banach spaces, and we will obtain existence and uniqueness of mild solution employing the analytic semigroup theory and stochastic equations in infinite dimensions [76, 91, 98, 191].

We introduce some notations. For an open set $\Omega \subset \mathbf{R}^n$, an integer m and a real number q such that $1 \leq q < \infty$, we denote by $W^{m,q}(\Omega)$ the usual Sobolev space on Ω and $H^m(\Omega) = W^{m,2}(\Omega)$. For a real number s, $W^{s,q}(\Omega)$ the usual fractional Sobolev space on Ω and $H^s(\Omega) = W^{s,2}(\Omega)$. $H^s(\Omega)$ is a separable Hilbert space. We denote by $W_0^{s,q}(\Omega)$ the closure of $C^\infty(\Omega)$ in $W^{s,q}(\Omega)$ and $H_0^m(\Omega) = W_0^{m,2}(\Omega)$. If $\partial\Omega$ is sufficiently smooth, $s > \frac{1}{2}$, then the trace operator Tr is a a bounded linear operator and surjective from $H^s(\Omega)$ to $H^{s-\frac{1}{2}}(\partial\Omega)$.

Solutions of the stochastic model will be stochastic processes on the probability space $(\mathbf{\Omega}, \mathcal{F}, \mathbf{P})$ with values in Hilbert space $H^m(\Omega)$ (or $H^{m-\frac{1}{2}}(\Gamma_0)$). For example, the glucose variable is a function $G : [0,T] \times \mathbf{\Omega} \to H^m(\Omega)$, denoted by $G(t,\xi,x), t \in [0,T], \xi \in \mathbf{\Omega}, x \in \Omega$; in the following section, we suppress the dependence on ξ without ambiguity and denote G by $G(t,x)$.

We assume that $\Gamma_0 \in H^{m-\frac{1}{2}}$, $m \geq 4$ is an integer.

Let ω be a variable point of Γ_0 and $n(\omega)$ the unit exterior normal to Γ_0 at ω.

Let γ_0 be a given sufficiently small positive number such that the mapping

$$x : \Gamma_0 \times [-\gamma_0, \gamma_0] \to N_0 \subset R^2, x(\omega,\lambda) = \omega + \lambda n(\omega)$$

is a $H^{m-\frac{3}{2}}$ diffeomorphism.

We define $\Gamma_{0,T} = \Gamma_0 \times [0,T]$ and $\Omega_{0,T} = \Omega_0 \times [0,T]$. For $\rho(t,\omega) \in C([0,T], H^{m-\frac{1}{2}}(\Gamma_0))$ with $\|\rho\|_{m-\frac{1}{2}} \leq \gamma_0$. Let

$$\Gamma_{\rho,T} = \{\omega + \rho(t,\omega)n(\omega); (\omega,t) \in \Gamma_{0,T}\}$$

and $\Omega_{\rho,T}$ be the domain bounded by $\Gamma_{\rho,T}$ and Γ_M.

Let δ_0 be sufficiently small so that $4\delta_0 < \gamma_0$. Choose a function $\chi(\lambda) \in C^\infty(R)$ so that

(1) $\chi(\lambda) = 1$, for $|\lambda| \leq \delta_0$.
(2) $\chi(\lambda) = 0$, for $\lambda > 3\delta_0$.
(3) $|\chi'(\lambda)| \leq \frac{3}{4\delta_0}$ for $\lambda \in R$.

For $\rho(t,\omega) \in C([0,T], H^{m-\frac{1}{2}}(\Gamma_0)) \cap C^1([0,T], H^{m-\frac{3}{2}}(\Gamma_0))$, with $|\rho|_{H^{\frac{5}{2}}} \leq \delta_0$ for any $t \in [0,T]$, we define Hanzawa diffeomorphism:

$$\begin{aligned} &e_\rho : R_y^2 \times [0,T] \to R_x^2 \times [0,T] \\ &e_\rho(y,t) = (x(\omega, \lambda + \chi(\lambda)\rho(t,\omega)), t) \\ &\qquad \text{for } (y,t) = (x(\omega,\lambda),t) \in N_0 \times [0,T] \\ &e_\rho(y,t) = (y,t) \text{ for } (y,t) \in (R^2 - N_0) \times [0,T] \end{aligned} \tag{2.301}$$

Note that $e_\rho(\Omega_{0,T}) = \Omega_{\rho,T}, e_\rho(\Gamma_{0,T}) = \Gamma_{\rho,T}$.

Define a function $\eta : R \times [-\delta_0, \delta_0] \to R$ by $\eta(\lambda,\mu) + \chi_0(\eta(\lambda,\mu))\mu = \lambda$ for $(\lambda,\mu) \in R \times [-\delta_0,\delta_0]$. Since $|\chi'(\lambda)| \leq \frac{3}{4\delta_0}$, the function η is well defined and C^∞. And we have

$$\begin{aligned} &e_\rho^{-1} : R_x^2 \times [0,T] \to R_y^2 \times [0,T] \\ &e_\rho^{-1}(x(\omega,\lambda),t) = (x(\omega, \eta(\lambda, \rho(t,\omega))), t) \\ &\qquad \text{for } (x,t) = (x(\omega,\lambda),t) \in N_0 \times [0,T] \\ &e_\rho^{-1}(t,x) = (x,t) \text{ for } (x,t) \in (R^2 - N_0) \times [0,T] \end{aligned} \tag{2.302}$$

We define the following operators: for $v \in C^2(\overline{\Omega_{0T}})$

$$\mathcal{L}_\rho v \equiv \Delta(v \circ e_\rho^{-1}) \circ e_\rho = \sum_{k,j=1}^{2} A_{\rho,kj}(y,t)\partial^2_{y_k y_j} v + \sum_{k=1}^{2} A_{\rho,k}\partial_{y_k} v,$$

$$\begin{aligned} &A_{\rho,kj}(y,t) = A_{kj}(y, \rho(t,\omega(y)); \partial_\omega \rho(t,\omega(y))), \\ &\quad \text{for } k,j = 1,2, \text{ and } (y,t) \in N_0 \times [0,T], \\ &A_{\rho,kj}(y,t) = \delta_{kj} \text{ for } k,j = 1,2, (y,t) \in (R^n - N_0) \times [0,T]. \end{aligned} \tag{2.303}$$

$$A_{\rho,k}(y,t) = A_k(y, \rho(t,\omega(y)), \partial_\omega \rho(t,\omega(y)), \partial^2_\omega \rho(t,\omega(y))) \quad k = 1,2; \tag{2.304}$$

$$S_\rho = 1 + \left|\partial_\omega \rho \nabla_x \omega(x(\omega, \rho(t,\omega)))\right|^2. \tag{2.305}$$

For $v \in C^1(\overline{\Omega_{0T}})$ we define the operator

$$\nabla_\rho v = \nabla(v \circ e_\rho^{-1}) \circ e_\rho. \tag{2.306}$$

For given $\rho(t,\omega) \in C^1([0,T] \times \Gamma_0)$, we define the function

$$\psi_\rho : N_0 \to R, \qquad \psi_\rho(x) = \lambda(x) - \rho(t,\omega(x)), \text{ for } x \in N_0. \tag{2.307}$$

So $\Gamma_\rho = \{x \in N_0 : \psi_\rho(x) = 0\}$, the unit outward normal vector on Γ_ρ is given by

$$\mathbf{n}_\rho(x) = \frac{\nabla \psi_\rho(x)}{|\nabla \psi_\rho(x)|} \text{ for } x \in \Gamma_\rho. \tag{2.308}$$

The normal velocity V_n is given by

$$V_n = \frac{\partial_t \rho(t,\omega(x))}{|\nabla \psi_\rho(x)|} \text{ for } x \in \Gamma_\rho. \tag{2.309}$$

For $v \in C^1(\overline{\Omega_{0T}})$ we define the operator

$$\mathcal{D}_\rho v = \left(\nabla(v \circ e_\rho^{-1})|_{\Gamma_\rho} \cdot \nabla \psi_\rho|_{\Gamma_\rho}\right) \circ e_\rho. \tag{2.310}$$

We define

$$\mathcal{M}_\rho(y) = \begin{cases} \chi(\lambda)\partial_\lambda x(\omega(y), \lambda + \chi(\lambda)\rho(t,\omega(y))), \\ \qquad \text{for } (y,t) = (x(\omega,\lambda),t) \in N_0 \times [0,T], \\ 0, \qquad \text{for } (y,t) = (x(\omega,\lambda),t) \in \Omega_{0T}/N_0 \times [0,T]. \end{cases} \tag{2.311}$$

Set

$$\tilde{G} = G \circ e_\rho,\ \tilde{I} = I \circ e_\rho,\ \tilde{\sigma} = \sigma \circ e_\rho,\ \tilde{\beta} = \beta \circ e_\rho,\ \tilde{R} = R \circ e_\rho,$$
$$\tilde{S} = S \circ e_\rho,\ \tilde{L} = I \circ e_\rho,\ \tilde{H} = H \circ e_\rho,\ \tilde{F} = F \circ e_\rho.$$

Then the system (2.283)–(2.287) and (2.294)–(2.297) become

$$\frac{d\tilde{G}}{dt} - (\mathcal{D}_\rho \tilde{\sigma})\mathcal{M}_\rho(y) \cdot \nabla_\rho \tilde{G} - D_G \mathcal{L}_\rho \tilde{G} = \tilde{G}_0 - (E_{G0} + S_I \tilde{I})\tilde{G} + \delta_G \tilde{G} \dot{W}_G(t), \tag{2.312}$$

$$\frac{d\tilde{I}}{dt}-(\mathcal{D}_\rho\tilde{\sigma})\mathcal{M}_\rho(y)\cdot\nabla_\rho\tilde{I}-D_I\mathcal{L}_\rho\tilde{I}=\frac{\sigma_0\tilde{G}^2\tilde{\beta}}{\alpha+\tilde{G}^2}-k\tilde{I}-\lambda_{RI}\tilde{R}\tilde{I}+\delta_I\tilde{I}\dot{W}_I(t); \quad (2.313)$$

$$\begin{aligned}-\mathcal{L}_\rho\tilde{\sigma}&=F_1(\tilde{G},\tilde{S},\tilde{\beta},\tilde{L},\tilde{H},\tilde{F})\\&+M_0^{-1}\delta_\beta\dot{W}_\beta(t)+M_0^{-1}\delta_F\dot{W}_F(t)+M_0^{-1}\delta_M\dot{W}_M(t),\end{aligned} \quad (2.314)$$

$$\frac{d\tilde{L}}{dt}-D_L\mathcal{L}_\rho\tilde{L}-(\mathcal{D}_\rho\tilde{\sigma})\mathcal{M}_\rho(y)\cdot\nabla_\rho\tilde{L}=F_4(\tilde{G},\tilde{L},\tilde{R},\tilde{\beta},\tilde{F})+\delta_L\tilde{L}\dot{W}_L(t), \quad (2.315)$$

where

$$F_4(\tilde{G},\tilde{L},\tilde{R},\tilde{\beta},\tilde{F})=-k_L\tilde{R}\tilde{L}+\lambda_{GL}(\tilde{G}-G_s)\tilde{L}-\lambda_{ML}\frac{(M_0-\tilde{\beta}-\tilde{F})\tilde{L}}{K_{ML}+\tilde{L}}, \quad (2.316)$$

$$\frac{d\tilde{H}}{dt}-D_H\mathcal{L}_\rho\tilde{H}-(\mathcal{D}_\rho\tilde{\sigma})\mathcal{M}_\rho(y)\cdot\nabla_\rho\tilde{H}=F_5(\tilde{H},\tilde{R},\tilde{F})+\delta_H\tilde{H}\dot{W}_H(t), \quad (2.317)$$

$$F_5(\tilde{H},\tilde{R},\tilde{F})=-k_H\tilde{R}\tilde{H}-\lambda_{HF}\frac{\tilde{H}\tilde{F}}{(K_{HF}+\tilde{H})}, \quad (2.318)$$

$$\frac{d\tilde{R}}{dt}-D_R\mathcal{L}_\rho\tilde{R}-(\mathcal{D}_\rho\tilde{\sigma})\mathcal{M}_\rho(y)\cdot\nabla_\rho\tilde{R}=F_6(\tilde{G},\tilde{I},\tilde{L},\tilde{H},\tilde{R})+\delta_R\tilde{R}\dot{W}_I(t), \quad (2.319)$$

where

$$F_6(\tilde{G},\tilde{I},\tilde{L},\tilde{H},\tilde{R})=\tilde{R}_0-\tilde{R}(k_L\tilde{L}+k_H\tilde{H})+\lambda_{GR}(\tilde{G}-G_S)\tilde{R}+\lambda_{IR}\tilde{I}\tilde{R}. \quad (2.320)$$

$$\begin{aligned}&\frac{d\tilde{\beta}}{dt}-(\nabla_\rho\tilde{\sigma}+(\mathcal{D}_\rho\tilde{\sigma})\mathcal{M}(y))\cdot\nabla_\rho\tilde{\beta}-D_\beta\mathcal{L}_\rho\tilde{\beta}=F_2(\tilde{G},\tilde{\beta},\tilde{I},\tilde{L},\tilde{F})\\&+\delta_\beta\dot{W}_\beta(t)-\tilde{\beta}[M_0^{-1}\delta_\beta\dot{W}_\beta(t)+M_0^{-1}\delta_F\dot{W}_F(t)+M_0^{-1}\delta_M\dot{W}_M(t)];\end{aligned} \quad (2.321)$$

$$\begin{aligned}&\frac{d\tilde{F}}{dt}-(\nabla_\rho\tilde{\sigma}+(\mathcal{D}_\rho\tilde{\sigma})\mathcal{M}_\rho(y))\cdot\nabla_\rho\tilde{F}-D_F\mathcal{L}_\rho\tilde{F}=F_3(\tilde{G},\tilde{\beta},\tilde{I},\tilde{L},\tilde{H},\tilde{F})\\&+\delta_F\dot{W}_F(t)-\tilde{F}[M_0^{-1}\delta_\beta\dot{W}_\beta(t)+M_0^{-1}\delta_F\dot{W}_F(t)+M_0^{-1}\delta_M\dot{W}_M(t)];;\end{aligned} \quad (2.322)$$

The boundary conditions (2.293) and (2.294) becomes the following conditions on $\Gamma\times[0,T]$:

$$\partial_t\rho+\mathcal{D}_\rho\tilde{\sigma}=0; \quad (2.323)$$

$$\tilde{\sigma}=\gamma\kappa_\rho(\omega,t)\text{ on }\Gamma_{0T}; \quad (2.324)$$

where

$$\kappa_\rho(\omega,t)=\nabla(|\nabla\psi_\rho|^{-1}\nabla\psi_\rho)(\omega,t). \quad (2.325)$$

$$\begin{aligned}
&\mathcal{D}_\rho \tilde{L} + S_\rho \alpha_L(\tilde{L} - L_0) = 0,\ \mathcal{D}_\rho \tilde{H} + S_\rho \alpha_H(\tilde{H} - H_0) = 0,\\
&\mathcal{D}_\rho \tilde{G} + S_\rho \alpha_G(\tilde{G} - G_0) = 0,\ \mathcal{D}_\rho \tilde{I} + S_\rho \alpha_I(\tilde{I} - I_0) = 0,\\
&\mathcal{D}_\rho \tilde{\beta} + S_\rho \alpha_M(\tilde{\beta} - \beta_0) = 0,\ \mathcal{D}_\rho \tilde{R} + S_\rho \alpha_R(\tilde{R} - R_0) = 0,\ \mathcal{D}_\rho \tilde{F} + S_\rho \alpha_M \tilde{F} = 0.
\end{aligned} \tag{2.326}$$

and on the fixed boundary Γ_M:

$$\begin{aligned}
&\frac{\partial \tilde{L}}{\partial n} = \frac{\partial \tilde{H}}{\partial n} = \frac{\partial \tilde{G}}{\partial n} = 0\\
&\frac{\partial \tilde{R}}{\partial n} = \frac{\partial \tilde{\beta}}{\partial n} = \frac{\partial \tilde{I}}{\partial n} = \frac{\partial \tilde{F}}{\partial n} = 0\\
&\tilde{\sigma} = 0.
\end{aligned} \tag{2.327}$$

The initial conditions are: for $x \in \Omega_0$,

$$\begin{aligned}
&\tilde{L}(0,x) = L_0(x),\ \tilde{H}(0,x) = H_0(x),\ \tilde{\beta}(0,x) = \beta_0(x),\\
&\tilde{G}(0,x) = G_0(x),\ \tilde{I}(0,x) = I_0(x),\\
&\tilde{R}(0,x) = R_0(x),\ \tilde{F}(0,x) = F_0(x),\ \rho(\omega,t)|_{t=0} = 0.
\end{aligned} \tag{2.328}$$

We rewrite the system (2.312)-(2.328) as a quasi-linear abstract evolution equation in Banach spaces.

Lemma 2.15 *If $\rho \in H^{m-\frac{1}{2}}(\Gamma_0), \tilde{h} \in H^{k-2}(\Omega_0), \phi \in H^{m-\frac{1}{2}}(\Gamma_0)$, then the problem*

$$\begin{cases} \mathcal{L}_\rho \tilde{\sigma} = \tilde{h} & \text{in } \Omega_0\\ \tilde{\sigma} = \tilde{\phi} & \text{on } \Gamma_0\\ \tilde{\sigma} = 0 & \text{on } \Gamma_M \end{cases} \tag{2.329}$$

has a unique solution $\tilde{\sigma} \in H^k(\Omega_0)$. Moreover there are operators $\mathcal{U}(\rho), \mathcal{V}(\rho), j = 1, 2$ such that

$$\mathcal{U}(\rho) \in \bigcap_{2\le k\le m} L(H^{k-2}(\Omega_0), H^{k,\alpha}(\Omega_0)),\ \mathcal{V}(\rho) \in \bigcap L(H^{k-\frac{1}{2}}(\Gamma_0), H^k(\Omega_0))$$

and

$$\tilde{\sigma} = \mathcal{U}(\rho)\tilde{h} + \mathcal{V}(\rho)\tilde{\phi}. \tag{2.330}$$

Furthermore we have

$$\mathcal{U} \in C^\infty(H^{m-\frac{1}{2}}(\Gamma_0), L(H^{k-2}(\Omega_0), H^k(\Omega_0))),$$

$$\mathcal{V} \in C^\infty(H^{m-\frac{1}{2}}(\Gamma_0), L(H^{k-\frac{1}{2}}(\Gamma_0), H^k(\Omega_0))).$$

$$\frac{d\rho}{dt}+\mathcal{B}(\rho)\rho=\mathcal{G}_8(\tilde{G},\tilde{I},\tilde{\beta},\tilde{L},\tilde{F})-M_0^{-1}\mathcal{D}_\rho(\mathcal{U}(\rho)1)[\delta_\beta\dot{W}_\beta(t)+\delta_F\dot{W}_F(t)+\delta_M\dot{W}_M(t)]; \tag{2.351}$$

where

$$\mathcal{G}_8(\tilde{G},\tilde{\beta},\tilde{L},\tilde{H},\tilde{F})=-\mathcal{D}_\rho\mathcal{A}_{1,\rho}(\tilde{G},\tilde{\beta},\tilde{L},\tilde{H},\tilde{F}). \tag{2.352}$$

Let

$$U=\left(\tilde{G},\tilde{I},\tilde{L},\tilde{H},\tilde{R},\tilde{\beta},\tilde{F},\rho\right),\ \mathcal{G}(U)=\left(\mathcal{G}_1,\mathcal{G}_2,\mathcal{G}_3,\mathcal{G}_4,\mathcal{E}_5,\mathcal{G}_6,\mathcal{G}_7,\mathcal{G}_8\right),$$

$$W(t)=\left(W_G(t),W_I(t),W_L(t),W_H(t),W_R(t),W_\beta(t),W_F(t),W_G(t)\right),$$

$$\mathcal{A}_1(U)=\begin{pmatrix}-D_G\mathcal{L}_\rho & 0 & 0 & 0\\ 0 & -D_I\mathcal{L}_\rho & 0 & 0\\ 0 & 0 & -D_L\mathcal{L}_\rho & 0\\ 0 & 0 & 0 & -D_H\mathcal{L}_\rho\\ 0 & 0 & 0 & 0\\ 0 & 0 & 0 & 0\\ 0 & 0 & 0 & 0\\ 0 & 0 & 0 & 0\end{pmatrix},$$

$$\mathcal{A}_2(U)=\begin{pmatrix}0 & 0 & 0 & -\mathcal{C}(\rho,\tilde{G})\\ 0 & 0 & 0 & -\mathcal{C}(\rho,\tilde{I})\\ 0 & 0 & 0 & -\mathcal{C}(\rho,\tilde{L})\\ 0 & 0 & 0 & -\mathcal{C}(\rho,\tilde{H})\\ -D_R\mathcal{L}_\rho & 0 & 0 & -\mathcal{C}(\rho,\tilde{R})\\ 0 & -D_\beta\mathcal{L}_\rho & 0 & -\mathcal{E}(\rho,\tilde{\beta})\\ 0 & 0 & -D_F\mathcal{L}_\rho & -\mathcal{E}(\rho,\tilde{F})\\ 0 & 0 & 0 & -\mathcal{B}(\rho)\end{pmatrix},$$

and we define a 8×8 matrix $\mathcal{A}(U)$ by

$$\mathcal{A}(U)=(\mathcal{A}_1(U)\ \ \mathcal{A}_2(U)), \tag{2.353}$$

and

$$\mathbf{B}(U)=\begin{pmatrix}\delta_G G & 0 & 0 & 0 & 0 & 0 & 0 & 0\\ 0 & \delta_I I & 0 & 0 & 0 & 0 & 0 & 0\\ 0 & 0 & \delta_L L & 0 & 0 & 0 & 0 & 0\\ 0 & 0 & 0 & \delta_H H & 0 & 0 & 0 & 0\\ 0 & 0 & 0 & 0 & \delta_R R & 0 & 0 & 0\\ 0 & 0 & 0 & 0 & 0 & \mathbf{B}_{66} & \mathbf{B}_{67} & \mathbf{B}_{68}\\ 0 & 0 & 0 & 0 & 0 & \mathbf{B}_{76} & \mathbf{B}_{77} & \mathbf{B}_{78}\\ 0 & 0 & 0 & 0 & 0 & \mathbf{B}_{86} & \mathbf{B}_{87} & \mathbf{B}_{88}\end{pmatrix} \tag{2.354}$$

where

$$\mathbf{B}_{66}=\delta_\beta-M_0^{-1}\delta_\beta\tilde{\beta}+M_0^{-1}\delta_\beta\nabla\tilde{\beta}\cdot[\nabla_\rho(\mathcal{U}(\rho)1)+\mathcal{D}_\rho(\mathcal{U}(\rho)1)\mathcal{M}(y)] \tag{2.355}$$

$$\mathbf{B}_{67}=-M_0^{-1}\delta_F\tilde{\beta}+M_0^{-1}\delta_F\nabla\tilde{\beta}\cdot[\nabla_\rho(\mathcal{U}(\rho)1)+\mathcal{D}_\rho(\mathcal{U}(\rho)1)\mathcal{M}(y)] \tag{2.356}$$

$$\mathbf{B}_{67} = -M_0^{-1}\delta_M\tilde{\beta} + M_0^{-1}\delta_M\nabla\tilde{\beta}\cdot[\nabla_\rho(\mathcal{U}(\rho)1) + \mathcal{D}_\rho(\mathcal{U}(\rho)1)\mathcal{M}(y)] \quad (2.357)$$

$$\mathbf{B}_{76} = -M_0^{-1}\delta_\beta\tilde{F} + M_0^{-1}\delta_\beta\nabla\tilde{F}\cdot[\nabla_\rho(\mathcal{U}(\rho)1) + \mathcal{D}_\rho(\mathcal{U}(\rho)1)\mathcal{M}(y)] \quad (2.358)$$

$$\mathbf{B}_{77} = \delta_F - M_0^{-1}\delta_F\tilde{F} + M_0^{-1}\delta_F\nabla\tilde{F}\cdot[\nabla_\rho(\mathcal{U}(\rho)1) + \mathcal{D}_\rho(\mathcal{U}(\rho)1)\mathcal{M}(y)], \quad (2.359)$$

$$\mathbf{B}_{78} = -M_0^{-1}\delta_M\tilde{F} + M_0^{-1}\delta_M\nabla\tilde{F}\cdot[\nabla_\rho(\mathcal{U}(\rho)1) + \mathcal{D}_\rho(\mathcal{U}(\rho)1)\mathcal{M}(y)], \quad (2.360)$$

$$\begin{aligned}&\mathbf{B}_{86} = -M_0^{-1}\delta_\beta\mathcal{D}_\rho(\mathcal{U}(\rho)1),\ \mathbf{B}_{87} = -M_0^{-1}\delta_F\mathcal{D}_\rho(\mathcal{U}(\rho)1),\\ &\mathbf{B}_{88} = -M_0^{-1}\delta_M\mathcal{D}_\rho(\mathcal{U}(\rho)1).\end{aligned} \quad (2.361)$$

Then

$$\begin{cases} dU^T + \mathcal{A}(U)U^T dt = \mathcal{G}(U)^T dt + \mathcal{B}(U)dW^T(t),\ t > 0 \\ U|_{t=0} = U_0; \end{cases} \quad (2.362)$$

where $U_0 = (G_0(x), I_0(x), L_0(x), H_0(x), R_0(x), \beta_0(x), F_0(x), 0)$.
Now we define Banach spaces by

$$\mathcal{H}_1^m(U) = \{\tilde{G} \in H^m(\Omega_0)\ |\mathcal{D}_\rho\tilde{G} + S_\rho\alpha_G(\tilde{G} - G_0) = 0 \text{ on } \Gamma_0,\ \frac{\partial\tilde{G}}{\partial n} = 0 \text{ on } \Gamma_M\};$$

$$\mathcal{H}_2^m(U) = \{\tilde{I} \in H^m(\Omega_0)\ |\mathcal{D}_\rho\tilde{I} + S_\rho\alpha_I(\tilde{I} - I_0) = 0 \text{ on } \Gamma_0,\ \frac{\partial\tilde{I}}{\partial n} = 0 \text{ on } \Gamma_M\};$$

$$\mathcal{H}_3^m(U) = \{\tilde{L} \in H^m(\Omega_0)\ |\mathcal{D}_\rho\tilde{L} + S_\rho\alpha_L(\tilde{L} - L_0) = 0 \text{ on } \Gamma_0,\ \frac{\partial\tilde{L}}{\partial n} = 0 \text{ on } \Gamma_M\};$$

$$\mathcal{H}_4^m(U) = \{\tilde{H} \in H^m(\Omega_0)\ |\mathcal{D}_\rho\tilde{H} + S_\rho\alpha_H(\tilde{H} - H_0) = 0 \text{ on } \Gamma_0,\ \frac{\partial\tilde{L}}{\partial n} = 0 \text{ on } \Gamma_M\};$$

$$\mathcal{H}_5^m(U) = \{\tilde{R} \in H^m(\Omega_0)\ |\mathcal{D}_\rho\tilde{R} + S_\rho\alpha_R(\tilde{R} - R_0) = 0 \text{ on } \Gamma_0,\ \frac{\partial\tilde{R}}{\partial n} = 0 \text{ on } \Gamma_M\};$$

$$\mathcal{H}_6^m(U) = \{\tilde{\beta} \in H^m(\Omega_0)\ |\mathcal{D}_\rho\tilde{\beta} + S_\rho\alpha_M(\tilde{\beta} - \beta_0) = 0 \text{ on } \Gamma_0,\ \frac{\partial\tilde{\beta}}{\partial n} = 0 \text{ on } \Gamma_M\};$$

$$\mathcal{H}_7^m(U) = \{\tilde{F} \in H^m(\Omega_0)\ |\mathcal{D}_\rho\tilde{F} + S_\rho\alpha_M\tilde{F} = 0 \text{ on } \Gamma_0,\ \frac{\partial\tilde{F}}{\partial n} = 0 \text{ on } \Gamma_M\}.$$

$$\mathcal{H} = \left(\bigotimes_{j=1}^{7} H^{m-3}(\Omega_0)\right) \otimes H^{m-\frac{7}{2}}(\Gamma_0);$$

$$\mathcal{H}_0(U) = \left(\bigotimes_{j=1}^{7} \mathcal{H}_j^{m-1}(U)\right) \otimes H^{m-\frac{1}{2}}(\Gamma_0);$$

$$\mathcal{H}_1(U) = \left(\bigotimes_{j=1}^{7} \mathcal{H}_j^{m-2}(U)\right) \otimes H^{m-\frac{5}{2}}(\Gamma_0);$$

$$\mathcal{O}_{\delta_0} = \left(\bigotimes_{j=1}^{7} \mathcal{H}_j^{m-1}(U)\right) \otimes H_{\delta_0}^{m-\frac{1}{2}}(\Gamma_0);$$

where $H_{\delta_0}^{m-\frac{1}{2}}(\Gamma_0) = \{\rho \in H^{m-\frac{1}{2}}(\Gamma_0) : \|\rho\|_{H^{\frac{5}{2}}} < \delta_0\}$. Obviously we have $\mathcal{H}_0 \hookrightarrow \mathcal{H}$. We denote by $\boldsymbol{H}(\mathcal{H}_0, \mathcal{H})$ the set of all linear operators $\mathcal{A}$, such that $\mathrm{dom}(\mathcal{A}) = \mathcal{H}_0$ and $-\mathcal{A}$ generates an analytic semigroup.

Lemma 2.17 *Let $U \in \mathcal{O}_{\delta_0}$, then $\mathcal{A}(U) \in \boldsymbol{H}(\mathcal{H}_0, \mathcal{H})$. Moreover*

$$\mathcal{A} \in C^\infty(\mathcal{O}_{\delta_0}, \boldsymbol{H}(\mathcal{H}_0, \mathcal{H})).$$

Proof. By adapting the proofs of Lemmas 4.1 and 4.2 in [76], we have the proof of the lemma. ∎

Next we are going to prove the existence and uniqueness of mild solution to the stochastic problem (2.362). To this end, we are going to use some of the techniques in [91]. We note that the system (2.362) is fully nonlinear due to the fact that $\mathcal{A}$ depends on ρ and its derivatives from (2.353). To using the techniques in [91], we rewrite the Eq. (2.362) as:

$$\begin{cases} dU^T + \mathcal{A}(U_0)U^T dt = (\mathcal{A}(U_0) - \mathcal{A}(U))U^T dt + \mathcal{G}(U)^T dt + \mathcal{B}(U)dW(t),\ t > 0 \\ U|_{t=0} = U_0. \end{cases} \tag{2.363}$$

$W(t)$ is a Wiener process on $(\boldsymbol{\Omega}, \mathcal{F}, \mathbf{P})$ with values in $\mathbf{R}^8$. There is a normal filtration $\{\mathcal{F}_t\}_{t\geq 0}$ in $\mathcal{F}$ generated by the Wiener process $W(t)$. We assume that $U_0 \in \mathcal{O}_{\delta_0}$, then $-\mathcal{A}(U_0)$ generates an analytic semigroup from Lemma 3.3. We denote by $S(t) = e^{-\mathcal{A}(U_0)t}$ the analytic semigroup generated by $-\mathcal{A}(U_0)$, the integral form of (2.363) is

$$\begin{aligned} U(t) = S(U)(t)U_0 &+ \int_0^t S(t-s)(\mathcal{A}(U_0) - \mathcal{A}(U))U^T ds \\ &+ \int_0^t S(t-s)\mathcal{G}(U)ds + \int_0^t S(U)(t-s)B(U)dW(s). \end{aligned} \tag{2.364}$$

We are going to use some notations and definitions as in [91]. Let Y_1 and Y_2 be two separable Hilbert spaces, we denote by $L_2(Y_1, Y_2)$ the set of all Hilbert-Schmidt operators from Y_1 to Y_2; $L_2(Y_1, Y_2)$ is a separable Hilbert space. We can see from (2.354) that $\mathbf{B}$ is a linear operator from $\mathcal{H}$ to $L_2(\mathbf{R}^8, \mathcal{H})$ with $D(\mathbf{B}) = \mathcal{H}_1$. An $\mathcal{H}$ valued predictable process $U(t), t \in [0, T]$ is said to be a mild solution to (2.364) if $U(t)$ takes values in $D(\mathbf{B}), \mathbf{P}$-a.s., (2.364) holds for arbitrary $t \in [0, T]$ and $U(t)$ satisfies the following equations for arbitrary $t \in [0, T]$.

$$\mathbf{P}\left(\int_0^t |U(s)|ds < \infty\right) = 1, \tag{2.365}$$

$$\mathbf{P}\left(\int_0^t \|B(U(s))\|_{L_2(\mathbf{R}^8, \mathcal{H})} ds < \infty\right) = 1. \tag{2.366}$$

We define space $\mathcal{N}^2(0,T;Y_1)$ as the set all Y_1 predictable process Φ such that $\|\Phi\|_{Y_1} < \infty$; where

$$\|\Phi\|_{Y_1} = \left(\mathbf{E}\left(\int_0^T \|\Phi(s)\|_{Y_1}^2 ds\right)\right)^{\frac{1}{2}}.$$

For $\theta \in (0, \frac{1}{4})$, we have two interpolation spaces [191]

$$D_{\mathcal{A}}(\theta, 2) = \left(\left(\bigotimes_{j=1}^{7} H_j^{m-3+2\theta}\right) \otimes H^{m-\frac{7}{2}+2\theta}(\Gamma_0)\right) \tag{2.367}$$

and

$$D_{\mathcal{A}}(\theta + \frac{1}{2}, 2) = \left(\bigotimes_{j=1}^{7} H_j^{m-2+2\theta}\right) \otimes H^{m-\frac{5}{2}+2\theta}(\Gamma_0) \cap \mathcal{H}_1(U). \tag{2.368}$$

We introduce

$$\eta = \max\{\delta_G, \delta_I, \delta_L, \delta_H, \delta_R, \delta_\beta, \delta_F, \delta_M\}. \tag{2.369}$$

We are going to prove the main result of the section.

Theorem 2.18 *For any $U_0 \in \mathcal{O}_{\delta_0}(U_0)$ and sufficiently small η, there exist $T > 0$ and a unique maximal mild solution U to (2.363). Further more this solution belongs to $\mathcal{N}^2(0,T; D_{\mathcal{A}}(\theta + \frac{1}{2}, 2))$ and has continuous sample paths in $D_{\mathcal{A}}(\theta, 2)$.*

The idea of proving the above theorem is essentially the same as in that in [91] (Theorems 6.19 and 7.4). Since the nonlinear term $\mathcal{G}(U)$ only satisfies the local Lipschitz condition, we can only obtain a local mild solution instead of a global solution. We denote the norm of $D_{\mathcal{A}}(\theta, 2)$ by $|\cdot|_\theta$. For $U \in D(\mathbf{B})$, we denote by $\|B(U)\|_\theta$ the Hilbert-Schmidt norm of the operator $\mathbf{B}(U)$ from $\mathbf{R}^8$ to $D_{\mathcal{A}}(\theta, 2)$).

Lemma 2.19 *There exists $C > 0$ such that for any $U \in D_{\mathcal{A}}(\theta + \frac{1}{2}, 2))$*

$$\|\mathbf{B}(U)\|_\theta^2 \leq C\eta\left(|U|_{\theta+\frac{1}{2}}^2 + |U|_\theta^2\right). \tag{2.370}$$

Proof. The lemma follows straightly from (2.354)-(2.361). ■

Now for $T > 0$, we define operator $\mathcal{K}_0, \mathcal{K}_1$ and stochastic convolution $\mathcal{K}_2$ in $\mathcal{N}^2(0,T; D_{\mathcal{A}}(\theta + \frac{1}{2}, 2))$ as

$$\mathcal{K}_0(U)(t) = \int_0^t S(t-s)(\mathcal{A}(U_0) - \mathcal{A}(U))U ds \tag{2.371}$$

$$\mathcal{K}_1(U)(t) = \int_0^t S(t-s)\mathcal{G}(U(s))ds \tag{2.372}$$

and

$$\mathcal{K}_2(U)(t) = \int_0^t S(t-s))\mathbf{B}(U(s))dW(s) \tag{2.373}$$

for $U \in \mathcal{N}^2(0,T;D_{\mathcal{A}}(\theta+\frac{1}{2},2))$. We define

$$\mathcal{K}(U)(t) = S(U)(t)U_0 + \mathcal{K}_0(U)(t) + \mathcal{K}_1(U)(t) + \mathcal{K}_2(U)(t). \tag{2.374}$$

It is clear that U satisfies (2.364) if and only if U is a fixed point of $\mathcal{K}(U)$. We are going to show that the mapping $\mathcal{K}$ is a contraction on $\mathcal{N}^2(0,T;D_{\mathcal{A}}(\theta+\frac{1}{2},2))$.

Lemma 2.20 *Let* $U \in \mathcal{N}^2(0,T;D_{\mathcal{A}}(\theta+\frac{1}{2},2))$, *then*

$$\mathbf{E}\int_0^T |\mathcal{K}_1(U)(s)|^2_{\theta+\frac{1}{2}} ds \le CTM^2\left(1+\mathbf{E}\int_0^T |U(s)|^2_{\theta+\frac{1}{2}} ds\right) \tag{2.375}$$

where $M = \sup_{t\in[0,T]}\|S\|_{D_{\mathcal{A}}(\theta+\frac{1}{2},2)}$.

Proof.

$$\begin{aligned}\mathbf{E}\int_0^T |\mathcal{K}_1(U)(s)|^2_{\theta+\frac{1}{2}} ds &\le \mathbf{E}\int_0^T \left|\int_0^t S(t-s)\mathcal{G}(U(s))ds\right|^2_{\theta+\frac{1}{2}} dt \\ &\le \mathbf{E}\int_0^T tdt\int_0^t |S(t-s)\mathcal{G}(U(s))|^2_{\theta+\frac{1}{2}} ds \\ &\le TM^2\mathbf{E}\int_0^T |\mathcal{G}(U(s))|^2_{\theta-\frac{1}{2}} ds \\ &\le CTM^2\left(1+\mathbf{E}\int_0^T |U(s)|^2_{\theta+\frac{1}{2}} ds\right)\end{aligned}$$

■

Lemma 2.21 *Let* $U_1, U_2 \in \mathcal{N}^2(0,T;D_{\mathcal{A}}(\theta+\frac{1}{2},2))$, *then*

$$\begin{aligned}&\mathbf{E}\int_0^T \left|\int_0^t S(t-s)[\mathcal{G}(U_1(s))-\mathcal{G}(U_2(s))]ds\right|^2_{\theta+\frac{1}{2}} dt \\ &\qquad \le CTM^2\mathbf{E}\int_0^T |[U_1(s)-U_2(s)]|^2_{\theta+\frac{1}{2}} ds.\end{aligned} \tag{2.376}$$

Proof. Since $\mathcal{G}(U)$ satisfies the local Lipschitz condition, we have for $t \in [0,T]$

$$|\mathcal{G}(U_1(t)) - \mathcal{G}(U_2(t))|^2_{\theta-\frac{1}{2}} \le C|U_1(t)-U_2(t)|^2_{\theta+\frac{1}{2}}. \tag{2.377}$$

The lemma then follows from the proof of the above lemma. ■

Lemma 2.22 *Let $\Phi \in \mathcal{N}^2(0,T;L_2(\mathbf{R}^8, D_{\mathcal{A}}(\theta,2)))$, then*

$$\left\|\int_0^t S(t-s))\Phi(s))dW(s)\right\|^2_{\theta+\frac{1}{2}} = \frac{1}{1-2\theta}\|\Phi\|_\theta. \tag{2.378}$$

Proof. This is Theorem 6.12 (i) in [91]. ∎

Lemma 2.23 *Let $U \in \mathcal{N}^2(0,T;D_{\mathcal{A}}(\theta+\frac{1}{2},2))$, then*

$$\mathbf{E}\int_0^T |\mathcal{K}_2(U)(s)|^2_{\theta+\frac{1}{2}}ds \le C\eta\left(\mathbf{E}\int_0^T |U(s)|^2_{\theta+\frac{1}{2}}ds + \mathbf{E}\int_0^T |U(s)|^2_\theta ds\right) \tag{2.379}$$

Proof. The lemma follows from Lemmas 2.19 and 2.22. ∎

Lemma 2.24 *Let $U_1, U_2 \in \mathcal{N}^2(0,T;D_{\mathcal{A}}(\theta+\frac{1}{2},2))$, then*

$$\begin{aligned}&\mathbf{E}\int_0^T |\mathcal{K}_2(U_1)(s) - \mathcal{K}_2(U_2)(s)|^2_{\theta+\frac{1}{2}}ds \\ &\le C\eta\left(\mathbf{E}\int_0^T |U_1(s)-U_2(s)|^2_{\theta+\frac{1}{2}}ds + \mathbf{E}\int_0^T |U_1(s)-U_2(s)|^2_\theta ds\right)\end{aligned} \tag{2.380}$$

Proof. From (2.354)-(2.361), we have for $t \in [0,T]$

$$\|\mathbf{B}(U_1(t)) - \mathbf{B}(U_2(t))\|^2_\theta \le C\eta\left(|U_1(t)-U_2(t)|^2_{\theta+\frac{1}{2}} + |U_1(t)-U_2(t)|^2_\theta\right) \tag{2.381}$$

Then the lemma follows from Lemmas 2.19 and 2.22. ∎

Lemma 2.25 *Let $U_1, U_2 \in L^2(0,T;D_{\mathcal{A}}(\theta+\frac{1}{2},2))$ a.s.; then $(\mathcal{K}_0(U_1) - \mathcal{K}_0(U_2)) \in L^2(0,T;D_{\mathcal{A}}(\theta+\frac{1}{2},2))$ and*

$$\begin{aligned}&\int_0^T |(\mathcal{K}_0(U_1) - \mathcal{K}_0(U_2))|^2_{\theta+\frac{1}{2}}ds \\ &\quad\le C\left(\int_0^T |U_1|^2_{\theta+\frac{1}{2}}ds + \int_0^T |U_2|^2_{\theta+\frac{1}{2}}ds\right)\int_0^T |(U_1-U_2)|^2_{\theta+\frac{1}{2}}ds\end{aligned} \tag{2.382}$$

Proof. We prove (2.382) componentwise. We only prove it for the first component, the other components are similar. Let u_1 be the first component of $\mathcal{K}_0(U_1) - \mathcal{K}_0(U_2)$. Then u_1 satisfies the following PDEs from (2.371):

$$\begin{aligned}\partial_t u_1 - \mathcal{L}_{\rho_0}u_1 - \mathcal{C}(\rho_0,G_0)u_1 &= [(\mathcal{A}(U_0) - \mathcal{A}(U_1))U_1 - (\mathcal{A}(U_0) - \mathcal{A}(U_2))U_2]_1 \\ &= [\mathcal{A}(U_0)(U_1-U_2)]_1 + [(\mathcal{A}(U_2) - \mathcal{A}(U_1))U_1]_1 + [\mathcal{A}(U_2)(U_2-U_1)]_1,\end{aligned} \tag{2.383}$$

where $[\cdot]_1$ denotes the first component of the vector. Using (2.303), (2.304), and (2.335), we have

$$\begin{aligned} &\partial_t u_1 - \mathcal{L}_{\rho_0} u_1 - \mathcal{C}(\rho_0, G_0) u_1 \\ &= \sum_{k,j=1}^{2} (A_{\rho_1,kj}(y,t) - A_{\rho_2,kj}(y,t)) \partial^2_{y_k y_j} \tilde{G}_1 + \sum_{k=1}^{2} (A_{\rho_1,k}(y,t) - A_{\rho_2,k}(y,t)) \partial_{y_k} \tilde{G}_1 \\ &\qquad + (\mathcal{C}(\rho_1, \tilde{G}_1) u_1 - \mathcal{C}(\rho_2, \tilde{G}_1)\rho_1 + \mathcal{C}(\rho_2, \tilde{G}_1)(\rho_1 - \rho_2) \\ &\qquad\qquad + [\mathcal{A}(U_0)(U_1 - U_2)]_1 + [\mathcal{A}(U_2)(U_2 - U_1)]_1, \end{aligned} \tag{2.384}$$

where

$$\begin{aligned} &|A_{\rho_1,kj}(y,t) - A_{\rho_2,kj}(y,t))|_{\theta-\frac{3}{2}} \le C|\rho_1 - \rho_2|_{\theta+\frac{1}{2}} \\ &|A_{\rho_1,k}(y,t) - A_{\rho_2,k}(y,t)|_{\theta-\frac{3}{2}} \le C|\rho_1 - \rho_2|_{\theta-\frac{1}{2}} \\ &|\mathcal{C}(\rho_1, \tilde{G}_1)\rho_1 - \mathcal{C}(\rho_2, \tilde{G}_1)\rho_1|_{\theta-\frac{3}{2}} \le C|\rho_1 - \rho_2|_{\theta-\frac{1}{2}} \\ &|\mathcal{A}(U_0)(U_1 - U_2)|_{\theta-\frac{3}{2}} \le C|\rho_1 - \rho_2|_{\theta+\frac{1}{2}} \\ &|\mathcal{A}(U_2)(U_1 - U_2)|_{\theta-\frac{3}{2}} \le C|U_2|_{\theta+\frac{1}{2}}|\rho_1 - \rho_2|_{\theta+\frac{1}{2}} \\ &\left|\mathcal{C}(\rho_2, \tilde{G}_1)(U_1 - U_2)\right|_{\theta-\frac{3}{2}} \le C|\rho_1 - \rho_2|_{\theta-\frac{1}{2}} \\ &|\partial^2_{y_k y_j} \tilde{G}_1|_{\theta-\frac{3}{2}} \le C|U_1|_{\theta+\frac{1}{2}}, \ |\partial_{y_k} \tilde{G}_1|_{\theta-\frac{3}{2}} \le C|U_1|_{\theta+\frac{1}{2}}. \end{aligned} \tag{2.385}$$

On the boundary Γ_0, from (2.326) we have

$$\mathcal{D}_{\rho_1} u_1 + S_{\rho_1} \alpha_G u_1 = (S_{\rho_1} - S_{\rho_2})(G_0 - \tilde{G}_2), \tag{2.386}$$

and from (2.305)

$$|(S_{\rho_1} - S_{\rho_2})(G_0 - G_2)|_{\theta-\frac{1}{2}} \le C|\tilde{G}_2|_{\theta+\frac{1}{2}}|\rho_1 - \rho_2|_{\theta+\frac{1}{2}}. \tag{2.387}$$

Now applying the classical regularity results [99,176] to the boundary problem (2.384)-(2.387) we obtain

$$\begin{aligned} \int_0^T |u_1(s)|^2_{\theta+\frac{1}{2}} ds &\le C \left(\int_0^T |U_1|^2_{\theta+\frac{1}{2}} ds + \int_0^T |U_2|^2_{\theta+\frac{1}{2}} ds \right) \int_0^T |\rho_1 - \rho_2|^2_{\theta+\frac{1}{2}} ds \\ &\le C \left(\int_0^T |U_1|^2_{\theta+\frac{1}{2}} ds + \int_0^T |U_2|^2_{\theta+\frac{1}{2}} ds \right) \int_0^T |U_1 - U_2|^2_{\theta+\frac{1}{2}} ds. \end{aligned} \tag{2.388}$$

Similarly the other components of $S(U_1)(t)\mathcal{G}(U_1)$ and $S(U_2)(t)\mathcal{G}(U_1)$ can be estimated as (2.388), hence the lemma follows.

■

Lemma 2.26 *Let $U \in \mathcal{N}^2(0,T; D_{\mathcal{A}}(\theta + \frac{1}{2}, 2))$, then*

$$\mathbf{E} \int_0^T |\mathcal{K}_0(U)(s)|^2_{\theta+\frac{1}{2}} ds \le C \left(\mathbf{E} \int_0^T |U(s)|^2_{\theta+\frac{1}{2}} ds \right) \left(\mathbf{E} \int_0^T |U(s) - U_0|^2_{\theta+\frac{1}{2}} ds \right) \tag{2.389}$$

Proof. The Lemma follows from Lemma 2.25 with $U_1 = U_0, U_2 = U$. ∎

Lemma 2.27 *Let* $U_1, U_2 \in \mathcal{N}^2(0,T; D_{\mathcal{A}}(\theta + \frac{1}{2}, 2))$ *a.s.; then* $(\mathcal{K}_0(U_1) - \mathcal{K}_0(U_2)) \in \mathcal{N}^2(0,T; D_{\mathcal{A}}(\theta + \frac{1}{2}, 2))$ *and*

$$\mathbf{E}\int_0^T |(\mathcal{K}_0(U_1) - \mathcal{K}_0(U_2))|^2_{\theta+\frac{1}{2}} ds \\ \leq C\left(\mathbf{E}\int_0^T |U_1|^2_{\theta+\frac{1}{2}} ds + \mathbf{E}\int_0^T |U_2|^2_{\theta+\frac{1}{2}} ds\right) \mathbf{E}\int_0^T |(U_1 - U_2)|^2_{\theta+\frac{1}{2}} ds \tag{2.390}$$

Proof. The lemma follows immediately from Lemma 2.25. ∎

Now we can prove the main theorem. We introduce the norm

$$\|U\|_T = \mathbf{E}\int_0^T |U(s)|^2_{\theta+\frac{1}{2}} ds + \mathbf{E}\int_0^T |U(s)|^2_{\theta} ds \tag{2.391}$$

We consider the Hilbert space $\mathbf{Z}$ defined by

$$\mathbf{Z} = \{U \in \mathcal{N}^2(0,T; D_{\mathcal{A}}(\theta + \frac{1}{2}, 2)) : \|U - U_0\|_T \leq C(\eta + T)\}$$

It is to be noted that for $U \in \mathbf{Z}$ then

$$\|U\|_T \leq \|U_0\|_T + C(\eta + T) \leq C_1(\eta + T), \tag{2.392}$$

since

$$\|U_0\|_T = T\left(\mathbf{E}|U_0|^2_{\theta+\frac{1}{2}} + \mathbf{E}|U_0|^2_{\theta}\right).$$

Then it follows, from Lemmas 2.20–2.27, that the mapping $\mathcal{K}$ in (2.374) is a contraction from $\mathbf{Z}$ to $\mathbf{Z}$ for sufficiently small T and η, so we have proved the existence and uniqueness of mild solution. The remaining part of the theorem can be proved by standard argument as in [91].

CHAPTER 3

Mathematical Modeling of Cancer and Therapy

Cancer is one of the leading causes to death in many parts of the world. Despite major scientific, medical and technological advances over the last few decades, a cure for cancer remains elusive. Although the focus historically has been to study these events through experimental and clinical observations, mathematical Modeling and simulation that enable analysis at multiple time and spatial scales have also complemented these efforts. A vast literature is reported in a few review papers devoted to modeling, analysis, numerical simulation and control of tumor immune system interactions [4, 19, 45, 56, 57, 72, 107, 110, 190]. Most models fall into two broad categories, based on how the tumor tissue is represented: discrete cell-based models and continuum models. Although continuum and discrete approaches have each provided important insight into cancer-related processes occurring at particular length and time scales, the complexity of cancer and the interactions among the cell- and tissue-level scales ideally call for a multiscale continuum-discrete (hybrid) approach, coupling biological phenomena from the molecular and cellular scales to the tumour scale [276].

In discrete modeling, individual cells are tracked and updated according to a specific set of biophysical rules. This approach is particularly useful for studying carcinogenesis, natural selection, genetic instability and interactions of individual cells with each other and the microenvironment. Analyses of cell population dynamics have also been employed in order to study biological characteristics applying to all cells in a particular population, such as response to therapy and in studies of immunology. There are two main types of discrete models, lattice based and lattice-free. The former describes the dynamics of discrete tumour cells as automata on a grid whose states are governed by a set of deterministic or probabilistic rules. The latter type describes the actions of discrete cells in arbitrary locations and their interactions. Because these methods are based on a series of rules for each cell, it is possible to translate

DOI: 10.1201/9781003376675-3

detailed biological processes (e.g. cell-cycle events, mutation pathways) into rules for the model. In this book we do not discuss discrete models.

In larger scale systems, continuum methods provide a good Modeling alternative. Continuum models treat tumours as a collection of tissue, where densities or volume fractions of cells are described. This approach draws upon principles from continuum mechanics to describe cancer related variables as continuous fields by means of partial differential and integro-differential equations. Individual cells and other elements are not tracked; model variables may include cell volume fractions and cell substrate concentrations, e.g. nutrient, oxygen and growth factors. In addition, fast numerical solvers can be developed. Continuum model parameters may be somewhat easier to obtain, analyze and control compared with the discrete case. They may also be more accessible through laboratory experimentation. Although these models are appropriate at the tissue scale where gross tumour behavior can be quantified, the limitations in scale prevent them from modeling individual cells and discrete events (e.g. epithelial to mesenchymal phenotypic transition that leads to individual cell migration).

Continuum tumour models are based on reaction-diffusion equations describing the tumour cell density, extracellular matrix (ECM), matrix-degrading enzymes (MDEs) and concentrations of cell substrates such as glucose, oxygen, and growth factors and inhibitors (e.g. [58]). Classical work [135,136] used ordinary differential equations to model tumours as a homogeneous population, as well as partial differential equation models confined to a spherical geometry. In the case of avascular tumours, growth has been modeled as a function of cell substrate concentration, usually oxygen. More recent work has incorporated cell movement, through diffusion (e.g. [59,255]), convection (e.g. [44,83,277,278]) and chemo/haptotaxis. Cell proliferation, death and pressure have also been considered (e.g. [46,73]). Linear and weakly nonlinear analysis have been performed to assess the stability of spherical tumours to asymmetric perturbations (e.g. [73, 186]) in order to characterize the degree of aggression. Various interactions with the microenvironment, such as nutrient-, inhibitory factor- or stress-induced limitations to growth, have also been studied (e.g. [82]).

Rigorous analysis has been done for aforementioned models. The well posedness of solutions has been proven by Friedman and Reitich [124] and Cui and Friedman [83] for radially symmetric solutions using the Darcy law model; Cui [74] for a model with inhibitors; Friedman and Reitich [125], Bazaliy and Friedman [15,16], Cui [75], Cui and Wei [85] and Cui [76] for non-symmetric solutions; Friedman [107] and Wu and Cui [286] for a Stokes model; Zhou, Escher and Cui [312] for a model of multilayer tumours and Cui [77] for a hyperbolic equation model of tumour growth. Bifurcations from spherically symmetric solutions have been studied by Friedman and Reitich [126], Friedman and Hu [115–117] and Zhou and Cui [311]. Xu and Gilbert [295] formulated and analyzed inverse problems that connect a tumour model for ductal carcinoma in situ with clinical data.

variables are radially symmetric and that the tumor domain $\Omega(t)$ is spherical:

$$\Omega(t) = \{x = (x_1, x_2, x_3) \in \mathbb{R}^3 : 0 \leq r < R(t) \; ; \; 0 < t < \infty\},$$

where $r = |x| = \sqrt{x_1^2 + x_2^2 + x_3^2}$ and $R(t)$ varies in time. We assume that the density of the cells is uniform throughout the tumor, that is

$$C(r,t) + N(r,t) + T(r,t) = \text{ Constant for } 0 \leq r \leq R(t), t > 0. \tag{3.1}$$

Since tumor cells grow abnormally fast, the condition (3.1) implies that there is an internal pressure among the cells, which give rise to a velocity field $\mathbf{u} = u(r,t)\mathbf{e}_r$ where $\mathbf{e}_r$ is the unit radial vector. From conservation of mass, C, N and T satisfy the following PDEs in $\Omega(t)$:

$$\frac{\partial C}{\partial t} + \frac{1}{r^2}\frac{\partial}{\partial r}(r^2 uC) - \frac{1}{r^2}\frac{\partial}{\partial r}(r^2\frac{\partial C}{\partial r}) = X_1(C,N,T,\eta), \tag{3.2}$$

$$\frac{\partial N}{\partial t} + \frac{1}{r^2}\frac{\partial}{\partial r}(r^2 uN) - \frac{1}{r^2}\frac{\partial}{\partial r}(r^2\frac{\partial N}{\partial r}) = X_2(C,N), \tag{3.3}$$

and

$$\frac{\partial T}{\partial t} + \frac{1}{r^2}\frac{\partial}{\partial r}(r^2 uT) - \frac{1}{r^2}\frac{\partial}{\partial r}(r^2\frac{\partial T}{\partial r}) = X_3(C,T), \tag{3.4}$$

where $X_k, k = 1,2,3$ account for the transition among the cells, and the parameter η is introduced to represents the killing rate of cancer cells by T cells. η can also account for a drug called checkpoint inhibitor [120, 121, 177]. The free boundary $r = R(t)$ is moving with velocity of the cells,

$$\frac{dR}{dt} = u(R(t),t). \tag{3.5}$$

In [110], the author considered the case where $T = constant$, and take

$$C(r,t) + N(r,t) = 1 \text{ for } 0 \leq r \leq R(t), t > 0. \tag{3.6}$$

C and N were assumed to satisfy the following equations [110]:

$$\frac{\partial C}{\partial t} + \frac{1}{r^2}\frac{\partial}{\partial r}(r^2 uC) - \frac{1}{r^2}\frac{\partial}{\partial r}(r^2\frac{\partial C}{\partial r}) = \lambda_C C\left(1 - \frac{C+N}{K}\right) - \delta_0 C - \eta C, \tag{3.7}$$

$$\frac{\partial N}{\partial t} + \frac{1}{r^2}\frac{\partial}{\partial r}(r^2 uN) - \frac{1}{r^2}\frac{\partial}{\partial r}(r^2\frac{\partial N}{\partial r}) = \lambda_N N\left(1 - \frac{C+N}{K}\right) - \delta_0 N, \tag{3.8}$$

where λ_C and λ_N are the growth constants of the cancer cell and normal cell in their logistic growth, $K > 1$ is the capacity constant in the logistic growth and δ_0 is the death rate of the cells. It is assumed that $\lambda_C > \lambda_N > \delta_0$. Under the assumption that $\frac{\partial C}{\partial r} = 0$, $\frac{\partial N}{\partial r} = 0$ on $r = R(t)$ and $\gamma_1 := \lambda_N\left(1 - \frac{1}{K}\right) - \delta_0 = 0$. It was obtained that the tumor volume will continuously decrease if the killing rate η exceeds the critical value $\gamma_0 := (\lambda_C - \lambda_N)\left(1 - \frac{1}{K}\right)$; while the tumor

volume will grow to ∞ if the killing rate η is smaller than the critical value γ_0; see Theorem 3.1 in [110].
In this section, we consider two cancer models. Model one in subsection 1 is the case where the density of normal cells is assumed to be a constant, so this model consists of PDEs for the cancer cell and the T cell. Model two in subsection 3 is the case where all C, N and T are present.

In the case where $N = constant = 0$, and we take

$$C(r,t) + T(r,t) = 1 \text{ for } 0 \leq r \leq R(t), t > 0. \tag{3.9}$$

We assume that C satisfies the following equation in the tumor domain $\Omega(t)$:

$$\frac{\partial C}{\partial t} + \frac{1}{r^2}\frac{\partial}{\partial r}(r^2 uC) - \frac{1}{r^2}\frac{\partial}{\partial r}(r^2\frac{\partial C}{\partial r}) = \lambda_c C\left(1 - \frac{C}{K}\right) - \delta_0 C - \eta TC. \tag{3.10}$$

To derive an equation for T, we note that cancer cells are recognized by dendritic cells and the dendritic cells then activate T cells. We represent the activation simply by introducing a production term $\lambda_T C$ in the following equation for T cells in the tumor domain $\Omega(t)$:

$$\frac{\partial T}{\partial t} + \frac{1}{r^2}\frac{\partial}{\partial r}(r^2 uT) - \frac{1}{r^2}\frac{\partial}{\partial r}(r^2\frac{\partial T}{\partial r}) = \lambda_T C - \delta_T T, \tag{3.11}$$

where λ_T is the production rate and δ_T is the death rate of T cells. Adding (3.10) to (3.11) and using (3.9), we get

$$\frac{1}{r^2}\frac{\partial}{\partial r}(r^2 u) = F(C), \tag{3.12}$$

where $F(C)$ is given by

$$F(C) = \left(\eta - \frac{\lambda_C}{K}\right)C^2 + (\lambda_C - \delta_0 + \lambda_T + \delta_T - \eta)C - \delta_T. \tag{3.13}$$

Using $\frac{dR}{dt} = u(R,t)$, we have

$$\frac{dR}{dt} = \frac{1}{R(t)^2}\int_0^{R(t)} s^2 F(C(s,t))ds. \tag{3.14}$$

Plugging (3.12) and (3.9) into (3.10) we get that C satisfies the following equation in the tumor domain $\Omega(t)$:

$$\frac{\partial C}{\partial t} + u\frac{\partial C}{\partial r} - \frac{1}{r^2}\frac{\partial}{\partial r}(r^2\frac{\partial C}{\partial r}) = G(C), \tag{3.15}$$

where $G(C)$ is given by

$$G(C) = \left[-\left(\eta - \frac{\lambda_C}{K}\right)C^2 + (2\eta - A)C - (\eta - B)\right]C, \tag{3.16}$$

where

$$A = \left(1 + \frac{1}{K}\right)\lambda_C - \delta_0 + \lambda_T + \delta_T, \qquad B = \lambda_C + \delta_T - \delta_0. \tag{3.17}$$

We impose either the flux boundary conditions:

$$\frac{\partial C}{\partial r} + \beta C \quad = \quad 0 \quad on \quad \partial\Omega(t) \tag{3.18}$$

and

$$\frac{\partial T}{\partial r} + \beta(T - 1) = 0 \quad on \quad \partial\Omega(t);$$

where β is a positive constant;
or zero-flux boundary condition

$$\frac{\partial C}{\partial r} = 0 \text{ on } \quad r = R(t). \tag{3.19}$$

So model one is the free boundary problem consisting of (3.14), (3.15) and either (3.18) or (3.19) with initial data for $C(r, 0)$ and $R(0)$.

3.1.2 Mathematical Analysis of Model One

In the following subsections, we are going to establish the global existence and uniqueness of solution to Model one and study the long time behavior of the solution [5, 6, 292].

3.1.2.1 Existence of Stationary Solution of Model one with flux Boundary Condition

For a steady solution, $C(r, t), u(r, t)$, and $R(t)$ will be independent of the time t, so the derivative with respect to t will be zero. So to find steady solutions, we need to solve the following ODE system:

$$u\frac{\partial C}{\partial r} - \frac{1}{r^2}\frac{\partial}{\partial r}\left(r^2\frac{\partial C}{\partial r}\right) = G(C); \tag{3.20}$$

$$\frac{1}{r^2}\frac{\partial}{\partial r}\left(r^2 u\right) = F(C); \tag{3.21}$$

$$\frac{\partial C}{\partial r}(0) = u(0) = 0; \tag{3.22}$$

$$\int_0^R s^2 F\big(C(s)\big)ds = 0; \tag{3.23}$$

$$0 < C(r) \leq 1 \quad and \quad u(r) > 0 \quad for\, 0 < r < R; \tag{3.24}$$

$$u(R) = 0; \tag{3.25}$$

$$\frac{\partial C}{\partial r}(R) + \beta C(R) = 0. \tag{3.26}$$

In this subsection we are going to prove the existence of solution to the system (3.20)–(3.26). Similar to [122], we will use a shooting method with $\sigma = C(0)$, the values of R, $C(R)$ and $C_r(R)$ will be determined by σ, so will β. Hence we denote

$$\sigma = C(0) \tag{3.27}$$

and then $\beta = \beta(\sigma)$ is determine by

$$\beta = -\frac{\partial C}{\partial r}(R)/C(R). \tag{3.28}$$

We assume that $\frac{\lambda_c}{K} < \eta < \lambda_c + \delta_T - \delta_0$.
We denote by σ_0 the positive root of the quadratic equation $F(\sigma) = 0$ that is

$$\sigma_0 = \frac{-\lambda_C + \delta_0 - \lambda_T - \delta_T + \eta + \sqrt{(\lambda_C - \delta_0 + \lambda_T + \delta_T - \eta)^2 + 4\delta_T(\eta - \frac{\lambda_C}{K})}}{2(\eta - \frac{\lambda_C}{K})}, \tag{3.29}$$

then $0 < \sigma_0 < 1$, and

$$F(\sigma) = \begin{cases} > 0 & \text{if} \quad \sigma > \sigma_0 \\ < 0 & \text{if} \quad 0 < \sigma < \sigma_0. \end{cases} \tag{3.30}$$

We introduce the function

$$F_1(C) = (\eta - \frac{\lambda_C}{K})C^2 + (A - 2\eta)C + \eta - B, \tag{3.31}$$

where

$$A = (1 + \frac{1}{K})\lambda_C - \delta_0 + \lambda_T + \delta_T, \quad B = \lambda_C + \delta_T - \delta_0.$$

Theorem 3.1 *There exists a sufficiently small $\epsilon_0 > 0$ such that for each $\sigma \in (\sigma_0, \sigma_0 + \epsilon_0)$, the system (3.20)–(3.26) has a unique solution $(C(\sigma, r), u(\sigma, r), R(\sigma))$. Furthermore, it holds*

$$R(\sigma) = R_0^{\frac{1}{2}}(\sigma - \sigma_0)^{\frac{1}{2}} + o\big[(\sigma - \sigma_0)^{\frac{3}{2}}\big]; \tag{3.32}$$

where

$$R_0 = \frac{-6}{\sigma_0 F_1(\sigma_0)} \cdot \frac{F'(\sigma_0)}{2(\eta - \frac{\lambda_C}{K})\sigma_0 + (\lambda_T - \delta_0 + \lambda_T + \delta_T - \eta)}. \tag{3.33}$$

Proof. It will be convenient to write (3.20) in the form

$$C_{rr} = -\frac{2}{r}C_r + uC_r + C^2\Big[-(\eta - \frac{\lambda_C}{K})C^2 + (2\eta - A)C - (\eta - B)\Big] \quad (3.34)$$

and Eq. (3.21) as

$$u_r = -\frac{2}{r}u + F(C). \quad (3.35)$$

Recalling that

$$C_r(0) = u(0) = 0 \quad and \quad C(0) = \sigma, \quad (3.36)$$

we claim that

$$C_{rr}(0) = \frac{\sigma}{3}\ F_1(\sigma) < 0 \quad if \quad \sigma_0 < \sigma < 1. \quad (3.37)$$

Indeed, the equality follows from (3.34) by taking r $\to$ 0 and applying L'Hospital's rule. We can write

$$F_1(\sigma) = F(\sigma) + (\frac{\lambda_C}{K} - \eta)\sigma + \eta - \lambda_C - \lambda_T + \delta_0 + \delta_T.$$

To prove that $F_1(\sigma) < 0$, we observe that $F_1(\sigma)$ is a quadratic polynomial of σ. Using (3.13) and (3.31), we have

$$F_1(1) = -\delta_T;$$

$$F_1'(1) = \lambda_C + \lambda_T + \delta_T - \delta_0 - \frac{\lambda_C}{K};$$

$$F_1(\sigma_0) = (\frac{\lambda_C}{K} - \eta)\sigma_0 + \eta - \lambda_C - \lambda_T + \delta_0 + \delta_T;$$

$$F_1(1) < 0 \qquad F_1'(1) < 0 \qquad F_1(\sigma_0) < 0;$$

so

$$F_1(\sigma) < 0 \quad if \quad \sigma_0 \le \sigma < 1.$$

We next expand $C(r)$ and $u(r)$ into power series in r

$$C(r) = \sum_{k=0}^{\infty} C_{2k} r^{2k}, \qquad u(r) = \sum_{k=0}^{\infty} u_{2k+1} r^{2k+1};$$

where $C_0 = \sigma$; substituting these series into $u_r = -\frac{2}{r}u + F(C)$, we have

$$\sum_{k=0}^{\infty}(2k+1)u_{2k+1}\ r^{2k} = -2\sum_{k=0}^{\infty} u_{2k+1}\ r^{2k} + F(C);$$

here

$$
\begin{aligned}
F(C) = (\eta - \frac{\lambda_C}{K})\Big(\sum_{k=0}^{\infty} C_{2k}\ \ r^{2k}\Big)^2 \\
+ (\lambda_C - \delta_0 + \lambda_T + \delta_T - \eta)\sum_{k=0}^{\infty} C_{2k}\ \ r^{2k} - \delta_T \ \ ; \\
= -\delta_T + (\lambda_C - \delta_0 + \lambda_T + \delta_T - \eta)\ \sum_{k=0}^{\infty} C_{2k}\ \ r^{2k} \\
+ (\eta - \frac{\lambda_C}{K})\ \sum_{k=0}^{\infty}\Big(\ \sum_{k=0}^{\infty} C_{2k}C_2(K-C)\Big)r^{2k}.
\end{aligned}
$$

So we have

$$u_1 = \frac{1}{3}F(\sigma);$$

$$u_{2k+1} = \frac{1}{2k+3}\Big[(\lambda_C - \delta_0 + \lambda_T + \delta_T - \eta)C_{2k} + (\eta - \frac{\lambda_C}{K})\sum_{L=0}^{k} C_{2L}C_{2(k-L)}\Big](k \geq 1).$$

In particular, we have

$$u_3 = \frac{1}{5}\big[(\lambda_C - \delta_0 + \lambda_T + \delta_T - \eta)C_2 + (\eta - \frac{\lambda_C}{K})(2C_0C_2)\big]$$

and

$$u_4 = \frac{C_2}{5}\big[\lambda_C - \delta_0 + \lambda_T + \delta_T - \eta + 2C_0(\eta - \frac{\lambda_C}{K})\big];$$

using $C_2 = \frac{1}{2}C_{rr}(0) = \frac{\sigma}{6}F_1(\sigma) < 0$, we obtain

$$u_3 = \frac{\sigma}{18}F_1(\sigma)\big[2(\eta - \frac{\lambda_c}{K})\sigma + (\lambda_c - \delta_0 + \lambda_T + \delta_T - \eta)\big] < 0. \tag{3.38}$$

For each $\sigma' \in (\sigma_0, 1)$ there is exists $\delta_1 > 0$ such that

$$u_3 < -\delta_1 < 0 \quad if \quad \sigma_0 \leq \sigma < 1.$$

On the other hand, if $\sigma = \sigma_0 + \epsilon, \epsilon$ positive and small enough, then

$$u_1 = \frac{1}{3}F'(\sigma_0)\epsilon + o(\epsilon^2)$$

$$= \frac{1}{3}\big[(\eta - \frac{\lambda_C}{K})\sigma^2 + (\lambda_C - \delta_0 + \lambda_T + \delta_T - \eta)\sigma - \delta_T\big]\Big|_{\sigma=\sigma_0} \epsilon + o(\epsilon^2).$$

In order to determine the smallest root of

$$u(r) = u_1 r + u_3 r^3 + o(r^5).$$

We set $\sigma = \sigma_0 + \epsilon$, and consider u as a function of two variables, r and ϵ, and introduce a function

$$w(\bar{r}, \epsilon) = \frac{u(\bar{r}^{1/2})}{(\bar{r}^{1/2})}.$$

Then

$$w(\bar{r}, \epsilon) = \frac{1}{3} f'(\sigma_0)\epsilon + u_3\Big|_{\sigma=\sigma_0} \bar{r} + o(\epsilon^2 + \bar{r}^2)$$

and note

$$w(0,0) = 0, \quad \frac{\partial w}{\partial \bar{r}}(0,0) < -\delta_1.$$

By the implicit function theorem it follows that the zero set of w near $(0,0)$ is given by a curve $(\overline{R_\epsilon}, \epsilon)$, where $\bar{R}_\epsilon$ is a smooth function of ϵ, and

$$\frac{d\overline{R_\epsilon}}{d\epsilon}\Big|_{\epsilon=0} = -\frac{\partial \overline{w}/\partial \epsilon}{\partial \overline{w}/\partial \bar{r}}\Big|_{\epsilon=0}.$$

Hence $\overline{R_\epsilon}$ is given by

$$\overline{R_\epsilon} = \frac{F'(\sigma_0)/3}{u_3\big|_{\sigma=\sigma_0}}\epsilon + O(\epsilon^2)$$

$$= -\frac{6F'(\sigma_0)\epsilon}{\sigma_0 F_1(\sigma_0)\big[2(\eta - \frac{\lambda_C}{K})\sigma_0 + (\lambda_C - \delta_0 + \lambda_T + \delta_T - \eta)\big]} + \epsilon + O(\epsilon^2).$$

Notice that the radius $R(\sigma)$ corresponding to $\sigma = \sigma_0 + \epsilon$ is equal to $\overline{R_\epsilon}^{\frac{1}{2}}$, we have

$$R(\sigma) = R_0^{\frac{1}{2}}(\sigma - \sigma_0)^{\frac{1}{2}} + o\big[(\sigma - \sigma_0)^{\frac{3}{2}}\big],$$

where $R_0 = \frac{-6}{\sigma_0 F_1(\sigma_0)} \cdot \frac{F'(\sigma_0)}{2(\eta - \frac{\lambda_C}{K})\sigma_0 + (\lambda_T - \delta_0 + \lambda_T + \delta_T - \eta)}$. ■

3.1.2.2 Stability of stationary solution

In this section, we are going to discuss the linear stability of the stationary solutions obtained in the previous section. Let us first recall some of the estimates obtained and denote the steady-state solution by (C_s, u_s, R) with $C_s(0) = \sigma$, $\sigma - \sigma_0$ positive and small, and $0 < r < R$, R is small:

$$\sigma - \sigma_0 = \frac{1}{R_0} R^2 + O(R^4) \equiv \sigma_1 R^2 + O(R^4); \tag{3.39}$$

$$C_s(r) = \sigma + \frac{\sigma_0}{6} F_1(\sigma) r^2 + O(r^4) = \sigma_0 + O(R^2); \tag{3.40}$$

$$\begin{aligned} \beta = -\frac{(C_s)_r(R)}{C_s(R)} &= -\frac{\frac{1}{3}\sigma F_1(\sigma) R + O(R^3)}{\sigma + \frac{\sigma}{6} F_1(\sigma) R^2 + O(R^4)} \\ &= -\frac{1}{3} F_1(\sigma_0) R + O(R^3) = \lambda_\beta R + O(R^3); \end{aligned} \tag{3.41}$$

$$
\begin{aligned}
& -u_s(r) = -\frac{1}{3}F(\sigma)r - u_3 r^3 + O(r^5) \\
&= -\frac{1}{3}F(\sigma)r - \frac{\sigma}{18}F_1(\sigma)r^3\big[2(\eta - \frac{\lambda_C}{K})\sigma + (\lambda_C - \delta_0 + \lambda_C + \delta_T - \eta)\big] + O(r^5) \\
&= -\frac{1}{3}\sigma_1 F'(\sigma_0)R^2 r - \frac{\sigma_0}{18}F_1(\sigma_0)\big[2(\eta - \frac{\lambda_C}{K})\sigma + (\lambda_C - \delta_0 + \lambda_C + \delta_T - \eta)\big]r^3 + O(r^5);
\end{aligned} \tag{3.42}
$$

$$
\begin{aligned}
& -u_s'(r) = -\frac{1}{3}\sigma_1 F'(\sigma_0)R^2 \\
& \quad - \frac{\sigma_0}{6}F_1(\sigma_0)\big[2(\eta - \frac{\lambda_C}{K})\sigma + (\lambda_C - \delta_0 + \lambda_C + \delta_T - \eta)\big]r^2 + O(r^4).
\end{aligned} \tag{3.43}
$$

Since $0 = u_s(R) = u_1 R + u_3 R^3 + O(R^5)$, we have

$$
u_3 R^2 = -u_1 + O(R^4) = -\frac{1}{3}F(\sigma) + O(R^4).
$$

Hence

$$
\begin{aligned}
-\frac{\partial u}{\partial r}(R) &= -u_1 - 3u_3 R^2 + O(R^4) \\
&= \frac{2}{3}\sigma_1 F'(\sigma_0)R^2 + O(R^4).
\end{aligned} \tag{3.44}
$$

Next we are going to derive the linearized system about the stationary solution $(C_s(r), u_s(r), R)$. Accordingly we set

$$
\begin{aligned}
C(r,t) &= C_s(r) + \epsilon w(r,t), \\
u(r,t) &= u_s(r) + \epsilon q(r,t), \\
R(t) &= R + \epsilon \rho(t).
\end{aligned} \tag{3.45}
$$

Plugging (3.45) into (3.15), we obtain

$$
\begin{aligned}
& \frac{\partial C_s}{\partial t} + \epsilon\frac{\partial w}{\partial t} + \left(u_s + \epsilon q\right)\left(\frac{\partial C_s}{\partial r} + \epsilon\frac{\partial w}{\partial r}\right) \\
& \qquad - \frac{1}{r^2}\frac{\partial}{\partial r}\left(r^2\left(\frac{\partial C_s}{\partial r} + \epsilon\frac{\partial w}{\partial r}\right)\right) = G(C_s + \epsilon w).
\end{aligned}
$$

Linearizing the above equation to obtain

$$
\frac{\partial w}{\partial t} + q\frac{\partial C_s}{\partial r} + u_s\frac{\partial w}{\partial r} - \frac{1}{r^2}\frac{\partial}{\partial r}\left(r^2\frac{\partial w}{\partial r}\right) = wG'(C_s), \qquad 0 < r < R \tag{3.46}
$$

Plugging (3.45) into (3.12), we have

$$
\frac{1}{r^2}\frac{\partial}{\partial r}\left(r^2(u_s + \epsilon q)\right) = F(C_s + \epsilon w).
$$

Linearizing the above equation to obtain

$$\frac{1}{r^2}\frac{\partial}{\partial r}(r^2 q) = F'(C_s)w \qquad 0 \le r \le R. \tag{3.47}$$

To obtain a boundary condition for $w(t,r)$, we use (3.18)

$$\left(\frac{\partial C_s}{\partial r} + \epsilon\frac{\partial w}{\partial r}\right)\Bigg|_{r=R(t)=R+\epsilon\rho} + \beta(C_s + \epsilon w)\Bigg|_{r=R+\epsilon\rho} = 0.$$

Linearizing the above equation, we have

$$\left(\frac{\partial C_s}{\partial r}\Bigg|_{r=R}\right) + \left(\frac{\partial^2 C_s}{\partial r^2}\Bigg|_{r=R}\right)(\epsilon\rho) + \epsilon\frac{\partial w}{\partial r}\Bigg|_{r=R} + \epsilon\rho^2\frac{\partial^2 w}{\partial r^2}\Bigg|_{r=R}$$
$$+\beta\left[\left(C_s\Bigg|_{r=R}\right) + \frac{\partial C_s}{\partial r}(\epsilon\rho) + \epsilon(w)\Bigg|_{r=R} + \left((\frac{\partial w}{\partial r}\Bigg|_{r=R})\epsilon\rho\right)\right] = 0.$$

So the linearized boundary condition is

$$\frac{\partial w}{\partial r} + \beta w + \beta\rho\frac{\partial C_s}{\partial r} + \rho\frac{\partial^2 C_s}{\partial r^2} = 0 \quad or \quad r = R. \tag{3.48}$$

Plugging (3.45) into (3.14), we have

$$\epsilon\frac{\partial \rho}{\partial t} = \frac{1}{(R+\epsilon\rho)^2}\int_0^{R+\epsilon\rho} s^2 F(C_s + \epsilon w)ds.$$

Linearizing the above equation, we have

$$\epsilon\frac{\partial \rho}{\partial t} = \left(\frac{-2\epsilon\rho}{R^3} + \frac{1}{R^2}\right)\times$$
$$\left[\int_0^R s^2\left(F(C_s) + F'(C_s)\epsilon w\right)ds + \left(R^2(F(c_s)) + F'(C_s) + \epsilon w\right)\epsilon\rho\right].$$

So the linearized equation for ρ is

$$\frac{\partial \rho}{\partial t} = \frac{1}{R^2}\int_0^R r^2 F'(C_s)w \quad dr + F(C_s)\rho - \frac{2\rho}{R^3}\int_0^R r^2 F(C_s)dr. \tag{3.49}$$

To study the stability of the stationary solution, we are going to study an eigenvalue problem. Set

$$w(r,t) = e^{at}\overline{w}(r) \quad q(r,t) = e^{at}\overline{q}(r) \quad \rho(t) = e^{at}, \tag{3.50}$$

where a is a complex number, a is the eigenvalue, and if Re $a < 0$ the stationary solution is stable. If Re $a > 0$, the stationary solution is unstable.
To find the eigenvalue a, plugging (3.50) into the linearized equation of $w(r,t)$, $q(r,t)$, and $\rho(t)$. Plugging (3.51) into (3.46) we have

$$-\frac{1}{r^2}\frac{\partial}{\partial r}(r^2\frac{\partial \overline{w}}{\partial r}) + u_s\frac{\partial \overline{w}}{\partial r} + \left(a - G'(C_s)\right)\overline{w} = -\frac{\partial C_s}{\partial r}\overline{q} \qquad 0 < r < R. \tag{3.51}$$

Plugging (3.50) into (3.48) to obtain

$$\frac{\partial \overline{w}}{\partial r} + \beta \overline{w} = -\frac{\partial^2 C_s}{\partial r} - \beta \frac{\partial C_s}{\partial r}, \quad r = R. \tag{3.52}$$

To simplify (3.51), we use (3.42), (3.50) to get

$$u_s = O(R^3), \qquad \frac{\partial C_s}{\partial r} = O(R).$$

Now using $C_s = \sigma_0 + O(R^2)$ we have

$$G'(C_s) = G'\big(\sigma_0 + O(R^2)\big) = G'(\sigma_0) + O(R^2).$$

(3.51) becomes

$$-\frac{1}{r^2}\frac{\partial}{\partial r}(r^2 \overline{w}) + \big(a - G'(\sigma_0)\big)\overline{w} = 0. \tag{3.53}$$

From (3.40)

$$\frac{\partial^2 C_s}{\partial r^2} = \frac{\sigma_0}{3} F_1(\sigma_0) + O(R^3).$$

(3.52) becomes

$$\frac{\partial \overline{w}}{\partial r} + \beta \overline{w} = -\frac{\sigma_0}{3} F_1(\sigma_0), \qquad r = R. \tag{3.54}$$

Also, $\overline{w}(0)$ is bounded.
To solve (3.53) and (3.54) we need to review modified Bessel function [209]. We consider the following Bessel's equation:

$$r^2 \overline{w}'' + r\overline{w}' - (r^2 + \nu^2)\overline{w} = 0. \tag{3.55}$$

The function $I_\nu(r)$, which is the modified Bessel function of the first kind, and $I_{-\nu}(r)$ are two linearly independent solutions of (3.55).
We can verify that the general solution of (3.53) is given by

$$\overline{w}(r) = Ar^{\frac{1}{2}} I_{\frac{1}{2}}\left(r\sqrt{a - G'(\sigma_0)}\right) + Br^{-\frac{1}{2}} I_{-\frac{1}{2}}\left(r\sqrt{a - G'(\sigma_0)}\right). \tag{3.56}$$

We review the properties of the modified Bessel function $I_m(\xi)$ [209]:

- Property 1. $I_m(\xi) = \left(\frac{\xi}{2}\right)^m \sum_{k=0}^{\infty} \frac{1}{k!\Gamma(m+k+1)} \left(\frac{\xi}{2}\right)^{2k}$
- Property 2. $I_{\frac{1}{2}}(\xi) = \sqrt{\frac{2}{\pi\xi}} \sinh\xi \sim \sqrt{\frac{2}{\pi}}\sqrt{\xi} \quad as \quad \xi \to 0$
- Property 3. $I_{\frac{3}{2}}(\xi) = \sqrt{\frac{2}{\pi\xi}}\left(\frac{-\sinh\xi}{\xi} + \cosh\xi\right) \sim \frac{1}{3}\sqrt{\frac{2}{\pi}}\xi^{\frac{3}{2}} \quad as \quad \xi \to 0$
- Property 4. $I'_m(\xi) - \frac{m}{\xi} I_m(\xi) = I_{m+1}(\xi)$, $m \geq 0$; $I'_{\frac{1}{2}}(\xi) = \frac{1}{2\xi} I_{\frac{1}{2}}(\xi) + I_{\frac{3}{2}}(\xi)$.

Now we go back to (3.56); since $I_{-1/2}(\xi)$ has a singularity at $\xi = 0$ from Property 1, and $\overline{w}(r)$ is bounded, we obtain $B = 0$ in (3.56).
Plugging (3.56) into (3.54), we have:

$$\begin{aligned}
&\frac{\partial \overline{w}}{\partial r} + \beta \overline{w}\Big|_{r=R} \\
&= A\Big[-\frac{1}{2}r^{-\frac{3}{2}}I_{\frac{1}{2}}(r\sqrt{a-G'(\sigma_0)}) + r^{-\frac{1}{2}}I'_{-\frac{1}{2}}(r\sqrt{a-G'(\sigma_0)})(\sqrt{a-G'(\sigma_0)})\Big] \\
&\qquad + \beta A r^{-\frac{1}{2}} I_{\frac{1}{2}}(r\sqrt{a-G'(\sigma_0)}) \\
&\quad = A\Big[-\frac{1}{2}r^{-\frac{3}{2}}I_{\frac{1}{2}}(r\sqrt{a-G'(\sigma_0)}) + r^{-\frac{1}{2}}(\sqrt{a-G'(\sigma_0)}) \\
&\times \Big(\frac{\frac{1}{2}}{r(\sqrt{a-G'(\sigma_0)})}I_{\frac{1}{2}}\Big(r\sqrt{a-G'(\sigma_0)}\Big) + I_{\frac{3}{2}}(r\sqrt{a-G'(\sigma_0)})\Big)\Big] \\
&\qquad + \beta A r^{-\frac{1}{2}} I_{\frac{1}{2}}(r\sqrt{a-G'(\sigma_0)}) \\
&= A\Big[\sqrt{a-G'(\sigma_0)}r^{-\frac{1}{2}}I_{\frac{3}{2}}(r\sqrt{a-G'(\sigma_0)}) + \beta r^{-\frac{1}{2}}I_{\frac{1}{2}}(r\sqrt{a-G'(\sigma_0)})\Big|_{r=R} \\
&\qquad = -\frac{\sigma_0 F_1(\sigma_0)}{3}.
\end{aligned}$$

So we obtain

$$A = \frac{-\frac{\sigma_0 F_1(\sigma_0)}{3}}{(\sqrt{a-G'(\sigma_0)})R^{-\frac{1}{2}}I_{\frac{3}{2}}(R(\sqrt{a-G'(\sigma_0)}) + \beta R^{-\frac{1}{2}}I_{\frac{1}{2}}(R(\sqrt{a-G'(\sigma_0)})}. \tag{3.57}$$

From (3.41), we have

$$\beta = -\frac{1}{3}F_1(\sigma_0)R + O(R^2) = \lambda_\beta R + O(R^3).$$

So

$$A = \frac{R^{\frac{1}{2}}(-\frac{1}{3}\sigma_0 F_1(\sigma_0))}{\sqrt{a-G'(\sigma_0)}I_{\frac{3}{2}}(R\sqrt{a-G'(\sigma_0)}) + \lambda_\beta R I_{\frac{1}{2}}(R\sqrt{a-G'(\sigma_0)})}. \tag{3.58}$$

Plugging (3.58) into (3.56) and $r = R$ to obtain

$$\overline{w}(R) = \frac{-\frac{1}{3}\sigma_0 F_1(\sigma_0) I_{\frac{1}{2}}(R\sqrt{a-G'(\sigma_0)})}{\sqrt{a-G'(\sigma_0)}I_{\frac{3}{2}}(R\sqrt{a-G'(\sigma_0)}) + \lambda_\beta R I_{\frac{1}{2}}(R\sqrt{a-G'(\sigma_0)})}. \tag{3.59}$$

We introduce

$$P_0(\xi) = \frac{I_{\frac{3}{2}}(\xi)}{\xi I_{\frac{1}{2}}(\xi)}. \tag{3.60}$$

Then (3.59) becomes

$$\overline{w}(R) = \frac{-\frac{1}{3}\sigma_0 F_1(\sigma_0)}{\lambda_\beta R + \big(a - G'(\sigma_0)\big) R P_0(R\sqrt{a - G'(\sigma_0)})} \tag{3.61}$$

To obtain an equation for a, we plug (3.50) into (3.49) to get

$$ae^{at} = \frac{1}{R^2}\int_0^R r^2 F'(C_s(r))\overline{w}(r)e^{at}dr + e^{at}F(C_s(R)) - \frac{2e^{at}}{R^3}\int_0^R r^2 F(C_s(r))dr;$$

so

$$a = \frac{1}{R^2}\int_0^R r^2 F'(C_s(r))\overline{w}(r)dr + F(C_s(R)) - \frac{2}{R^3}\int_0^R r^2 F(C_s(r))dr. \tag{3.62}$$

To simplify (3.62), we recall

$$C_s(r) = \sigma + \frac{\sigma_0}{\sigma}F_1(\sigma)r^2 + O(r^4) = \sigma_0 + O(R^2),$$

$$F(C_s(R)) = F(\sigma_0 + O(R^2)) = F(\sigma_0) + O(R^2) = O(R^2). \tag{3.63}$$

Now

$$-\frac{2}{R^3}\int_0^R r^2 F(C_s(r))dr = -\frac{2}{R^3}\int_0^R r^2 O(R^2)dr = O(R^2) \tag{3.64}$$

and

$$\begin{aligned}
&\frac{1}{R^2}\int_0^R r^2 F'(C_s(r))\overline{w}(r)dr \\
&\quad = \frac{1}{R^2}\int_0^R r^2 (F'(\sigma_0))Ar^{-\frac{1}{2}} I_{\frac{1}{2}}(r\sqrt{a - G'(\sigma_0)})dr \\
&\quad = \frac{1}{R^2}F'(\sigma_0)A\int_0^R r^2 r^{-\frac{1}{2}}\sqrt{\frac{2}{\pi}}\sqrt{\sqrt{a - G'(\sigma_0)}}r^{\frac{1}{2}}dr \\
&\quad = \frac{1}{3}F'(\sigma_0)A\sqrt{\frac{2}{\pi}}(a - G'(\sigma_0))^{\frac{1}{4}},
\end{aligned} \tag{3.65}$$

so (3.62) becomes

$$a = \frac{1}{3}F'(\sigma_0)A\sqrt{\frac{2}{\pi}}(a - G'(\sigma_0))^{\frac{1}{4}}. \tag{3.66}$$

In (3.58), we have

$$A = \frac{R^{\frac{1}{2}}\big(-\frac{1}{3}\sigma_0 F_1(\sigma_0)\big)}{\sqrt{a - G'(\sigma_0)}\sqrt{\frac{2}{\pi}}\frac{1}{3}(\sqrt{a - G'(\sigma_0)}R)^{\frac{3}{2}} + \lambda_\beta R\sqrt{\frac{2}{\pi}}(\sqrt{a - G'(\sigma_0)}R)^{\frac{1}{2}}};$$

$$= \frac{-\sigma_0 F_1(\sigma_0)\sqrt{\frac{\pi}{2}}}{\left[\sqrt{a - G'(\sigma_0)}^{\frac{5}{2}} + \lambda_\beta \sqrt{a - G'(\sigma_0)}^{\frac{1}{2}}\right] R}. \tag{3.67}$$

Plugging (3.67) into (3.66), we have

$$a = \frac{-\frac{1}{3}\sigma_0 F'(\sigma_0) F_1(\sigma_0)}{a - G'(\sigma_0) + 3\lambda_\beta}. \tag{3.68}$$

Now solving for a in (3.68), we obtain

$$a = \frac{-(3\lambda_\beta - G'(\sigma_0)) \pm \sqrt{(3\lambda_\beta - G'(\sigma_0))^2 - \frac{4}{3}\sigma_0 F'(\sigma_0) F_1(\sigma_0)}}{2}. \tag{3.69}$$

From (3.13) and (3.31), we $F'(\sigma_0) > 0, F_1(\sigma_0) < 0$. Consequently we can see from (3.69) that there are two eigenvalues a, one is positive, and the other one is negative, so the stationary solution is unstable; hence we have proved the following theorem:

Theorem 3.2 *If R is sufficiently small, then there exists solution $(e^{at}w(r), e^{at}q(r), e^{at})$ to the linearized system (3.46)–(3.49) with $a > 0$. Thus the stationary solution is unstable.*

Biologically, these results imply that if the initial cancer cell density is at the level of the steady state, the cancer will not grow. However, if the initial cancer density is a little different than the level of steady state, the cancer will grow indefinitely.

3.1.2.3 Global Solution of Model one with Flux Boundary Condition

In this subsection, we are going to prove the existence and uniqueness of global solution to Model one with flux boundary condition (3.18) and the following initial conditions:

$$\begin{aligned} R(t)|_{t=0} &= R_0 > 0 \\ C(0, r) &= C_0(r) \text{ for } 0 \le r \le R_0. \end{aligned} \tag{3.70}$$

Lemma 3.3 *If $C(t, r)$ is a solution of Model one in $\Omega(\tau)$ with the boundary condition (3.18) and the initial condition (3.70), where $\tau > 0$ and $1 \ge C_0(r) \ge 0$ for $0 \le r < R_0, R_0 = R(0) > 0$, then $1 \ge C(t, r) \ge 0$ for $(t, r) \in \Omega(\tau)$.*

Proof. The theorem follows from the maximum principle. ■

Let

$$M(C) = \Big[-(\eta - \frac{\lambda_c}{K})C^2 + (2\eta - A)C - (\eta - B)\Big], \tag{3.71}$$

then $G(C) = M(C)C$. We define the global solution as the following

Definition 3.1 *A smooth solution* $C(r,t) \in C^{2+\alpha,1+\alpha/2}(\Omega_\tau(t)), \dot{R}(t) \in C^{1+\alpha/2}[0,\tau)$ *is said to be global, if either* $\tau = \infty$ *or* $\tau < \infty$ *and* $\limsup_{t\to\tau} R(t) = 0$. *Here* $\Omega_\tau(t) = \{0 \le r \le R(t), 0 \le t \le \tau\}$.

Theorem 3.4 *If* $C_0 \in C^{2+\alpha}[0,R_0], 0 < \alpha < 1$ *where* $1 \ge C_0(r) \ge 0$ *for* $0 \le r < R_0$ *and* $\frac{\partial C_0}{\partial r} + \beta C_0 = 0$ *at* $r = R_0 = R(0) > 0$, *then there exists a unique global solution* $(C(r,t), R(t))$ *of Model one with (3.18) and (3.70), and* $C(r,t) \in C^{2+\alpha,1+\alpha/2}(\Omega_\infty(t)), R(t) \in C^{1+\alpha/2}[0,\infty)$.

Proof. For given positive constants T, L_1, L_2, Let

$$X_\tau = \Big[R(t):\ R(0) = R_0\ ,\ \| \dot{R}(t) \|_{C^{\alpha/2}_{(0,\tau)}}\ ,\ \le L_1\Big]$$

$$Y_\tau = \Big[C(r,t) : 0 \le C(r,t) \le 1,$$

$$C(r,0) = C_0(r),\ \ \| C \| = |C|_{C^{\alpha,\frac{\alpha}{2}}_{r,t}} + |C_r|_{C^{\alpha,\frac{\alpha}{2}}_{r,t}} \le L_2\Big] \quad (3.72)$$

First we fix $R(t)$ in X_τ. Define for $C(r,t) \in Y_\tau$, $\hat{C} = S(C) \in Y_\tau$ to be the solution of

$$\frac{\partial \hat{C}}{\partial t} + u\frac{\partial \hat{C}}{\partial r} - \frac{1}{r^2}\frac{\partial}{\partial r}\Big(r^2\frac{\partial \hat{C}}{\partial r}\Big) - M(C)\hat{C} \ = \ 0; \quad (3.73)$$

here u is obtained from (3.14) for C, and boundary condition

$$\frac{\partial \hat{C}}{\partial r} + \beta\hat{C} \ = 0 \quad on \quad \partial\Omega(t) \qquad 0 \le t \le \tau. \quad (3.74)$$

We observe (3.73) with Robin boundary condition (3.74) is linear in $\hat{C}$, with coefficients $M(C)$ and u in $C^{\alpha_r,\frac{\alpha}{2}}$. Applying Schauder estimates to (3.73) and (3.74) we have a solution $\hat{C}$ with

$$|\hat{C}|_{C^{2+\alpha,1+\frac{\alpha}{2}}_{r,t}} \le L = L(\tau, L_1, L_2). \quad (3.75)$$

Let

$$v(r,t) = \hat{C}(r,t) - C_0(r)$$

Since $\hat{C}$ satisfies (3.75), we have a bound on $\frac{\partial \hat{C}}{\partial t}$ and hence on $\frac{\partial}{\partial t}u(r,t)$

Since $v(r,0) = \hat{C}(r,0) - C_0(r) = 0$ we conclude

$$\| v \|_{L^\infty} \le C_1\tau$$

with C_1 a function of L increasing. From now on, we assume $L \ge 1$ as this will simplify estimates on expressions.

For any smooth function v, we have the following interpolation inequality [188]:

$$|v|_{C^{\alpha,\frac{\alpha}{2}}_{r,t}} \le |v|^{\frac{\alpha}{1+\beta}}_{C^{1+\beta,\frac{1+\beta}{2}}_{r,t}} \qquad \| v \|^{\frac{1+\beta-\alpha}{1+\beta}}_{L^\infty}, \text{ for } \beta > 0. \quad (3.76)$$

With $\beta = 1 + \alpha$ in the interpolation inequality for v to obtain

$$\begin{aligned}|v|_{C_{r,t}^{\alpha,\frac{\alpha}{2}}} &\le |v|^{\frac{\alpha}{2+\alpha}}_{C_{r,t}^{2+\alpha;1+\frac{\alpha}{2}}} \qquad \| v \|^{\frac{2}{2+\alpha}}_{L^\infty} \\ &\le L^{\frac{\alpha}{2+\alpha}} \big(C_1 \tau\big)^{\frac{2}{2+\alpha}} \\ &\le L\big(C_1\tau\big)^{\frac{2}{2+\alpha}}.\end{aligned}$$

Therefore

$$\begin{aligned}|\hat{C}|_{C_{r,t}^{\alpha,\frac{\alpha}{2}}} &\le |C_0|_{C_{r,t}^{\alpha,\frac{\alpha}{2}}} + |u|_{C_{r,t}^{\alpha,\frac{\alpha}{2}}} \\ &\le |C_0|_{C^{2+\alpha}} + L\big(C_1\tau\big)^{\frac{2}{2+\alpha}}.\end{aligned}$$

Similarly as

$$\frac{\partial v}{\partial r}(0,r) = 0$$

$$\|\frac{\partial v}{\partial r}\|_{L^\infty} \le C_2\tau.$$

With $\beta = \alpha$ in (3.76), we have

$$\begin{aligned}\left|\frac{\partial v}{\partial r}\right|_{C_{r,t}^{\alpha,\frac{\alpha}{2}}} &\le \left|\frac{\partial v}{\partial r}\right|^{\frac{\alpha}{1+\alpha}}_{C_{r,t}^{1+\alpha,\frac{\alpha}{2}}} \cdot \| \frac{\partial v}{\partial r} \|^{\frac{1}{1+\alpha}}_{L^\infty} \\ &\le |v|^{\frac{\alpha}{1+\alpha}}_{C_{r,t}^{2+\alpha,1+\frac{\alpha}{2}}} \big(C_2\tau\big)^{\frac{1}{1+\alpha}} \\ &\le L^{\frac{\alpha}{1+\alpha}} \big(C_2\tau\big)^{\frac{1}{1+\alpha}} \\ &\le L\big(C_2\tau\big)^{\frac{1}{1+\alpha}}.\end{aligned}$$

Therefore

$$\left|\frac{\partial \hat{C}}{\partial r}\right|_{C_{r,t}^{\alpha,\frac{\alpha}{2}}} \le \left|\frac{\partial C_0}{\partial r}\right|_{C_r^\alpha} + \left|\frac{\partial v}{\partial r}\right|_{C_{r,t}^{\alpha,\frac{\alpha}{2}}} \le |C_0|_{r^{2+\alpha}} + L\big(C_2\tau\big)^{\frac{1}{1+\alpha}}.$$

We conclude

$$|\hat{C}|_{C^{\alpha,\frac{\alpha}{2}}} + |\hat{C}_r|_{C^{\alpha,\frac{\alpha}{2}}} \le 2|C_0|_{C_r^{2+\alpha}} + L\bigg((C_1\tau)^{\frac{2}{2+\alpha}} + (C_2\tau)^{\frac{1}{1+\alpha}}\bigg)$$

Let L_2 in the definition of Y_τ be defined as $L_2 = 2|C_0|_{C_r^{2+\alpha}} + 1$. Then for τ small enough, $\| \hat{C} \| \le L_2$ so we have shown that $\hat{C} = S(C) \in Y_\tau$ with L_2 as above and τ small enough if $C \in Y_\tau$.

To show that for τ small enough $S : Y_\tau \longrightarrow Y_\tau$ is a contraction recall that u in (3.73) depends on C as in (3.12). So, For C_i, $i = 1, 2$ $\hat{C}_i = S(C_i)$ satisfies

$$\frac{\partial \hat{C}_i}{\partial t} + u(C_i)\frac{\partial \hat{C}_i}{\partial r} - \frac{1}{r^2}\frac{\partial}{\partial r}\left(r^2\frac{\partial}{\partial r}\hat{C}_i\right) - M(C_i)C_i = 0;$$

$$\frac{\partial \hat{C}_i}{\partial r} + \beta\hat{C}_i = 0 \quad on \quad \partial\Omega(t).$$

Subtract these for $i = 1, 2$ to obtain

$$\frac{\partial}{\partial t}(\hat{C}_1 - \hat{C}_2) + u(C_1)\frac{\partial}{\partial r}(\hat{C}_1 - \hat{C}_2) - \frac{1}{r^2}\frac{\partial}{\partial r}\left(r^2\frac{\partial}{\partial r}(\hat{C}_1 - \hat{C}_2)\right)$$

$$-M(C_1)(\hat{C}_1 - \hat{C}_2) = -\Big(u(C_1) - u(C_2)\Big)\frac{\partial}{\partial r}\hat{C}_2 + \Big(M(C_1) - M(C_2)\Big)\hat{C}_2;$$

$$\frac{\partial}{\partial r}(\hat{C}_1 - \hat{C}_2) + \beta(\hat{C}_1 - \hat{C}_2) = 0 \quad on \quad \partial\Omega(t)$$

From (3.71) for the definition of $M(C)$,

$$M(C_1) - M(C_2) = \Big[-(\eta - \frac{\lambda_c}{K})(C_1 - C_2)(C_1 + C_2) + (2\eta - A)(C_1 - C_2)\Big].$$

Therefore $\exists$ constant $C_3(T, L_2, C_0)$ if $C_1, C_2 \in Y_\tau$

$$\parallel M(C_1) - M(C_2) \parallel \leq C_3 \parallel C_1 - C_2 \parallel .$$

From (3.12)

$$\frac{1}{r^2}\frac{\partial}{\partial r}(r^2 u) = F(C).$$

We obtain

$$\frac{1}{r^2}\frac{\partial}{\partial r}\left(r^2\big(u(C_1) - u(C_2)\big)\right) = F(C_1) - F(C_2)$$

$$= (\eta - \frac{\lambda_c}{K})(C_1 - C_2)(C_1 + C_2) + (\lambda_c - \delta_0 + \lambda_T + \delta_T - \eta)(C_1 - C_2)$$

and there exists $C_4(T, L_2, C_0)$ so that

$$\parallel u(C_1) - u(C_2) \parallel \leq C_4 \parallel C_1 - C_2 \parallel .$$

Applying the Schauder estimates to the above in homogeneous equation with Robin boundary condition, we obtain an estimate for $\hat{C}_1 - \hat{C}_2$ on Y_τ for some positive constants C_4, C_5

$$|\hat{C}_1 - \hat{C}_2|_{C_{T,t}^{2+\alpha, 1+\frac{\alpha}{2}}} \leq C_4 \parallel C_1 - C_2 \parallel$$

$$|\hat{C}_1 - \hat{C}_2|_\infty \leq C_5\tau \parallel C_1 - C_2 \parallel$$

Therefore, using the interpolation inequality with $\beta = 1+\alpha$, we obtain:

$$|\hat{C}_1 - \hat{C}_2|_{C^{\alpha,\frac{\alpha}{2}}_{r,t}} \le \Big(C_4 \parallel C_1 - C_2 \parallel\Big)^{\frac{\alpha}{2+\alpha}} \cdot \Big(C_5\tau \parallel C_1 - C_2 \parallel\Big)^{\frac{2}{2+\alpha}}$$

$$= C_4^{\frac{\alpha}{2+\alpha}} (C_5\tau)^{\frac{2}{2+\alpha}} \parallel C_1 - C_2 \parallel$$

and similarly with $\beta = \alpha$

$$\left|\frac{\partial}{\partial r}(\hat{C}_1 - \hat{C}_2)\right|_{C^{\alpha,\frac{\alpha}{2}}_{r,t}} \le C_6^{\frac{\alpha}{1+\alpha}} (C_5\tau)^{\frac{1}{1+\alpha}} \parallel C_1 - C_2 \parallel .$$

Therefore, there exist constants C_7, $\gamma > 0$. By choosing τ sufficiently small so that $K = C_7\tau^\gamma < 1$. We obtain

$$\parallel \hat{C}_1 - \hat{C}_2 \parallel \le K \parallel C_1 - C_2 \parallel$$

So we have shown that given $R(t) \in X_\tau$, and τ sufficiently small, $S : Y_\tau \longrightarrow Y_\tau$, $S(C) = \hat{C}$ is contraction. Applying the Banach fixed point theorem, we obtain that for $R(t) \in X_\tau$, τ small enough there exists a fixed point C of S and C in Y_τ. Let us denote this fixed point as $C_{R(t)}$. Given $R(t) \in X_\tau$, and τ sufficiently small we define a mapping V by $\hat{R} = V(R)$ which solves

$$\frac{d\hat{R}}{dt} = \frac{1}{R(t)^2}\int_0^{R(t)} s^2 F\Big(C_{R(t)}(s.t)\Big)ds.$$

with initial condition $\hat{R}(0) = R_0$.

Given R_1 and $R_2 \in X_\tau$ we now need to compare $C_{R_1(t)}(r,t)$ and $C_{R_2(t)}(r,t)$ on domains $\Omega_1(t), \Omega_2(t)$. These domains are different and in order to make a comparison convert problems to a fixed boundary problem on the domain $e \le 1$ via the change of coordinates $e = \frac{r}{R_1(t)}$, resp $e = \frac{r}{R_2(t)}$

Let

$$\hat{C}_1(e,t) = C_{R_1(t)}(r,t),$$
$$\hat{u}_1(e,t) = u_1(r,t),$$
$$\hat{C}_2(e,t) = C_{R_2(t)}(r,t),$$
$$\hat{u}_2(e,t) = u_2(r,t).$$

Then we obtain for $i = 1,2$

$$\frac{\partial \hat{C}_i}{\partial t} + \hat{u}_i \frac{1}{R_i}\frac{\partial \hat{C}_i}{\partial e} - \frac{1}{e^2 R_i(t)^2}\frac{\partial}{\partial e}\left(e^2 \frac{\partial \hat{C}_i}{\partial e}\right) - e\frac{\dot{R}_i}{R_i}\frac{\partial \hat{C}_i}{\partial e} = M(\hat{C}_i)\hat{C}_i. \quad (3.77)$$

Subtracting there equations, one obtains from Schauder estimate

$$|\hat{C}_1 - \hat{C}_2|_{C^{2+\alpha,1+\frac{\alpha}{2}}_{e,t}} \le C_8|\dot{R}_1 - \dot{R}_2|_{C^{\frac{\alpha}{2}}}.$$

As $R_1(0) = R_2(0)$, using the interpolation inequality on domain $e \leq 1$, there exists constants $C_9 > 0$ and $\gamma > 0$

$$|\partial_e \hat{C}_1 - \partial_e \hat{C}_2|_{C^{\alpha,\frac{\alpha}{2}}_{r,t}} \leq (C_9\tau)^\gamma |C_1 - C_2|_{C^{2+\alpha,1+\frac{\alpha}{2}}_{r,t}}$$

$$\leq C_8(C_9\tau)^\gamma |\dot{R}_1 - \dot{R}_2|^{\frac{\alpha}{2}}_{C}.$$

Since

$$\frac{\partial}{\partial t}\hat{R}_i(t) = \hat{u}_i(1,t) \ ; \ i = 1, 2$$

with

$$\hat{u}_i(e,t) = R_i(t) \int_0^1 s^2 F\Big(\hat{C}_i(s,t)\Big) ds,$$

we have

$$\frac{d}{dt}|\hat{R}(t_1) - \hat{R}(t_2)|_{C_t^{\frac{\alpha}{2}}} \leq C\tau^\gamma |R_1 - R_2|_{C_t^{\frac{\alpha}{2}}}. \tag{3.78}$$

Since $R_1(0) = R_2(0)$, $\quad R_i = \int_0^t \dot{R}_i(s)ds$

$$|R_1 - R_2|_{C_t^{\frac{\alpha}{2}}} \leq C|\dot{R}|_{C_t^{\frac{\alpha}{2}}} = C|R_1 - R_2|_{C_t^{\frac{\alpha}{2}}}$$

So if L_1 in the definition of X_τ is sufficiently small then for $K = C\tau^\gamma < 1$, if $R_i \in X_\tau$, $\hat{R}_i \in X_\tau$, and

$$|\hat{R}_1 - \hat{R}_2|_{C_t^\alpha} \leq K|R_1 - R_2|_{C_t^\alpha}$$

So the map: $R \longrightarrow \hat{R} = V(R)$ is a contraction of X_τ. So we have proven that there exists a unique solution for τ is small enough.
In order to extend the local solution, we need to estimate $\frac{dR}{dt}$. Using the same steps as (3.78), using Lemma 3.3, we have

$$\left|\frac{dR}{dt}\right| \leq F_M R(t) \text{ for } 0 \leq t < \tau; \tag{3.79}$$

where $F_M = \max_{[0,1]} |F(C)$. which implies

$$R(0)e^{-F_M t} \leq R(t) \leq R(0)e^{F_M t}. \tag{3.80}$$

(3.79) and (3.80) implies that the local solution can be extended infinitely in t, so the global solution exists. ■

3.1.2.4 Long Time Behavior of Solution to Model one with Zero Flux Boundary Condition

In this section, we consider model one with zero flux boundary condition (3.19). The similar to the proof of Theorem 3.4, we can obtain the global

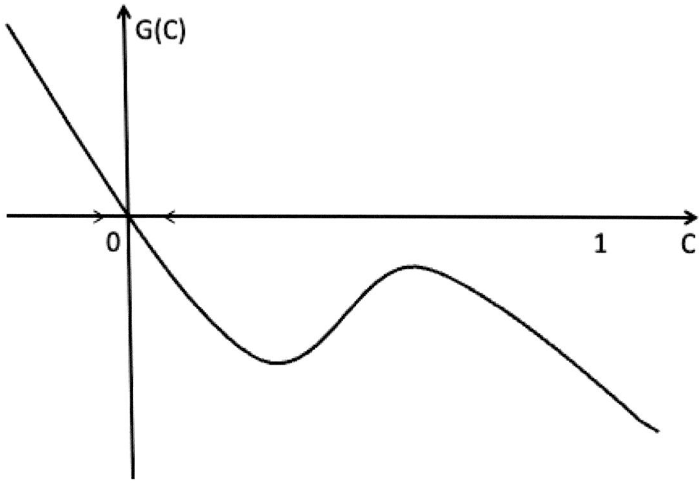

Figure 3.1 The graph of $G(C)$ for $\eta > \frac{\lambda_C}{K} + \frac{\left[\left(1-\frac{1}{K}\right)\lambda_C - \delta_0 + \lambda_T + \delta_T\right]^2}{4\lambda_T}$, $G(C)$ has only one zero at $C = 0$, which is a stable fixed point of the ODE $\frac{dC}{dt} = G(C)$.

existence and uniqueness of solution to model one with zero flux boundary condition (3.19). We will only discuss the asymptotic properties of the solution.

We denote by D the discriminant of the quadratic factor in $G(C)$ in (3.16). By straight computation, we get

$$\begin{aligned} D &= (2\eta - A)^2 - 4\left(\eta - \frac{\lambda_C}{K}\right)(\eta - B) \\ &= -4\lambda_T\left(\eta - \frac{\lambda_C}{K}\right) + \left[\left(1 - \frac{1}{K}\right)\lambda_C - \delta_0 + \lambda_T + \delta_T\right]^2. \end{aligned} \tag{3.81}$$

Theorem 3.5 *Consider the system (3.14), (3.15), and (3.19), and with initial condition* $0 < C(r, 0) < 1$ *for* $0 < r < R(0)$.
If $\eta > \frac{\lambda_C}{K} + \frac{\left[\left(1-\frac{1}{K}\right)\lambda_C - \delta_0 + \lambda_T + \delta_T\right]^2}{4\lambda_T}$, *then* $R(t) \to 0$ *and* $C(r, t) \to 0$ *uniformly as* $t \to \infty$.

Proof. Since $D < 0$ for $\eta > \frac{\lambda_C}{K} + \frac{\left[\left(1-\frac{1}{K}\right)\lambda_C - \delta_0 + \lambda_T + \delta_T\right]^2}{4\lambda_T}$, $G(C)$ has only one zero $C = 0$. Since $\eta > \frac{\lambda_C}{K}$, $G(C) > 0$ on the interval $(-\infty, 0)$ while $G(C) < 0$ on the interval $(0, \infty)$, the fixed point $C = 0$ is asymptotically stable; see Fig. 3.1. Let $\hat{C}(t)$ be the solution of ODE $\frac{d\hat{C}}{dt} = G(\hat{C}), \hat{C}(0) = \sup_{0<r<R(0)} C(r, 0)$, then $\hat{C}(t) \to 0$ as $t \to \infty$.

Using comparison theorem (see chapter 2 in [105]), we then obtain $0 \leq C(r,t) \leq \hat{C}(t)$ hence $C(r,t) \to 0$ as $t \to \infty$, which implies that $F(C) \to -\delta_T$ from (3.5). Using (3.6) we get $\frac{dR}{dt} \leq -\frac{\delta_T}{6} R(t)$ for large t. So $R(t) \leq c_1 e^{-\frac{\delta_T}{6} t}$ for some positive constant c_1.

■

We assume in the following theorem

$$\gamma_2 := \left(1 - \frac{1}{K}\right) \lambda_C - \delta_0 > 0. \tag{3.82}$$

Theorem 3.6 *Consider the system (3.14), (3.15), and (3.19) with* λ_C *as in (3.82), and with initial condition* $0 < C(r,0) < 1$ *for* $0 < r < R(0)$. *If* $\eta < \frac{\lambda_C}{K}$, *then* $R(t) \to \infty$.

Proof. If $\eta < \frac{\lambda_C}{K}$, then it follows from (3.81) that $D > 0$ and

$$\sqrt{D} > \left(1 - \frac{1}{K}\right) \lambda_C - \delta_0 + \lambda_T + \delta_T. \tag{3.83}$$

$G(C)$ has three zeros $C = 0$, $C = C_1$, and $C = C_2$, where

$$\begin{aligned} C_1 &= \frac{2\eta - A + \sqrt{D}}{2\left(\eta - \frac{\lambda_C}{K}\right)}, \\ C_2 &= \frac{2\eta - A - \sqrt{D}}{2\left(\eta - \frac{\lambda_C}{K}\right)}. \end{aligned} \tag{3.84}$$

It follows from (3.17) and (3.83) that $0 < C_1 < 1 < C_2$. Since $\eta < \frac{\lambda_C}{K}$, $G(C) < 0$ on the interval $(-\infty, 0)$ while $G(C) > 0$ on the interval $(0, C_1)$ and $G(C) < 0$ on the interval (C_1, C_2), see Figure 3.2. Let $\hat{C}(t)$ be a solution of ODE $\frac{d\hat{C}}{dt} = G(\hat{C})$ with initial condition $0 < \hat{C}(0) < 1$, then $\hat{C}(t) \to C_1$ as $t \to \infty$. Using comparison theorem [105], we then obtain $C(r,t) \to C_1$ uniformly in r as $t \to \infty$; hence $F(C) \to F(C_1)$. It follows from (3.5) (3.16) and straight computation

$$F(C_1) = \frac{1}{2}\left[\left(1 - \frac{1}{K}\right) \lambda_C - \delta_0 - \lambda_T - \delta_T\right] + \frac{1}{2}\sqrt{D}. \tag{3.85}$$

Using (3.83) we get $F(C_1) > \gamma_2 > 0$. It follows from (3.14) that $\frac{dR}{dt} \geq \frac{\gamma_2}{6} R(t)$ for large t. So $R(t) \geq c_1 e^{\frac{\gamma_2}{6} t}$ for some positive constant c_1. ■

Theorem 3.7 *Consider the system (3.14), (3.15), and (3.19) with* $\gamma_2 > \lambda_T$, *and with initial condition* $0 < C(r,0) < 1$ *for* $0 < r < R(0)$. *If* $\frac{\lambda_C}{K} < \eta < \lambda_C + \delta_T - \delta_0$, *then* $R(t) \to \infty$.

Proof. If $\frac{\lambda_C}{K} < \eta < \lambda_C + \delta_T - \delta_0$, then it follows from (3.13) that $D > 0$ and

$$\left(1 - \frac{1}{K}\right) \lambda_C - \delta_0 - \lambda_T + \delta_T < \sqrt{D} < \left(1 - \frac{1}{K}\right) \lambda_C - \delta_0 + \lambda_T + \delta_T. \tag{3.86}$$

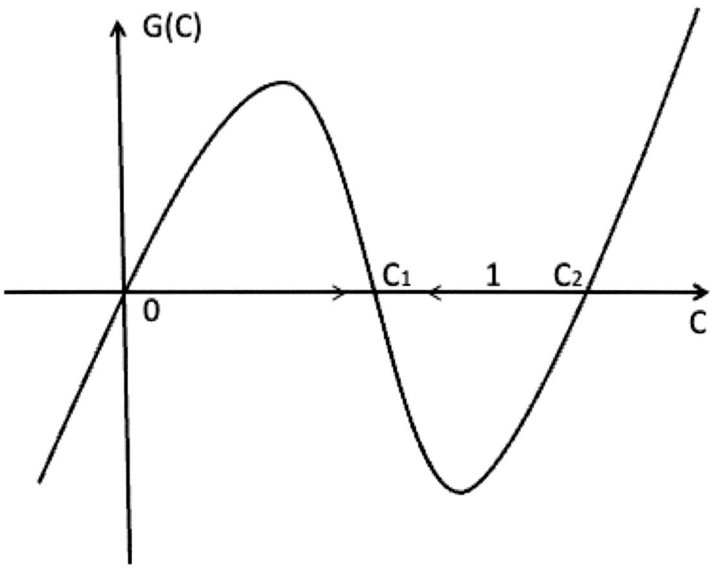

Figure 3.2 The graph of $G(C)$ for $\eta < \frac{\lambda_C}{K}$. $G(C)$ has three zeros at $C = 0, C_1, C_2$, C_1 is a stable fixed point of the ODE $\frac{dC}{dt} = G(C)$.

$G(C)$ has three zeros $C = 0$, $C = C_1$, and $C = C_2$. It follows from (3.84) and (3.86) that $C_2 < 0 < C_1 < 1$. Since $\eta > \frac{\lambda_C}{K}$, $G(C) > 0$ on the interval $(-\infty, C_2)$ while $G(C) < 0$ on the interval $(C_2, 0)$ and $G(C) > 0$ on the interval $(0, C_1)$, see Figure 3.3. Let $\hat{C}(t)$ be a solution of ODE $\frac{d\hat{C}}{dt} = G(\hat{C})$ with initial condition $0 < \hat{C}(0) < 1$, then $\hat{C}(t) \to C_1$ as $t \to \infty$. Using comparison theorem [105], we then obtain $C(r,t) \to C_1$ uniformly in r as $t \to \infty$; hence $F(C) \to F(C_1)$, where $F(C_1)$ is given by (3.85). Using (3.86) we get $F(C_1) > \gamma_2 - \lambda_T > 0$. It follows from (3.16) that $\frac{dR}{dt} \geq \frac{\gamma_2 - \lambda_T}{6} R(t)$ for large t. So $R(t) \geq c_1 e^{\frac{\gamma_2 - \lambda_T}{6} t}$ for some positive constant c_1. ∎

Remark 3.8 *It follows from Theorems 3.4–3.7 that the tumor volume will continuously decrease to zero if the killing rate η is large enough; while the tumor volume will grow to ∞ if the killing rate η is small.*

Theorem 3.9 *Consider the system (3.14), (3.15), and (3.19) with $\gamma_2 > \lambda_T + \delta_T$. If*

$$\lambda_C + \delta_T - \delta_0 < \eta < \frac{\lambda_C}{K} + \frac{\left[\left(1 - \frac{1}{K}\right)\lambda_C - \delta_0 + \lambda_T + \delta_T\right]^2}{4\lambda_T}, \tag{3.87}$$

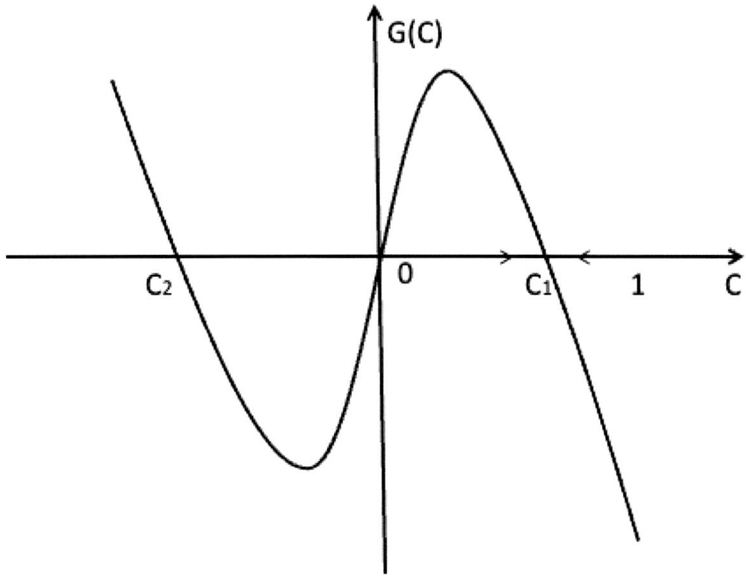

Figure 3.3 The graph of $G(C)$ for $\frac{\lambda_C}{K} < \eta < \lambda_C + \delta_T - \delta_0$. $G(C)$ has three zeros at $C = 0, C_1 > 0, C_2 < 0$, C_1 is a stable fixed point of the ODE $\frac{dC}{dt} = G(C)$.

then the following holds:
(i) If $\sup\limits_{0<r<R(0)} C(r, 0) < C_2$, *then* $R(t) \to 0$ *as* $t \to \infty$,
(ii) If $\inf\limits_{0<r<R(0)} C(r, 0) > C_2$, *then* $R(t) \to \infty$ *as* $t \to \infty$,
where C_2 *is given by (3.84).*

Proof. If η satisfies (3.87), then it follows from (3.81) that $D > 0$ and $\sqrt{D} < \left(1 - \frac{1}{K}\right) \lambda_C - \delta_0 + \lambda_T + \delta_T$. $G(C)$ has three zeros $C = 0$, $C = C_1$, and $C = C_2$. It follows from (3.84) and (3.87) that $0 < C_2 < C_1 < 1$. Since $\eta > \frac{\lambda_C}{K}$, $G(C) > 0$ on the interval $(-\infty, 0)$ while $G(C) < 0$ on the interval $(0, C_2)$ and $G(C) > 0$ on the interval (C_2, C_1), see Fig. 3.4.

(i) Let $\hat{C}(t)$ be a solution of ODE $\frac{d\hat{C}}{dt} = G(\hat{C})$ with initial condition $\hat{C}(0) = \sup\limits_{0<r<R(0)} C(r, 0)$, then $\hat{C}(t) \to 0$ as $t \to \infty$. Using comparison theorem [105], we get $C(r, t) \leq \hat{C}(t)$. We then obtain $C(r, t) \to 0$, hence $F(C) \to F(0) = -\delta_T$. It follows from (3.6) that $\frac{dR}{dt} \leq -\frac{\lambda_T}{6} R(t)$ for large t. So $R(t) \leq c_1 e^{-\frac{\lambda_T}{6} t}$ for some positive constant c_1.

(ii) Let $\hat{C}(t)$ be a solution of ODE $\frac{d\hat{C}}{dt} = G(\hat{C})$ with initial condition $\hat{C}(0) = \inf\limits_{0<r<R(0)} C(r, 0)$, then $\hat{C}(t) \to C_1$ as $t \to \infty$. Using comparison theorem [105],

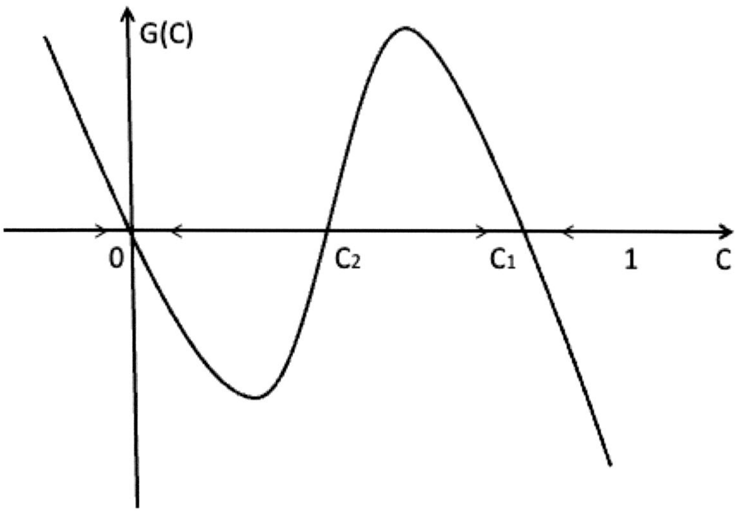

Figure 3.4 The graph of $G(C)$ for $\lambda_C + \delta_T - \delta_0 < \eta < \frac{\lambda_C}{K} + \frac{\left[(1-\frac{1}{K})\lambda_C - \delta_0 + \lambda_T + \delta_T\right]^2}{4\lambda_T}$. $G(C)$ has three zeros at $C = 0, C_1 > 0, C_2 > 0$, 0 and C_1 are stable fixed points of the ODE $\frac{dC}{dt} = G(C)$.

we then obtain $C(r,t) \geq \hat{C}(t)$. From (3.13), $F(C)$ is quadratic function of C and $F'(C_1) > 0$, hence for large t, $F(C) \geq F(C_1) \geq \frac{1}{2}[\gamma_2 - (\lambda_T + \delta_T)] > 0$ from (3.85). It follows from (3.14) that $\frac{dR}{dt} \geq \frac{\gamma_2 - (\lambda_T + \delta_T)}{12} R(t)$ for large t. So $R(t) \geq c_1 e^{\frac{\gamma_2 - (\lambda_T + \delta_T)}{12} t}$ for some positive constant c_1. ■

Remark 3.10 *Theorem 3.9 shows that when the killing rate η falls in certain interval, the asymptotic behavior of the tumor depends on the initial density level of the cancer cells.*

3.1.2.5 Long Time Behavior of Solution to Model one with Flux Boundary Condition and Numerical Simulations

In this subsection, we discuss the long time property of the solution of model one with flux boundary condition (3.14), (3.15), and (3.18)

Theorem 3.11 *Consider the system (3.14), (3.15), and (3.18), and with initial condition $0 < C(r,0) < 1$ for $0 < r < R(0)$. If we have*

$$\eta > \frac{\lambda_C}{K} + \frac{\left((1 - \frac{1}{K})\lambda_C - \delta_0 + \lambda_T + \delta_T\right)^2}{4\lambda_T},$$

then $R(t) \longmapsto 0$ and $C(r,t) \longmapsto 0$ uniformly as $t \longmapsto \infty$.

Proof. The proof is similar to that for Theorem 3.5. ■

Theorem 3.12 *Consider the system (3.14), (3.15), and (3.18) with* $\gamma_2 > \lambda_T + \delta_T$. *If*

$$\lambda_T + \delta_T - \delta_0 < \eta < \frac{\lambda_C}{K} + \frac{\left[(1-\frac{1}{K})\lambda_C - \delta_0 + \lambda_T + \delta_T\right]^2}{4\lambda_T}$$

and if $\sup_{0<r<R(0)} C(r,0) < C_2$, *then* $R(t) \longmapsto 0$ *as* $t \longmapsto \infty$.

Proof. The proof is similar to that for Theorem 3.9 (i). ■

When η is small, we cannot prove a result similar to Theorem 3.6, since the comparison technique cannot be applied due to the Robin boundary condition. However we believe the result is still true based on numerical simulation [6] that we are going to describe in the following.

We now rewrite these equations in the rescaled variable $\rho = \frac{r}{R(t)}$, on the fixed domain $0 \leq \rho \leq 1$. Let $\hat{C}(\rho,t) = C(r,t) = C(\rho R(t),t)$, and $\hat{u}(\rho,t) = u(r,t) = u(\rho R(t),t)$. Then:

$$\frac{\partial}{\partial r}C = \frac{1}{R(t)}\frac{\partial}{\partial \rho}\hat{C},$$

$$\frac{\partial^2}{\partial r^2}C = \frac{1}{R(t)^2}\frac{\partial^2}{\partial \rho^2}\hat{C}.$$

Similarly:

$$\frac{\partial}{\partial t}\hat{C}(\rho,t) = \frac{\rho\dot{R}}{R(t)}\frac{\partial}{\partial \rho}\hat{C}(\rho,t) + \frac{\partial}{\partial t}C(r,t).$$

This produces the equation for $\hat{C}(\rho,t)$:

$$\frac{\partial \hat{C}}{\partial t} + \left(\frac{\hat{u}-\rho\dot{R}(t)}{R(t)} - \frac{2\delta_C}{\rho R(t)^2}\right)\frac{\partial \hat{C}}{\partial \rho} - \frac{\delta_C}{R^2}\frac{\partial^2 \hat{C}}{\partial \rho^2} = G(\hat{C}). \tag{3.88}$$

To derive the corresponding equation for $\hat{u}(\rho,t)$, observe that:

$$\frac{\partial}{\partial r}(r^2 u(r,t)) = \frac{1}{R(t)}\frac{\partial}{\partial \rho}(R(t)^2\rho^2\hat{u}(\rho,t))$$

while

$$r^2 F(C) = R(t)^2\rho^2 F(\hat{C}).$$

We then obtain:

$$\frac{\partial}{\partial \rho}\left(\rho^2\hat{u}(\rho,t)\right) = \rho^2 R(t) F(\hat{C}(\rho,t)). \tag{3.89}$$

In what follows, we will rewrite $\hat{C}$ as C and $\hat{u}$ as u.

we discretize the mathematical model using the finite difference method in order to derive a numerical algorithm for its implementation. The goal is to approximate the solution of the partial differential equations governing the tumor evolution by constructing a fully discrete scheme on a fixed computational domain.

Denote the numerical solution at the n-th time step at the grid points $\rho_j = (j-1)\Delta\rho$, $1 \leqslant j \leqslant J$ with $(J-1)\Delta\rho = 1$.

We define the components of the discretized solution of the model as follows as:

$$(C_j^n, U_j^n, R^n) = (C(t_n, \rho_j), u(t_n, \rho_j), R(t_n)); \text{ for } j = 1, \cdots, J, \text{ and } n = 1, \cdots. \tag{3.90}$$

where $t_n = n\Delta t$ denotes the discrete time points, and ρ_j denotes the spatial grid points.
To properly define the initialization of the numerical algorithm, we specify the initial condition for the system as follows:
At $t = 0$, the initial condition is:

$$C_0(r) = A_0(r - R_0)^2 + \bar{A}_0(r - R_0) + \bar{B}_0. \tag{3.91}$$

Since

$$r = R_0\rho,$$

$$C_0(\rho) = A_0R_0^2(\rho - 1)^2 + \bar{A}_0R_0(\rho - 1) + \bar{B}_0 \tag{3.92}$$

which, for $j = 1, \cdots, J$, is discretized as

$$C_j^1 = A_0R_0^2(\rho_j - 1)^2 + \bar{A}_0R_0(\rho_j - 1) + \bar{B}_0. \tag{3.93}$$

The initial condition for the radius $R(0)$ is defined by

$$R(0) = R_0 \quad \Longleftrightarrow \quad R^0 = R_0. \tag{3.94}$$

For the initial condition to satisfy the robin boundary solution, we choose that $\bar{A}_0 = \beta\bar{B}_0$, $\bar{B}_0$= constant be chosen, $A_0 = -\frac{\beta\bar{B}_0}{2R_0}$, and, $R_0 = 0.5$. cm

Given the data at the n-th time step, the algorithm first computes the velocity at the next time step U_j^{n+1} $j = 1, ..., J$ using the trapezoidal rule with left boundary condition at $\rho = 0$: $U_1^{n+1} = 0$, for $j = 1, ..., J-1$ from the relation:

$$\rho_{j+1}^2U_{j+1}^{n+1} - \rho_j^2U_j^{n+1} = \frac{R^n}{2}\Delta\rho\left[\rho_{j+1}^2F_{j+1}^n + \rho_j^2F_j^n\right]. \tag{3.95}$$

We define $F_j^n = F(C_j^n)$, where F is evaluated at C_j^n, the concentration at the n-th time step and j-th spatial point. The next step is to use the Euler method to update the radius at time step $n+1$, R^{n+1} and its rate of change $\dot{R}^{n+1}$ as:

$$\begin{aligned} R^{n+1} &= R^n + \Delta t U_J^{n+1} \\ \dot{R}^{n+1} &= U_J^{n+1}. \end{aligned} \tag{3.96}$$

We write the advection-diffusion-reaction equation as:

$$\frac{\partial C}{\partial t} + A_1 \frac{\partial C}{\partial \rho} + A_2 \frac{\partial^2 C}{\partial \rho^2} = G_1(C)C. \tag{3.97}$$

where

$$\begin{aligned} A_1 &= A_1(\rho, u, R(t), \dot{R}(t)) = \frac{u - \rho \dot{R}(t)}{R(t)} - \frac{2\delta_C}{\rho R(t)^2}, \\ A_2 &= A_2(R(t)) = -\frac{\delta_C}{R(t)^2}. \end{aligned} \tag{3.98}$$

We discretize Eq. (3.97) as

$$\begin{aligned} &\frac{C_j^{n+1} - C_j^n}{\Delta t} + (A_1)_j^{n+1} \frac{C_{j+1}^{n+1} - C_{j-1}^{n+1}}{2\Delta\rho} \\ &\qquad + (A_2)_j^{n+1} \frac{C_{j+1}^{n+1} - 2C_j^{n+1} + C_{j-1}^{n+1}}{(\Delta\rho)^2} = G_1(C_j^n) C_j^{n+1} \end{aligned} \tag{3.99}$$

for $j = 1, \ldots, J$, where

$$G_1(C_j^n) = -\Big(\eta - \frac{\lambda_C}{K}\Big)(C_j^n)^2 + (2\eta - A)C_j^n - (\eta - B) \tag{3.100}$$

The coefficients $(A_1)_j^{n+1}$ and $(A_2)_j^{n+1}$ are

$$\begin{aligned} (A_1)_j^{n+1} &= \frac{U_j^{n+1} - \rho_j \dot{R}^{n+1}(t)}{R^{n+1}(t)} - \frac{2\delta_C}{\rho_j R^{n+1}(t)^2} \\ (A_2)_j^{n+1} &= -\frac{\delta_C}{R^{n+1}(t)^2}. \end{aligned} \tag{3.101}$$

We multiply Eq. (3.99) by $2\Delta t$, and we simplify as follows and write these equations as:

$$b_j C_{j-1}^{n+1} + d_j C_j^{n+1} + a_j C_{j+1}^{n+1} = S_j, \quad j = 2, \ldots, J-1. \tag{3.102}$$

For the internal nodes $j = 2, \ldots, J-1$:

$$\begin{aligned} a_j &= \left(\frac{(A_1)_j^{n+1}}{\Delta\rho} + 2\frac{(A_2)_j^{n+1}}{\Delta\rho^2} \right) \Delta t \\ b_j &= \left(-\frac{(A_1)_j^{n+1}}{\Delta\rho} + 2\frac{(A_2)_j^{n+1}}{(\Delta\rho)^2} \right) \Delta t \\ d_j &= 2 - 2\left(2\frac{(A_2)_j^{n+1}}{(\Delta\rho)^2} + G_1(C_j^n) \right) \Delta t \\ S_j &= 2C_j^n. \end{aligned} \tag{3.103}$$

For $j = 1$, we have as boundary condition:

$$C_0^{n+1} = C_2^{n+1}. \tag{3.104}$$

Using the above boundary condition, (3.99) becomes

$$\begin{aligned} d_1 C_1^{n+1} + a_1 C_2^{n+1} &= S_1 \\ a_1 &= \left(4\frac{(A_2)_1^{n+1}}{(\Delta\rho)^2} \right) \Delta t \\ d_1 &= 2 - 2\left(2\frac{(A_2)_1^{n+1}}{(\Delta\rho)^2} + G_1(C_1^n) \right) \Delta t \\ S_1 &= 2C_1^n. \end{aligned} \tag{3.105}$$

For $j = J$, we have as discretization of the boundary condition $\frac{\partial C}{\partial r} = -\beta C$ and therefore $\frac{1}{R(t)}\frac{\partial \hat{C}}{\partial \rho} = -\beta \hat{C}$:

$$\frac{1}{R^{n+1}} \left(\frac{C_{J+1}^{n+1} - C_{J-1}^{n+1}}{2\Delta\rho} \right) = -\beta C_J^{n+1}. \tag{3.106}$$

Hence:

$$C_{J+1}^{n+1} = C_{J-1}^{n+1} - 2R^{n+1}\Delta\rho\beta C_J^{n+1}. \tag{3.107}$$

Inserting that into the discretized equation yields:

$$\begin{aligned} &2(C_J^{n+1} - C_J^n) + 2\Delta t (A_1)_J^{n+1}(R^{n+1}(-\beta)C_J^{n+1}) \\ &+ 2\frac{\Delta t (A_2)_J^{n+1}}{\Delta\rho^2}(2C_{J-1}^{n+1} - 2C_J^{n+1} - 2R^{n+1}\Delta\rho\beta C_J^{n+1}) \\ &= 2\Delta t G_1(C_J^n) C_J^{n+1}. \end{aligned} \tag{3.108}$$

Rearranging yields:

$$b_J C_{J-1}^{n+1} + d_J C_J^{n+1} = 2C_J^n \tag{3.109}$$

with:

$$b_J = 4\frac{(A_2)_J^{n+1}}{\Delta\rho^2}\Delta t \tag{3.110}$$

$$d_J = 2 - 2\left(\frac{2(A_2)_J^{n+1}}{\Delta\rho^2}(1 + R^{n+1}\Delta\rho\beta) + G_1(C_J^n) + (A_1)_J^{n+1}\beta R^{n+1} \right) \Delta t. \tag{3.111}$$

With this, the discretized system writes in matrix form as:

$$BC^{n+1} = S, \tag{3.112}$$

where matrix B is a tridiagonal matrix defined as:

$$B = \begin{bmatrix} d_1 & a_1 & 0 & \cdots & 0 \\ b_2 & d_2 & a_2 & \cdots & 0 \\ 0 & b_3 & d_3 & \cdots & 0 \\ \vdots & \vdots & \vdots & \ddots & \vdots \\ 0 & 0 & 0 & b_J & d_J \end{bmatrix} \tag{3.113}$$

and

$$\mathbf{C^{n+1}} = \begin{bmatrix} C_1^{n+1} \\ C_2^{n+1} \\ \vdots \\ C_{J-1}^{n+1} \\ C_J^{n+1} \end{bmatrix}, \quad \text{and} \quad S = \begin{bmatrix} S_1 \\ S_2 \\ \vdots \\ S_{J-1} \\ S_J \end{bmatrix} = 2\mathbf{C^n}. \tag{3.114}$$

The above finite difference algorithm is proved to be stable in [6].

In the following, we present numerical simulations of the tumor evolution model one to illustrate the effects of varying key parameters on tumor dynamics. By solving the discretized system, we examine how changes in the T-cell killing rate (η) and activation rate (λ_T) influence the tumor radius, cancer cell concentration, and cell velocity over time. Table 3.1 summarizes the parameter values used in these simulations, indicating both literature-sourced and chosen values. These simulations provide visual validation of the theoretical results, demonstrating how stronger immune responses can effectively suppress tumor growth or even drive regression.

Figures 3.5–3.8 demonstrates that when the killing rate η is small (e.g., $\eta = 0$ or $\eta = 1$), the tumor radius $R(t) \to \infty$ grows unboundedly as $t \to \infty$, indicating uncontrolled tumor growth. In contrast, when η is sufficiently large

TABLE 3.1 Model Parameters Used in Numerical Simulation

Parameter	Description	Value (Reference)
η	T-cell killing rate (varied in simulations)	$\{0, 1, 3\}$ cm^3/g·day (Chosen in simulation)
λ_T	Activation rate of T-cells (varied)	$\{2\times10^{-2}, \ 3\times10^{-2}, \ 4\times10^{-2}\}$ day^{-1} (Chosen in simulation)
K	Carrying capacity of cancer cells	0.8 (Chosen in simulation)
λ_C	Proliferation rate of cancer cells	2.24 day^{-1} ([178])
δ_T	Death rate of T-cells	0.18 day^{-1} ([178])
δ_0	Death rate of cancer cells	0.17 day^{-1} ([178])
δ_c	Diffusion coefficient	8.64×10^{-7} cm^2/day ([178])
R_0	Initial tumor radius	0.5 cm (Chosen in simulation)
β	Robin boundary condition parameter	0.1 (Chosen in simulation)
$\overline{B}_0$	Initial cancer cell concentration	$\{0.5, 0.7, 1\}$ g/cm^3 (Chosen in simulation)

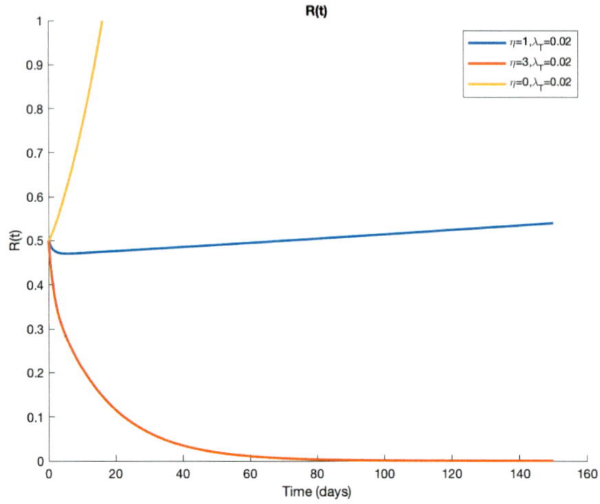

Figure 3.5 Tumor radius $R(t)$ over time for fixed $\lambda_T = 0.02$ and varying η: 0, 1, and 3 and $\overline{B}_0 = 0.7$.

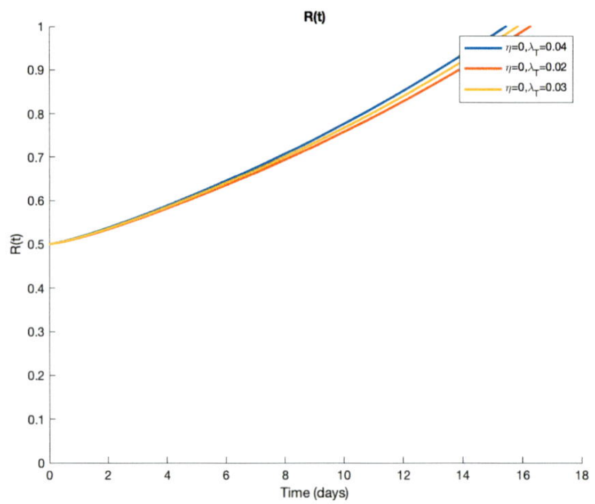

Figure 3.6 Tumor radius $R(t)$ over time for fixed $\eta = 0$ and varying $\lambda_T =$ 0.02, 0.03, and 0.04 and $\overline{B}_0 = 0.7$.

(e.g., $\eta = 3$), $R(t)$ decreases to zero as $t \to \infty$, representing complete tumor eradication by the immune system. Furthermore, for a fixed η, changes in the activation rate of T cells λ_T do not impact whether $R(t)$ increases or decreases, showing that the tumor's fate is governed primarily by the strength of the immune response. Similarly, for a fixed η, changes in the initial conditions of the system do not impact whether $R(t)$ ultimately grows or shrinks, but only influence the transient dynamics before reaching the long-term outcome. It is

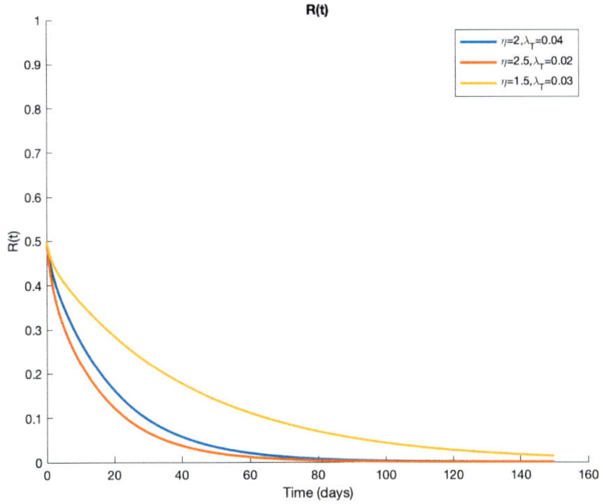

Figure 3.7 Tumor radius $R(t)$ over time for different values of η and λ_T. The curves show $\eta = 2,\ \lambda_T = 0.04$; $\eta = 2.5,\ \lambda_T = 0.02$; and $\eta = 1.5,\ \lambda_T = 0.03$. and $\overline{B}_0 = 0.7$.

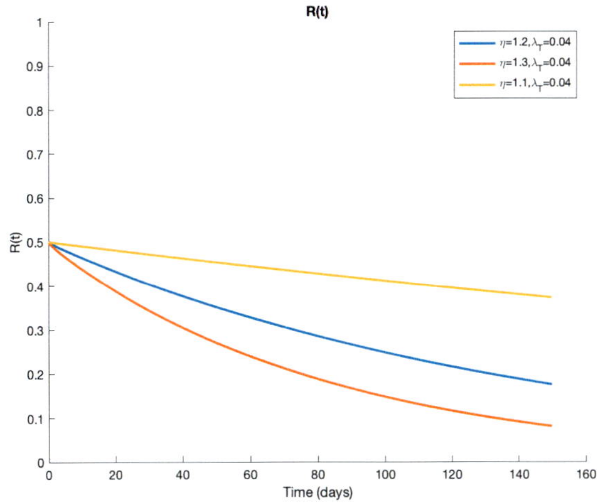

Figure 3.8 $R(t)$ over time for $\eta = 1.1$, 1.2, and 1.3 with fixed $\lambda_T = 0.04$ and and $\overline{B}_0 = 0.5$.

interesting to conduct a detailed analysis to determine a critical value η^* of the killing rate η that separates two distinct behaviors of the tumor:

$$\text{if } \eta > \eta^*, \quad R(t) \to 0 \quad \text{(tumor eradication)},$$

$$\text{if } \eta < \eta^*, \quad R(t) \to \infty \quad \text{(uncontrolled tumor growth)}.$$

While our current simulations already suggest the presence of such a threshold, a more rigorous mathematical and numerical bifurcation analysis would provide a precise characterization of η^* and offer insights into the transition between tumor persistence and elimination.

3.1.3 Model Two: Model with Cancer Cell, T-Cell and Normal Cell

In the case where both N and T are present, and we take

$$C + T + N = 1. \tag{3.115}$$

We assume that C, N and T satisfy the following equations in the domain $\Omega(t)$:

$$\frac{\partial C}{\partial t} + \frac{1}{r^2}\frac{\partial}{\partial r}(r^2 uC) - \frac{1}{r^2}\frac{\partial}{\partial r}(r^2\frac{\partial C}{\partial r}) = \lambda_c C\left(1 - \frac{C+N}{K}\right) - \delta_0 C - \eta TC, \tag{3.116}$$

$$\frac{\partial N}{\partial t} + \frac{1}{r^2}\frac{\partial}{\partial r}(r^2 uN) - \frac{1}{r^2}\frac{\partial}{\partial r}(r^2\frac{\partial N}{\partial r}) = \lambda_N N\left(1 - \frac{C+N}{K}\right) - \delta_0 N, \tag{3.117}$$

$$\frac{\partial T}{\partial t} + \frac{1}{r^2}\frac{\partial}{\partial r}(r^2 uT) - \frac{1}{r^2}\frac{\partial}{\partial r}(r^2\frac{\partial T}{\partial r}) = \lambda_T C - \delta_T T. \tag{3.118}$$

Adding (3.116), (3.117), and (3.118), we get

$$\frac{1}{r^2}\frac{\partial(r^2 u)}{\partial r} = H(C,T), \tag{3.119}$$

where

$$H(C,T) = (\frac{\lambda_C}{K} - \eta - \frac{\lambda_N}{K})CT - \frac{\lambda_N}{K}T^2 + (\lambda_C - \frac{\lambda_C}{K} + \lambda_T - \lambda_N + \frac{\lambda_N}{K})C + (\frac{2\lambda_N}{K} - \lambda_N + \delta_0 - \delta_T)T + (\lambda_N - \frac{\lambda_N}{K} - \delta_0). \tag{3.120}$$

Using $\frac{dR}{dt} = u(R,t)$, we have

$$\frac{dR}{dt} = \frac{1}{R(t)^2}\int_0^{R(t)} s^2 H(C(s,t),T(s,t))ds. \tag{3.121}$$

We assume $\lambda_C > \lambda_N$ and by scaling (3.118), we can set

$$\delta_T = \delta_0. \tag{3.122}$$

Plugging (3.115), and (3.119) into (3.116), and (3.118) we get

$$\frac{\partial C}{\partial t} + u\frac{\partial C}{\partial r} - \frac{1}{r^2}\frac{\partial}{\partial r}(r^2\frac{\partial C}{\partial r}) = G_1(C,T), \tag{3.123}$$

$$\frac{\partial T}{\partial t} + u\frac{\partial T}{\partial r} - \frac{1}{r^2}\frac{\partial}{\partial r}(r^2\frac{\partial T}{\partial r}) = G_2(C,T), \tag{3.124}$$

where $G_1(C,T)$ and $G_2(C,T)$ are given by

$$G_1(C,T) = \frac{\lambda_N}{K}T^2C - (\frac{\lambda_C}{K} - \eta - \frac{\lambda_N}{K})TC^2 - (\lambda_C - \frac{\lambda_C}{K} + \lambda_T - \lambda_N + \frac{\lambda_N}{K})C^2$$
$$+ (\frac{\lambda_C}{K} - \eta - \frac{2\lambda_N}{K} + \lambda_N)TC + (\lambda_C - \lambda_N + \frac{\lambda_N}{K} - \frac{\lambda_C}{K})C. \quad (3.125)$$

$$G_2(C,T) = \frac{\lambda_N}{K}T^3 - (\frac{\lambda_C}{K} - \eta - \frac{\lambda_N}{K})CT^2 - (\lambda_C - \frac{\lambda_C}{K} + \lambda_T - \lambda_N + \frac{\lambda_N}{K})CT$$
$$- (\frac{2\lambda_N}{K} - \lambda_N)T^2 - (\lambda_N - \frac{\lambda_N}{K})T + \lambda_T C. \quad (3.126)$$

We impose zero-flux boundary conditions

$$\frac{\partial C}{\partial r} = 0, \quad \frac{\partial T}{\partial r} = 0 \quad \text{on } r = R(t). \quad (3.127)$$

So Model two is the free boundary problem consisting of (3.121), (3.123), (3.124), and (3.127).

3.1.4 Mathematical Analysis of Model Two

Consider the solution $(C(r,t), T(r,t))$ of the system (3.121)–(3.127). If the initial conditions $C(r,0)$ and $T(r,0)$ are constant in $[0, R(0)]$, then $C(r,t)$ and $T(r,t)$ are independent of r, hence $(C(r,t), T(r,t))$ satisfy the following dynamical system of ODEs:

$$\frac{dC}{dt} = G_1(C,T), \quad \frac{dT}{dt} = G_2(C,T), \quad (3.128)$$

Solving (3.121) we have

$$R(t) = R(t_0)e^{\frac{1}{3}\int_{t_0}^{t} H(C(s),T(s))ds}, \quad (3.129)$$

for any $t_0 \geq 0$. To obtain the phase portraits of the nonlinear dynamical system (3.128), we need to find all fixed points of the system and study their linear stability. Due to the complexity of the system, we focus our analysis for the case where the killing rate η is large.

It is easy to see from (3.125) and (3.126) that $(C = 0, T = 0)$ is a fixed point for all η. Since $\frac{\partial G_1}{\partial C}(0,0) = \left(1 - \frac{1}{K}\right)(\lambda_C - \lambda_N)$, $\frac{\partial G_1}{\partial T}(0,0) = 0, \frac{\partial G_2}{\partial C}(0,0) = \lambda_T$ and $\frac{\partial G_2}{\partial T}(0,0) = \frac{\lambda_N}{K} - \lambda_N$, we find that the Jacobian matrix of the fixed point $(0,0)$ has a positive and negative eigenvalues; hence $(0,0)$ is a saddle point.

Plugging $C = 0$ into $G_2(C,T) = 0$ in (3.126) to obtain:

$$\frac{\lambda_N}{K}T^2 - (\frac{2\lambda_N}{K} - \lambda_N)T - (\lambda_N - \frac{\lambda_N}{K}) = 0$$

We solve the above quadratic equation and obtain $T = 1$ and $T = 1 - K < 0$ which should be dismissed because T has to be positive. Hence $(C = 0, T = 1)$ is the second fixed point.
The Jacobian at the fixed point $(0, 1)$ is

$$J_{(0,1)} = \begin{bmatrix} \lambda_C - \eta & 0 \\ \lambda_N - \lambda_C + \eta & \lambda_N \end{bmatrix}_{(0,1)}$$

which has one positive eigenvalue λ_N and one negative eigenvalue $\lambda_C - \eta$. So the fixed point $(0, 1)$ is also a saddle point.

To find the remaining fixed points, we can write $G_1(C, T) = CL(C, T)$, where

$$\begin{aligned} L(C,T) := \frac{\lambda_N}{K}T^2 - (\frac{\lambda_C}{K} - \eta - \frac{\lambda_N}{K})TC - (\lambda_C - \frac{\lambda_C}{K} + \lambda_T - \lambda_N + \frac{\lambda_N}{K})C \\ +(\frac{\lambda_C}{K} - \eta - \frac{2\lambda_N}{K} + \lambda_N)T + (\lambda_C - \lambda_N + \frac{\lambda_N}{K} - \frac{\lambda_C}{K}). \end{aligned}$$

$L(C, T) = 0$ implies

$$\begin{aligned} \frac{\lambda_N}{K}T^2 = (\frac{\lambda_C}{K} - \eta - \frac{\lambda_N}{K})TC + (\lambda_C - \frac{\lambda_C}{K} + \lambda_T - \lambda_N + \frac{\lambda_N}{K})C \\ -(\frac{\lambda_C}{K} - \eta - \frac{2\lambda_N}{K} + \lambda_N)T - (\lambda_C - \lambda_N + \frac{\lambda_N}{K} - \frac{\lambda_C}{K}) \end{aligned}$$

By plugging the above expression for $\frac{\lambda_N}{K}T^2$ into $G_2(C, T)$ we get

$$-(\frac{\lambda_C}{K} - \eta)T^2 - (\lambda_C - \frac{\lambda_C}{K})T + \lambda_T C = 0.$$

From this equation we get

$$C = \frac{(\frac{\lambda_C}{K} - \eta)T^2 + (\lambda_C - \frac{\lambda_C}{K})T}{\lambda_T}. \tag{3.130}$$

We substitute C value into $L(C, T) = 0$ and obtain

$$\begin{aligned} \frac{\lambda_N}{K}T^2 - (\frac{\lambda_C}{K} - \eta - \frac{\lambda_N}{K})T\Big[\frac{(\frac{\lambda_C}{K} - \eta)T^2 + (\lambda_C - \frac{\lambda_C}{K})T}{\lambda_T}\Big] \\ -(\lambda_C - \frac{\lambda_C}{K} + \lambda_T - \lambda_N + \frac{\lambda_N}{K})\Big[\frac{(\frac{\lambda_C}{K} - \eta)T^2 + (\lambda_C - \frac{\lambda_C}{K})T}{\lambda_T}\Big] \\ +(\frac{\lambda_C}{K} - \eta - \frac{2\lambda_N}{K} + \lambda_N)T + (\lambda_C - \lambda_N + \frac{\lambda_N}{K} - \frac{\lambda_C}{K}) = 0. \end{aligned} \tag{3.131}$$

By using ansatz $T = \beta + \frac{\gamma}{\eta} + \frac{\omega}{\eta^2} + O(\frac{1}{\eta^3})$ as $\eta \to \infty$, we find that (3.131) has a solution

$$T_0 = \frac{(\lambda_C - \lambda_N)(1 - \frac{1}{K})}{\eta} + \frac{(\lambda_C - \lambda_N)^2 \frac{1}{K}(1 - \frac{1}{K})}{\eta^2} + O(\frac{1}{\eta^3}). \tag{3.132}$$

Plugging T_0 into (3.130), we obtain that

$$C_0 = \frac{(\lambda_C - \lambda_N)(1-\frac{1}{K})^2\lambda_N}{\lambda_T\eta} + \frac{\frac{2\lambda_N}{K}(\lambda_C-\lambda_N)^2(1-\frac{1}{K})^2}{\lambda_T\eta^2} + O(\frac{1}{\eta^3}). \quad (3.133)$$

So (C_0, T_0) is the third fixed point if η is sufficiently large and $\lambda_C > \lambda_N$.

Taking partial derivatives of $G_1(C,T)$ and $G_2(C,T)$ in (3.125) and (3.126), and using (3.132) and (3.133), we obtain the Jacobian at the third fixed point (C_0, T_0):

$$J = \begin{pmatrix} -\frac{(\lambda_C-\lambda_N)\lambda_N(1-\frac{1}{K})^2}{\eta} + O(\frac{1}{\eta^2}) & -\frac{(\lambda_C-\lambda_N)(1-\frac{1}{K})^2\lambda_N}{\lambda_T} + O(\frac{1}{\eta}) \\ \lambda_T - \frac{(\lambda_C-\lambda_N)\lambda_T(1-\frac{1}{K})}{\eta} + O(\frac{1}{\eta^2}) & -(1-\frac{1}{K})\lambda_N + O(\frac{1}{\eta}) \end{pmatrix}.$$

By straight computation, we have

$$\left|\rho I - J_{(C_0,T_0)}\right| = \rho^2 + \tilde{A}\rho + \tilde{B}; \quad (3.134)$$

where

$$\tilde{A} = (1-\frac{1}{K})\lambda_N + O(\frac{1}{\eta}), \quad (3.135)$$

and

$$\tilde{B} = \lambda_N(\lambda_C - \lambda_N)(1-\frac{1}{K})^2 + O(\frac{1}{\eta}). \quad (3.136)$$

So the two eigenvalues of $J_{(C_0,T_0)}$ are

$$\rho_1 = -\frac{\tilde{A}}{2} - \frac{\sqrt{\tilde{A}^2 - 4\tilde{A}\tilde{B}}}{2}, \quad \rho_2 = -\frac{\tilde{A}}{2} + \frac{\sqrt{\tilde{A}^2 - 4\tilde{A}\tilde{B}}}{2}, \quad (3.137)$$

We can easily see from (3.135) and (3.136) that $\tilde{A} > 0$ and $\tilde{B} > 0$ for sufficiently large η, so $Re\ \rho_1 < 0$ and $Re\ \rho_2 < 0$ from (3.137); therefore the fixed point (C_0, T_0) is asymptotically stable.

Theorem 3.13 *For any sufficiently large η, there exists a small $\epsilon > 0$ such that if $C(t), T(t)$ and $R(t)$ is a solution of the system (3.128)–(3.129) with $|C(0) - C_0| < \epsilon$ and $|T(0) - T_0| < \epsilon$, then $C(t) \to C_0, T(t) \to T_0$ and*
(1) $R(t) \to 0$ as $t \to \infty$, if $\lambda_N(1-\frac{1}{K}) - \delta_0 < 0$;
(2) $R(t) \to \infty$ as $t \to \infty$, if $\lambda_N(1-\frac{1}{K}) - \delta_0 > 0$.

Proof. Since the fixed point (C_0, T_0) is stable, there exists a small $\epsilon > 0$ such that if $(C(t), T(t))$ is a solution of the system (3.128)–(3.129) with $C(0) = C_0 < \epsilon$ and $T(0) < \epsilon$, then $C(t) \to C_0, T(t) \to T_0$ as $t \to \infty$. Using (3.120), we have $H(C(t), T(t)) \to H(C_0, T_0) = \lambda_N(1-\frac{1}{K}) - \delta_0$. so there exists large $t_0 > 0$ so that $H(C(t), T(t)) \le \frac{\lambda_N(1-\frac{1}{K})-\delta_0}{2}$ as $t > t_0$ if $\lambda_N(1-\frac{1}{K}) - \delta_0 < 0$; or $H(C(t), T(t)) \ge \frac{\lambda_N(1-\frac{1}{K})-\delta_0}{2}$ as $t > t_0$ if $\lambda_N(1-\frac{1}{K}) - \delta_0 > 0$. It follows from (3.128) that $R(t) \to 0$ as $t \to \infty$ if $\lambda_N(1-\frac{1}{K}) - \delta_0 < 0$; or $R(t) \to \infty$ as $t \to \infty$, if $\lambda_N(1-\frac{1}{K}) - \delta_0 > 0$. ■

Remark 3.14 *The above theorem shows that if the initial density of the cancer cells is small and the density of T cells is small, then the tumor will eventually disappear if the kill rate η is large and the growth rate of the normal cell is larger than the death rate of the cancer cell. However, if the growth rate of the normal cell is less than the death rate of the cancer cell, then the tumor will eventually grow exponentially even if the killing rate is large.*

It is to be noted that Theorem 3.13 seems to be a surprise in contrast with Theorem 3.5. Theorem says that as long as η is large enough, the T cells in model one always kill the cancer cell and the tumor will shrink for any initial condition. As established for models in [120, 121], increasing the killing rate does not always decrease the cancer; on the contrary, it may increase the cancer. Theorem 3.8 demonstrates the same point for the model two.

Figure 3.9 shows the phase portrait of the system (3.128) with $\lambda_C = 1$, $\lambda_N = 0.5$, $\lambda_T = 0.1$, $K = 10$, $\eta = 10$ on the (C, T)-plane using MATLAB. The three fixed points are $(0,\ 0)$, $(0,\ 1)$ and $(C_0,\ T_0) = (0.2045,\ 0.0452)$. Numerical simulation confirms the local stability analysis of the fixed points. Moreover, when the initial conditions are in the range $0.05 < C(0) \leq 0.4$, $0.2 < T(0) < 0.5$, the trajectories go to the fixed point $(0, 0)$ as $t \to \infty$. When the initial conditions are in the range $0.05 < C(0) \leq 0.4$, $0.7 < T(0) < 0.9$, the trajectories go to the fixed point $(0, 1)$ as $t \to \infty$. The trajectories go to the fixed point (C_0, T_0) as $t \to \infty$ if the initial conditions are in the range $0.025 < C(0) \leq 0.4$, $0.1 < T(0) < 0.2$.

3.1.5 A More Comprehensive Cancer Model

We should point out that Model one and Model two in previous sections are relatively simple, they only include a limited variables such as the cancer cells, T cells and normal cells. The interaction between cancer and immune system is complex. T lymphocytes are usually divided into two types: $CD4^+$ T cells and $CD8^+$ T cells. $CD8^+$ T cells are involved in killing cancer cells while $CD4^+$ T cells affect other cells and cytokines of the immune system such as IL-12, IL-2, and TGF-β. We refer to [110, 120, 121, 177] for more comprehensive cancer models. Nevertheless, the simple models are suitable for rigorous analysis and can shed new lights on certain biological processes.
As discussed in [110], a comprehensive cancer model can be described by a system of parabolic equation in a domain $\{(x, t) : x \in \Omega(t), t > 0\}$:

$$\frac{\partial X_i}{\partial t} + \nabla \cdot (\mathbf{u} X_i) - \delta_{X_i} \nabla^2 X_i = F_i(X, c), \tag{3.138}$$

$$\frac{\partial c}{\partial t} - \delta_c \nabla^2 c = -\Sigma_{i=1}^{m} \lambda_i X_i c, \tag{3.139}$$

where $X = (X_1, X_1 \ldots, X_n), \theta_i = 1$ for $1 \geq i \leq m$ and $\theta_i = 0$ for $m+1 \geq i \leq n$. Here X_i for $1 \geq i \leq m$, represents the density of a species of cells, and X_i for $m + 1 \geq i \leq n$ is the concentration of species of cytokines or other molecules;

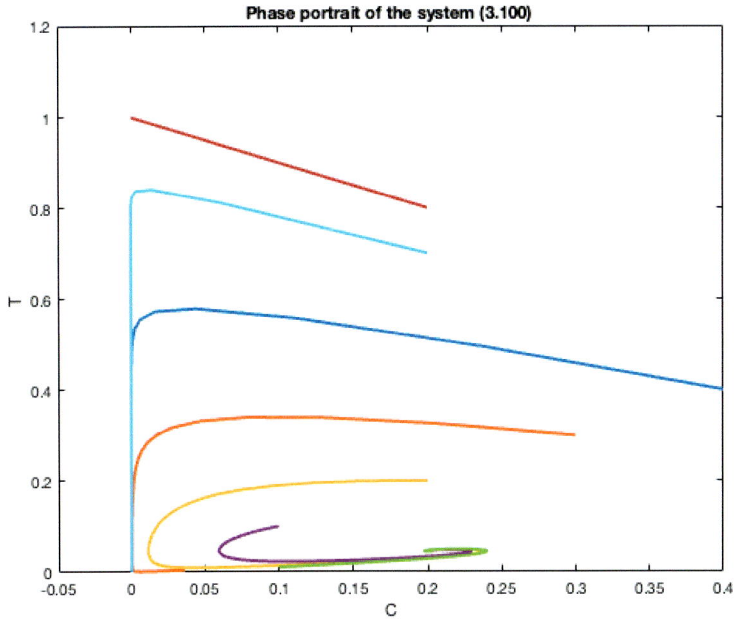

Figure 3.9 The phase portrait of the system (3.128) with $\lambda_C = 1, \lambda_N = 0.5, \lambda_T = 0.1, K = 10, \eta = 10; C_0 = 0.2045, T_0 = 0.0452$.

c is the concentration of nutrients consumed by the cells. We assume that all the cells move with the same velocity $\mathbf{u}$ and that the total density of all cells in $\Omega(t)$ is constant

$$\Sigma_{i=1}^{m} X_i(x,t) = 1 \text{ for } x \in \Omega(t), t > 0. \tag{3.140}$$

By adding Eq. (3.138) for $1 \geq i \leq m$ and using (3.140), we have

$$\nabla \cdot \mathbf{u} = H(X,c), \tag{3.141}$$

where

$$H(X,c) = \Sigma_{i=1}^{m} F_i(X,c). \tag{3.142}$$

The velocity $\mathbf{u}$ results from that Eq. (3.140) gives rise to an internal pressure among the cells. We assume that this pressure, p, is related to $\mathbf{u}$ by Darcy's law

$$\mathbf{u} = -\nabla p. \tag{3.143}$$

From Eqs. (3.141) and (3.143) we conclude that

$$-\nabla^2 p = H(X,c). \tag{3.144}$$

We prescribe boundary conditions on the free boundary $\partial\Omega(t)$:

$$\alpha_i \delta_{X_i} \frac{\partial X_i}{\partial n} + (1-\alpha_i)(X_i - \bar{X}_i) = 0 (1 \le i \le n) \tag{3.145}$$

$$\alpha_c \frac{\partial c}{\partial n} + (1-\alpha_c)(c - \bar{c}_i) = 0, \tag{3.146}$$

where $\frac{\partial}{\partial n}$ is the derivative in the direction of outward normal $\mathbf{n}$, $0 \le \alpha_i \le 1$, $0 \le \alpha_c \le 1$, $\bar{X}_i(x,t) \ge 0, \bar{c}(x,t) \ge 0$ for all $x \in \mathbf{R}^3, t > 0$, and, to be consistent with (3.143),

$$\Sigma_{i=1}^m \bar{X}_i(x,t) = 1 \text{ for } x \in \mathbf{R}^3, t > 0. \tag{3.147}$$

We prescribe the boundary condition for the pressure p:

$$p = \gamma\kappa \ (\gamma > 0) \tag{3.148}$$

where κ is the mean curvature on $\partial\Omega(t)$; $\kappa > 0$ if $\Omega(t)$ is a sphere.
we assume that the boundary $\partial\Omega(t)$ is moving with the velocity of the cells, so that

$$V_n = \mathbf{u} \cdot \mathbf{n} = -\frac{\partial p}{\partial n}. \tag{3.149}$$

We next prescribe the initial conditions:

$$X_i|_{t=0} = X_i^0(x), c|_{t=0} = c_0 \text{ for } x \in \Omega(0), \tag{3.150}$$

and assume that $X_i^0(x) \ge 0, c_0 \ge 0$ and, to be consistent with (3.143),

$$\Sigma_{i=1}^m \bar{X}_i^0(x) = 1 \text{ for } x \in \Omega(0). \tag{3.151}$$

In the case where $\Omega(t)$ and all the variables are radially symmetric, so that

$$X_i = X(r,t), c = c(r,t), \Omega(t) = \{0 \le r \le R(t)\}$$

and $\mathbf{u} = u\mathbf{e}_r = \frac{x}{|x|}$. In this case

$$\frac{dR(t)}{dt} = u(R(t),t), \tag{3.152}$$

and

$$\frac{1}{r^2}\frac{\partial}{\partial r}(r^2 u) = H(X,c). \tag{3.153}$$

So far we assumed that the tumor tissue has the structure of a porous media. But some cancer tissues are more fluid-like, so it makes more sense to assume that they satisfy the Stokes equations for viscous fluid rather than the Darcy law. The relation between the velocity $\mathbf{u}$ and the pressure p is

$$\nabla p - \mu\nabla^2\mathbf{u} - \frac{1}{3}\nabla(\text{ div } \mathbf{u}) = 0 \text{ in } \Omega(t), t > 0 \tag{3.154}$$

where μ is the viscosity coefficient. Introducing the stress sensor

$$T = \mu(\nabla \mathbf{u} + (\nabla \mathbf{u})^*) - (p + \frac{2\mu}{3}\nabla \cdot \mathbf{u})I, \tag{3.155}$$

where $*$ means the transpose of a matrix and I is the identity matrix, the boundary condition (3.148) is replaced by

$$T\mathbf{n} = -\kappa\, \mathbf{n}. \tag{3.156}$$

$$V_n = \mathbf{u} \cdot \mathbf{n} = -\frac{\partial p}{\partial n}. \tag{3.157}$$

We next prescribe the initial conditions:

$$X_i|_{t=0} = X_i^0(x), c|_{t=0} = c_0 \text{ for } x \in \Omega(0), \tag{3.158}$$

3.1.6 Analysis and Simulation of the Comprehensive Cancer Model

There are several mathematical issues to analyze the comprehensive model (3.138)–(3.151):

- Prove existense, uniqueness, and regularity for the model
- Study the regularity and geometric features of the free boundary $\partial\Omega(t), t > 0$.
- Determine whether there exist steady solutions, and study their asymptotic stability.

Theorem 3.15 *Given any smooth functions $F_i(X, c)$, smooth surface $\partial(0)$ and smooth initial and boundary conditions satisfying the standard compability conditions at $\partial\Omega(0)$, there exists a unique smooth solution of the system (3.138)–(3.151) for some time interval $0 \le t \le T, T > 0$.*

There are two ways to prove the theorem. One way of proof is to use fixed point argument as in [62] and we used the same way to prove Theorem 3.4 in section 3.1.2.3. The another way to prove this theorem is to use the analytic semigroup theory as in [76, 81, 191], and we used this way to obtain the existence theorem of the diabetic atherosclerosis model in Chapter two. To prove the non-negativeness of the solution, we can apply the maximum principal or the comparison principal if the $F_i(X, c)$ have some specific structure. The global existence will depend on whether priori bounds can be found for the derivatives of the variables and the free boundary.
The existence of steady solutions to the comprehensive system and their stability is difficult for the case where $n \ge 2$. In the following we review some results for simplified systems.

Special system (n=1)

When $n = 1$, we take that $X_1 = C = 1$, C is the density of the cancer cell, and we assume that

$$F_1(C, c) = C\lambda_C(c), \lambda_C(c) = \mu(c - \tilde{c}), \tag{3.159}$$

where $\mu > 0$.

From (3.142), $H(X, c) = \lambda_C(c) = \mu(c-\tilde{c})$. By (3.139) with $\delta_c = 1$ and (3.144), we have

$$\frac{\partial c}{\partial t} - \nabla^2 c = -c, \tag{3.160}$$

$$-\nabla^2 p = \mu(c - \tilde{c}). \tag{3.161}$$

We prescribe the boundary conditions on $\partial\Omega(t)$:

$$c = \bar{c}, \tag{3.162}$$

$$p = \kappa \ (\gamma = 1) \tag{3.163}$$

$$V_n = -\frac{\partial p}{\partial n}. \tag{3.164}$$

We next prescribe the initial conditions:

$$c|_{t=0} = c_0(x), 0 \leq c_0(x) \leq \bar{c}, \text{ for } x \in \Omega(0). \tag{3.165}$$

In the radially symmetric case,we get the following equation for the free boundary:

$$\frac{dR(t)}{dt} = \frac{\mu}{R^2(t)} \int_0^{R(t)} r^2(c(r,t) - \tilde{c})dr. \tag{3.166}$$

Theorem 3.16 *[124] In the radially case, the system (3.160)–(3.166) has a unique global solution.*

In the stationary case, $c = c(r), p = p(r)$ and (3.166) becomes a equation for R:

$$\int_0^R r^2(c(r,t) - \tilde{c})dr. \tag{3.167}$$

Theorem 3.17 *[124] There exists a unique radially symmetric steady solution of the system (3.160)–(3.166), given by*

$$c(r) = \bar{c}\frac{R}{\sinh R}\frac{\sinh r}{r}, p(r) = A - \mu c(r) + \frac{\mu}{6}\tilde{c}r^2, \tag{3.168}$$

where $A = \frac{1}{R} + \mu - \frac{mu}{6}\tilde{c}R^2$, *and the radius* R *is the unique solution of the equation*

$$\tanh R = \frac{R}{1 + BR^2}, B = \frac{\tilde{c}}{3\bar{c}}. \tag{3.169}$$

Note that R is independent of μ. Hence there is a family of radially symmetric steady solutions $(c(r), p(r,\mu), R)$ depending on the parameter μ with the same tumor radius R. The following questions arise: For which values of μ the spherical tumor is stable? are there bifurcation branches of non-spherical solutions iniating from some values of μ? The answers are given in the following two theorems.

Theorem 3.18 *[125,126] For any integer $m \geq 2$ there is a bifurcation branch of stationary solutions with free boundary*

$$r = R + \epsilon Y_{m,0}(\theta) + O(\epsilon^2)$$

and parameter

$$\mu = M_m + \epsilon M_{m,1} + O(\epsilon^2),$$

for any small ϵ, where $Y_{m,0}(\theta)$ is the spherical harmonics of mode $(m, 0)$,

$$M_m = \frac{1}{2} \frac{(m-1)(m+2)}{R^5 P_0(R)[P_1(R) - P_m(R)]},$$

$$P_k(r) = I_{k+3/2}(r)/[rI_{k+1/2}(y)],$$

and $I_n(r)$ is the modified Bessel function of order n.

Theorem 3.19 *[115,117] There exists a positive number μ such that a radially symmetric steady solution, in (3.168), is asymptotically stable if $\mu < \mu_*$ and not linearly stable if $\mu > \mu_*$. Furthermore*

$$\mu_* < M_2 \text{ if } R < R_* \text{ and } \mu_* = M_2 \text{ if } R > R_*$$

for some $R_* > 0$, and in the first case the linearized problem about the steady solution exhibits a Hopf bifurcation type behavior.
The numbers μ_* and R_* are solutions of explicit transcendental equations. In the case where $\mu_* = M_2$ the ϵ-bifurcation branch is linearly stable if $\epsilon > 0$ and unstable if $\epsilon < 0$.

Theorems 3.13–3.15 have been extended in [155, 156] to the case where the boundary condition $c = \bar{c}$ in (3.162) is replaced by the flux condition

$$\frac{\partial c}{\partial n} + \alpha(c - \bar{c}) = 0(\alpha > 0)$$

We now consider the case where the boundary condition $c = \bar{c}$ in (3.162) is replaced by the flux condition

$$\frac{\partial c}{\partial n} + \alpha(t)(c - \bar{c}) = 0 \text{ on } \partial\Omega(t), t > 0 \tag{3.170}$$

where $\alpha(t) > 0$. The interpretation of the condition is that nutrients with concentration $\bar{c}$ outside the tumor are attracted to and fluxed into the tumor, for example by angiogenesis promoted by VEGF.

Theorem 3.20 *[123] Consider the radially symmetric solution of the system (3.159)–(3.164) with (3.162) replaced by (3.170). Then, the following assertions hold: (i) if* $\mu(\bar{c}-\tilde{c}) < 1$ *then* $R(t) \in L^\infty[0,\infty)$ *whenever* $\alpha(t) \in L^\infty[0,\infty)$, *and* $\lim_{t\to\infty} R(t) = 0$ *whenever* $\lim_{t\to\infty} \alpha(t) = 0$.
(ii) if $\liminf t \to \infty\alpha(t) > 0$ *then* $\liminf t \to \infty R(t) > \delta_0$, *where* δ_0 *is a positive constant independent of the initial data.*

It is to be noted that for similar systems (including multi-layer problem,elliptic system, elliptic-hyperbolic system) to (3.159)–(3.164) under various boundary conditions (including nonlinear boundary conditions), there have been a plenty of recent literature on stationary solutions, their bifurcation and their stability [86, 181, 241, 285, 287, 306–310, 313].

There have been also works on the stationary solutions for systems with Stokes equations (3.154)–(3.157), see [116, 286].

There are fewer rigorous analysis for the case where $n > 1$, instead numerical simulations are important tools to gain insights into these systems [120, 177, 178, 190].

3.2 CANCER THERAPY

Cancer remains one of the leading causes of death worldwide, prompting the exploration of innovative treatment strategies. Among these, immunotherapy and oncolytic virotherapy have shown remarkable clinical success. Mathematical models provide a systematic framework for studying complex biological interactions within tumors, immune responses, and therapeutic interventions. The integration of such models with experimental and clinical data holds promise for enhancing treatment efficacy and personalizing cancer care.

Mathematical models of cancer immunotherapy commonly employ ordinary differential equations (ODEs)or partial differential equations (PDEs) to describe the interactions between tumor cells, immune cells, and cytokines. Checkpoint inhibitors (e.g., anti-TEGF, anti-PD1, anti-CTLA4) enhance T-cell responses. Inhibitor Models incorporate inhibition of tumor-induced immune suppression. Models of CAR-T cell therapy include dynamics of engineered T-cell proliferation, exhaustion, and cytotoxicity against tumor cells. Cytokine therapy models explore the effects of agents such as IL-2 on immune activation and associated toxicities.

Oncolytic virotherapy employs viruses engineered to selectively infect and kill cancer cells. Mathematical models typically involve variables such as uninfected tumor cells, infected tumor cells and free virus particles. ODE and PDE models of these variables incorporate the immune response to both the tumor and the virus, modeling innate and adaptive immunity, which can significantly influence therapy outcomes.

Combining immunotherapy with oncolytic virotherapy can produce synergistic effects: viruses lyse tumor cells and release antigens, enhancing immune recognition and response. Combined models feature virus-induced oncolysis, immune system priming and amplification, and interactions between viral dynamics, immune activation, and tumor growth.

3.2.1 Immunotherapy

In this section, we introduce two models in immunotherapy. One PDE model describes anti-vascular endothelial growth factor (anti-VEGF) which is a drug commonly used as anticancer agent; One ODE model decribes IL-2-based cancer immunotherapy [95].

3.2.1.1 VEGF Inhibitor Model

We are going to introduce a VEGF inhibitor model which is a simplified version of the model in [178].

The mathematical model is based on the network shown in Fig. 3.10. The variables are as follows:
D: density of dendritic cells; E: density of endothelial cells; C: density of cancer cells; T: density of T cells; W: oxygen concentration; G: VEGF concentration; B: anti-VEGF concentration.

We assume that the total density of cells within the tumor remains constant throughout the tumor tissue, for all time:

$$D + T + E + C = constant, \tag{3.171}$$

Equation for DCs
Dendritic cells are activated by HMGB-1. Hence, the activation rate of immature dendritic cells, with density D_0, is proportional to $\frac{C}{K_C+C}$. Here, the Michaelis-Menten law was used to account for the limited rate of receptor recycling which takes place in the process of DCs activation. The dynamics of DCs is given by the following equation:

$$\frac{\partial D}{\partial t} + \nabla \cdot (\mathbf{u}D) - \delta_D \nabla^2 D = D_0 \frac{C}{K_C + C} \cdot \frac{1}{(1 + G/K_{DG})} - d_D D, \tag{3.172}$$

where δ_D is the diffusion coefficient, d_D is the death rate of DCs, and $1/(1 + G/K_{DG})$ represents the impairment of maturation of dendritic cells by VEGF.

Equations for T cells
Both processes of activation and proliferation of T cell are assumed to be inhibited by VEGF, but is enhanced by IL-2. Hence T1 satisfies the following equation:

$$\frac{\partial T}{\partial t} + \nabla \cdot (\mathbf{u}T) - \delta_T \nabla^2 T = \hat{T}_{10} \frac{1}{(1 + G/K_{TG})} + \hat{\lambda}_{TI_2} T - d_T T, \tag{3.173}$$

where $\hat{T}_{10}$ is the density of T cells impacted by IL-12.

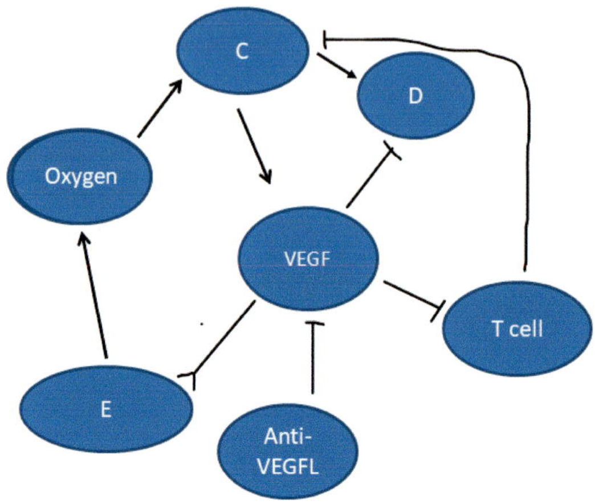

Figure 3.10 Interaction of immune cells with cancer cells. Sharp arrows indicate proliferation/activation, blocked arrows indicate killing/blocking, and the inverted arrow indicates recruitment/chemoattraction. C: cancer cells, D: dentritic cells, T cells, E: endothelial cells.

Equation for endothelial cells (E)

Endothelial cells are chemoattracted by VEGF, and their proliferation is increased by VEGF. The equation for the density of endothelial cells is given by

$$\frac{\partial E}{\partial t}+\nabla\cdot(\mathbf{u}E)-\delta_E\nabla^2E=\lambda_E(G)E(1-E/E_M)+\nabla\cdot(\chi_G E\nabla G)-d_ET, \quad (3.174)$$

where E_M is the carrying capacity of endothelial cells, $\lambda_E(G) = \lambda_{EG}(G-G_0)^+$, and G_0 is a threshold below which endothelial cells do not proliferate. Here we used the notion: $X^+ = X$ if $X \geq 0$ and $X^+ = 0$ if $X < 0$.

Equation for cancer cells

We assume a logistic growth for cancer cells, with carrying capacity (C_M), in order to account for competition for space among these cells. The proliferation rate depends on the density of oxygen (W). The equation for C takes the following form:

$$\frac{\partial C}{\partial t}+\nabla\cdot(\mathbf{u}C)-\delta_C\nabla^2C=\lambda_C(W)C(1-C/C_M)-\eta TC-d_CC, \quad (3.175)$$

where η is the killing rates of cancer cells by T cells, d_C is the natural death rate of cancer cells, and

$$\lambda_C(W) = \lambda_{CW} \times \begin{cases} W/W_0 \text{ if } W \leq W_0 \\ 1 \text{ if } W_0 < W, \end{cases} \tag{3.176}$$

where W_0 is the normal level of oxygen concentration in the blood.

Equation for oxygen (W)

Oxygen is infused through the blood. We identify the blood concentration with the density of endothelial cells and, accordingly, write the equation for W in the following form:

$$\frac{\partial W}{\partial t} - \delta_W \nabla^2 W = \lambda_{WE} E - d_W W, \tag{3.177}$$

where $d_W W$ represents the take-up rate of oxygen by all the cells.

Equation for VEGF (G)

VEGF is produced by cancer cells and is depleted by anti-VEGF. Hence G satisfies the following equation:

$$\frac{\partial G}{\partial t} - \delta_G \nabla^2 G = \lambda_G(W)C - \mu_{GB} GB - d_G G, \tag{3.178}$$

where B is the effective anti-VEGF concentration in the tumor, and

$$\lambda_G(W) = \lambda_{GW} \times \begin{cases} W/W^* \text{ if } 0 \leq W \leq W^* \\ 1 - 0.7\frac{W-W^*}{W_0-W^*} \text{ if } W^* < W \leq W_0 \\ 0.3 \text{ if } W > W_0. \end{cases} \tag{3.179}$$

Here we assumed that the secretion rate of VEGF by cancer cells increases with the oxygen level, but falls off when oxygen level exceeds a certain level, W^*.

Equation for anti-VEGF (B)

We denote by γ_B the concentration of the injected drug B during the dosing period, and by μ_{BG} the depletion rate of B blocking VEGF. The equation for B is then given by

$$\frac{\partial B}{\partial t} - \delta_B \nabla^2 B = \gamma_B I_B(t) - \mu_{BG} GB - d_B B, \tag{3.180}$$

where $I_B(t) = 1$ during dosing, and $I_B(t) = 0$ otherwise.

Equation for cells velocity (u)

We assume that the density of each cell type in the growing tumor tends to a steady state, and take the density of the extracellular matrix (ECM) in steady state to be 0.6 g/cm3. We take the steady state density of endothelial cells to be $E = 2.5 \times 10^{-3}$ g/cm3. The steady state densities of the immune cells D, T and C (in units of g/cm3) are taken to be (see Parameter estimation)

$$D = 4 \times 10^{-4}, T = 1 \times 10^{-3}, C = 0.4. \tag{3.181}$$

With these choices, the constant in Eq. (3.171) equal to 0.4014. We further assume that all cells have approximately the same diffusion coefficient. Adding Eqs. (3.172)–(3.176), we get

$$0.4014\nabla \cdot \mathbf{u} = \text{ Sum of RHS of Eqs. (3.172)–(3.176)} \tag{3.182}$$

To simplify the computations, we assume that the tumor is spherical and denote its radius by $r = R(t)$. We also assume that all the densities and concentrations are radially symmetric, that is, they are functions of (r, t), where $0 \geq r \leq R(t)$. In particular, $\mathbf{u} = u(r, t)\mathbf{e}_r$, where $\mathbf{e}_r$ is the unit radial vector.

Equation for free boundary (R)

We assume that the free boundary r = R(t) moves with the velocity of the cells, so that

$$\frac{dR(t)}{dt} = u(R(t), t). \tag{3.183}$$

Boundary conditions

We assume that the naive T cells which migrated from the lymph nodes into the tumor microenvironment have constant densitie $\hat{T}$ at the tumor's boundary, and, that upon crossing the tumor boundary, T are activated by IL-12. We then have the following flux conditions at the tumor's boundary:

$$\frac{\partial T}{\partial r} + \sigma_T(T - \hat{T}) = 0, \text{ at } r = R(t), \tag{3.184}$$

where $\sigma_T > 0$ is constant.

We assume that the endothelial cells that are attracted by the VEGF into the tumor microenvironment have constant density $\hat{E}$ at the tumor's boundary, and take

$$\frac{\partial E}{\partial r} + \sigma_E \frac{G}{K_G + G}(E - \hat{E}) = 0, \text{ at } r = R(t), \tag{3.185}$$

The boundary condition for the oxygen is given by

$$\frac{\partial W}{\partial r} + \sigma_W(W - W_0) = 0, \text{ at } r = R(t), \tag{3.186}$$

where W_0 is the normal level of oxygen concentration in the blood. We impose no-flux boundary condition for all the remaining variables:

$$\text{No-flux for D,C,G, and B at } r = R(t). \tag{3.187}$$

Initial conditions
We take the following initial values (in units of g/cm3):

$$\begin{aligned} &D = 2 \times 10^{-3}, T = 4 \times 10^{-3}, E = 2.45 \times 10^{-3}, C = 0.39565, \\ &W = 1.52 \times 10^{-4}, G = 6.3 \times 10^{-8}, R(0) = 0.01cm. \end{aligned} \tag{3.188}$$

Note that the total density of cells at time t = 0 satisfies Eq. (3.171) with the already chosen constant 0.4014. We also mention that the choice of initial conditions does not affect the simulation results after a few days.

3.2.1.2 IL-2-Based Cancer Immunotherapy

The cytokine interleukin-2 (IL-2) was discovered more than 40 years ago as a T cell growth factor. IL-2-based immunotherapies are currently in clinical trials for many types of cancer and autoimmune diseases.

We choose four basic and significant components in IL-2 immunotherapy, namely, IL-2, $CD4^+$ T cells, $CD8^+$ T cells , and tumor cells; We denote these variables by
$I(t)$ (IUs—international units): the concentration of IL-2 at time t,
$C(t)$ (cells): the number of tumor cells at time t,
$T_1(t)$ (cells): the number of $CD4^+$ T cells at time t,
$T_2(t)$ (cells): the number of $CD8^+$ T cells and Natural Killer (NK) cells at time t.

$CD4^+$ T cells have seven subsets, and their main function is the production of IL-2. $CD8^+$ T cells have two subsets and their main function is to kill tumor cells. Natural killer cells (NK) express intermediate affinity receptors, as do $CD8^+$ T cells, and natural killer cells will also directly kill tumor cells. Therefore, we consider natural killer cells and $CD8^+$ T cells as a single population and call them CD8+ T cells for convenience.

In the absence of immune responses and treatments, tumor growth is modeled by a logistic function. Killing tumor cells by CD8+ T cells and natural killer cells is modeled by the law of mass action, a quadratic term. CD4+ T cells produce IL-2, and the production rate is assumed to be proportional to the number of CD4+ T cells. The average lifetime of IL-2 is indicated by $\frac{1}{\mu_0}$. IL-2 treatment is indicated by s. Stimulation of immune cells including $CD4^+$ and $CD8^+$ T cells by tumor cells is also modeled by the law of mass action. IL-2 enhances the activities of $CD8^+$ T cells and natural killer cells; we model this enhanced effect by the Michaelis-Menten law. These interactions are illustrated in Fig. 3.11.

The following system of ordinary differential equations is proposed for IL-2 immunotherapy.

TABLE 3.2 Parameters' description and value

Parameters	Description	Value
δ_D	diffusion coefficient for DCs	$8.64 \times 10^{-7}\, cm^2\ d^{-1}$ [178]
δ_T	diffusion coefficient for T cells	$8.64 \times 10^{-7}\, cm^2\ d^{-1}$ [178]
δ_E	diffusion coefficient for endothelial cells	$8.64 \times 10^{-7}\, cm^2\ d^{-1}$ [178]
δ_C	diffusion coefficient for cancer cells	$8.64 \times 10^{-7}\, cm^2\ d^{-1}$ [178]
δ_W	diffusion coefficient for Oxygen	$0.8\, cm^2\ d^{-1}$ [178]
δ_G	diffusion coefficient for VGEF	$8.64 \times 10^{-2}\, cm^2\ d^{-1}$ [178]
δ_B	diffusion coefficient for anti-VGEF	$4.70 \times 10^{-2}\, cm^2\ d^{-1}$ [178]
χ_G	Chemoattraction coefficient of VEGF	$10, g^{-1}\, cm^5\ d^{-1}$ [178]
σ_T	Flux rate of T cells at the boundary	$1 cm^{-1}$ [178]
σ_E	Flux rate of endothelial cells at the boundary	$1 cm^{-1}$ [178]
σ_W	Flux rate of Oxygen at the boundary	$1 cm^{-1}$ [178]
λ_{DC}	Activation rate of DCs by tumor cells (mice)	$17.5\ d^{-1}$ estimated
λ_{DC}	Activation rate of DCs by tumor cells (humans)	$7.5\ d^{-1}$ estimated
$\hat{\lambda}_{TI_2}$	Activation rate of T cells by IL-2	$4.16 \times 10^{-2}\ d^{-1}$ estimated
λ_{EG}	Growth rate of endothelial cells (mice)	$2.77 \times 10^7\ cm^3\, g^{-1}\ d^{-1}$ estimated
λ_{EG}	Growth rate of endothelial cells (humans)	$2.08 \times 10^7\ cm^3\, g^{-1}\ d^{-1}$ estimated
λ_{CW}	Growth rate of cancer cells (mice)	$2.24\ d^{-1}$ estimated
λ_{CW}	Growth rate of cancer cells (humans)	$1.76\ d^{-1}$ estimated
λ_{WE}	Production rate of oxygen by endothelial cells	$0.07\ d^{-1}$ estimated
λ_{GW}	Production rate of VEGF by cancer cells	$2.21 \times 10^{-6}\ d^{-1}$ [147]

TABLE 3.3 Parameters' description and value

Parameters	Description	Value
d_D	death rate of DCs	$0.1\ d^{-1}$ [178]
d_T	death rate of T cells	$0.197\ d^{-1}$ [178]
d_E	death rate of endothelial cells	$0.69\ d^{-1}$ [178]
d_C	death rate of tumor cells	$0.17\ d^{-1}$ [178]
d_W	take up rate by cells	$1.04\ d^{-1}$ [178]
d_G	degradation rate of VEGF	$0.17\ d^{-1}$ [178]
K_C	half saturation for tumor cell	$0.4\,g\ cm^{-3}$ [178]
K_G	half saturation for VEGF	$7 \times 10^{-8}\,g\ cm^{-3}$ [178]
K_{DG}	Inhibition of dentritic cell by VEGF	$4 \times 10^{-4}\,g\ cm^{-3}$ [178]
K_{TG}	Inhibition of T cell by VEGF	$2 \times 10^{-3}\,g\ cm^{-3}$ [178]
D_0	Density of immature DCs	$2 \times 10^{-5}\,g\,cm^{-3}$ [178]
E_M	Carrying capacity of endothelial cells	$5 \times 10^{-3}\,g\,cm^{-3}$ [178]
C_M	Carrying capacity of cancer cells	$0.8\,g\,cm^{-3}$ [178]
G_0	Threshold VEGF concentration	$3.65 \times 10^{-10}\,g\,cm^{-3}$ [178]
$\hat{T}$	Density of T cells from lymph node	$4 \times 10^{-3}\,g\,cm^{-3}$ [178]
$\hat{E}$	Density of endothelial cells from outside tumor	$5 \times 10^{-3}\,g\,cm^{-3}$ [178]
W^*	Hypoxia threshold oxygen level	$1.69 \times 10^{-4}\,g\,cm^{-3}$ [178]
W_0	Normal threshold oxygen level	$4.65 \times 10^{-4}\,g\,cm^{-3}$ [178]
μ_{GB}	Blocking rate of VEGF by anti-VEGF	2.19×10^7 $cm^3\,g^{-1}\,day^{-1}$ [178]
μ_{BG}	Degradation rate of anti-VEGF in blocking VEGF	1.31×10^8 $cm^3\,g^{-1}\,day^{-1}$ [178]
$\hat{T}_{10}$	Density of T cells impacted by IL-12	$3.88 \times 10^{-4}\,g\,cm^{-3}\,day^{-1}$ Estimated

$$
\begin{aligned}
\frac{dI}{dt} &= \beta T_1 - \mu_0 I + s \\
\frac{dT_1}{dt} &= k_1 C T_1 - \mu_1 T_1 \\
\frac{dT_2}{dt} &= k_2 C T_2 + \frac{\sigma T_2 I}{g + I} - \mu_2 T_2 \\
\frac{dC}{dt} &= \lambda C \left(1 - \frac{C}{K}\right) - \alpha T_2 C,
\end{aligned}
\tag{3.189}
$$

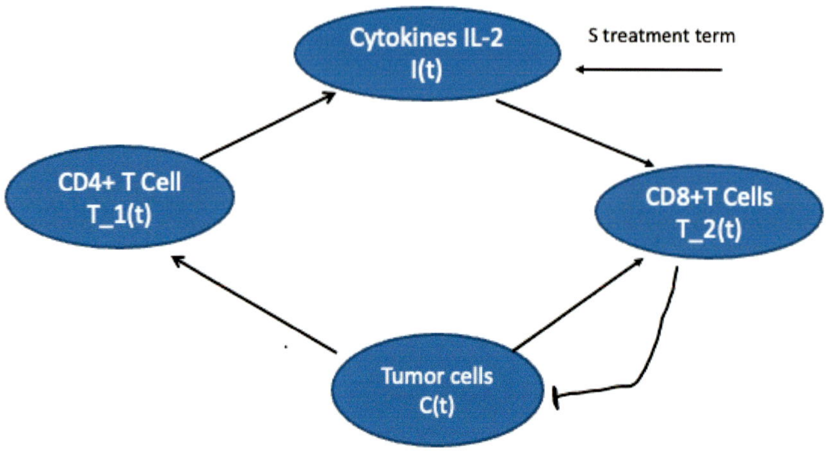

Figure 3.11 Schematic diagram of the IL-2 based model. Tumor cells $C(t)$ reproduce themselves by logistic growth and are killed by CD8$^+$ T cells and NK cells $T_2(t)$. Both CD4$^+$ T cells $T_1(t)$ and CD8$^+$ T cells, NK cells $T_2(t)$ are stimulated by cancer cells. These cells also decay. The cytokine IL-2 $I(t)$ is elicited by CD4$^+$ T cells $T_1(t)$ and, at the same time, provided by the treatment term s. IL-2 induces the growth of CD8$^+$ T cells and NK cells. It also degrades.

in which
β is the rate at which IL-2 is produced by one CD4$^+$ T cell in a unit of time;
μ_0 is the degradation rate of IL-2, in other words, $\frac{1}{\mu_0}$ is the average life time of IL-2;
s is the IL-2 treatment term. We can take this term to be piece-wise constant for simplicity;
k_1 is the stimulation rate of CD4$^+$ T cells by tumor cells, that is, $k_1 T_1$ CD4$^+$ T cells are recruited to the tumor site by one tumor cell in a unit of time;
μ_1 is the clearance rate of CD4$^+$ T cells, also called the death rate of CD4$^+$ T cells. $\frac{1}{\mu_1}$ is the average lifetime of CD4$^+$ T cells;
k_2 is the stimulation rate of CD8$^+$ T cells by tumor cells, that is, $k_2 T_2$ CD8$^+$ T cells are recruited to the tumor site by one tumor cell in a unit of time;
μ_2 is the clearance rate of CD8$^+$ T cells, also called the death rate of CD8+ T cells. $\frac{1}{\mu_2}$ is the average lifetime of CD8$^+$ T cells;
λ is the per capita growth rate of tumor cells;
K is the carrying capacity of the tumor;
α is the immune killing rate of tumor cells by CD8$^+$ T cells, the rate at which

TABLE 3.4 Dimensional Parameters' Ranges

Parameters	Ranges	Units	Reference
β	[0,1]	$IU\ cell^{-1}\ day^{-1}$	[95]
μ_0	[0,10]	day^{-1}	[95]
s		$IU\ day^{-1}$	[95]
k_1	$[3 \times 10^{-11}, 1.1 \times 10^{-7}]$	$cell^{-1}\ day^{-1}$	[95]
k_2	$[3 \times 10^{-11}, 1.1 \times 10^{-7}]$	$cell^{-1}\ day^{-1}$	[95]
μ_1	[0.03, 0.33]	day^{-1}	[95]
μ_2	[0.01, 0.93]	day^{-1}	[95]
σ	[0.124, 2.971]	day^{-1}	[95]
g	$[10^3, 2 \times 10^7]$	IU	[95]
λ	[0.01, 0.52]	day^{-1}	[95]
K	$[10^4, 10^{14}]$	$cells$	[95]
α	$[3.4 \times 10^{-10}, 3 \times 10^{-7}]$	$cell^{-1}\ day^{-1}$	[95]

each $CD8^+$ T cell suppresses a tumor cell in a unit of time.

We use the Michaelis-Menten term, $\frac{\sigma T_2 I}{g+I}$, to model the enhancement effect of $CD8^+$ T cells by IL-2 where σ is the maximum strength of IL-2 that enhances $CD8^+$ T cell in a unit of time, and g is the concentration of IL-2 at which the enhancement strength of IL-2 achieves $\frac{\sigma}{2}$.
The ranges of the dimensional parameters are given in Table 3.3.

3.2.2 Checkpoint Inhibitor and Virotherapy

In this section, we present several ODE models for virotherapy [262, 283, 284] and PDE models for combination of checkpoint inhibitor and virotherapy [120, 121, 127].

3.2.2.1 *ODE Models for Virotherapy*

Wodarz [283] proposed a three population model

$$\begin{aligned} \frac{dx}{dt} &= rx\left(1 - \frac{x+y}{K}\right) - dx - \beta xv \\ \frac{dy}{dt} &= \beta xv - \delta y \\ \frac{dv}{dt} &= \alpha y - \gamma v, \end{aligned} \tag{3.190}$$

where x stands for the uninfected tumor cell population and y the infected tumor cell population, v stands for the free virus population. The tumor growth is modeled by logistic growth, and K is maximal tumor size. The coefficient β represents the infectivity of the virus. The infected tumor cells die with a rate δy. The term αy models the release of virions by infected tumor cells, and γv

is the clearance rate of free virus particles by various causes including non-specific binding and generation of defective interfering particles. The death rate of tumor cells dx seems redundant, since it is included in the logistic model.

Dingli et al [94] proposed a similar model by replacing the first equation in (3.190) by a generalized logistic model,

$$\begin{aligned}\frac{dx}{dt} &= rx\left(1 - \frac{(x+y)^{\epsilon}}{K^{\epsilon}}\right) - \beta xv \\ \frac{dy}{dt} &= \beta xv - \delta y \\ \frac{dv}{dt} &= \alpha y - \gamma v,\end{aligned} \tag{3.191}$$

here, ϵ is a constant.

In order to consider the recombinant effect of measles virus, Bajzer et al [13] proposed the following model

$$\begin{aligned}\frac{dx}{dt} &= rx\left(1 - \frac{(x+y)^{\epsilon}}{K^{\epsilon}}\right) - \beta xv - \rho xy \\ \frac{dy}{dt} &= \beta xv - \delta y \\ \frac{dv}{dt} &= \alpha y - \gamma v - \beta xv,\end{aligned} \tag{3.192}$$

where ρxy describes cell-cell fusion effect during the virotherapy. This model includes an important fact that tumor cells and free virus both decrease due to infection.

Tian [262] modeled virus replication ability by its burst size. The burst size of a virus is the number of new viruses released from a lysis of an infected cell. Different types of viruses have different burst sizes. Viruses of the same type have almost the same burst size. The burst size is an important parameter of virus replicability. Including the burst size b, a common basic model for virotherapy is:

$$\begin{aligned}\frac{dx}{dt} &= \lambda x\left(1 - \frac{x+y}{K}\right) - \beta xv \\ \frac{dy}{dt} &= \beta xv - \delta y \\ \frac{dv}{dt} &= b\delta y - \beta xv - \gamma v.\end{aligned} \tag{3.193}$$

3.2.2.2 PDE Models for Combination Treatment

We present two PDE models in [121], one for co-treatment with oncolytic virus and one for co-treatment with vaccine.

Model one for co-treatment with oncolytic virus
We denote by C and C_i the densities of uninfected and virus-infected cancer cells, respectively, and consider the following system in the tumor $\Omega_\infty = \{0 \leq r < R(t); 0 < t < \infty$:

$$\frac{\partial C}{\partial t} + \nabla \cdot (\mathbf{u}C) - \nabla^2 C = \lambda C \left(1 - \frac{C}{K}\right) - \gamma_V C - \gamma_A TC, \tag{3.194}$$

$$\frac{\partial C_i}{\partial t} + \nabla \cdot (\mathbf{u}C_i) - \nabla^2 C_i = \gamma_V C - \gamma_A (1+\delta) TC_i, \tag{3.195}$$

where T is the density of T cells,

$$C + C_i = 1 \text{ in } \Omega_\infty, \tag{3.196}$$

$$\frac{\partial C}{\partial r} = \frac{\partial C_i}{\partial r} = 0 \text{ on } r = R(t), \tag{3.197}$$

$$\frac{dR}{dt} = u(R(t), t), t > 0 \tag{3.198}$$

where $\mathbf{u} = u\mathbf{e}_r$. It is assumed that

$$T = 1, K \geq 2, \text{ and } \lambda + \gamma_A \delta > \gamma_V. \tag{3.199}$$

The parameter γ_V represents the oncolytic virus therapy, which transforms cancer cells into infected cancer cells. The killing rate γ_A of cancer cells consist of $\gamma_0 + \gamma_1$where γ_0 is fixed, and γ_1 is the dose level of the checkpoint inhibitor. For simplicity, we shall refer to γ_A as the checkpoint inhibitor drug. The parameter δ is positive and reflects the fact that infected cells are more easily detected and killed by T cells than uninfected cancer cells. The parameter K is the carrying capacity of the tissue: cancer cells' density cannot exceed K. We note that the boundary conditions in (3.197) mean that there is no flux of cancer cells across the tumor boundary.

Model Two for co-treatment with cancer vaccine
We consider the model with cancer cells (C) and T cells (T),

$$\frac{\partial C}{\partial t} + \nabla \cdot (\mathbf{u}C) - \nabla^2 C = \lambda C - \gamma_A TC, \tag{3.200}$$

$$\frac{\partial T}{\partial t} + \nabla \cdot (\mathbf{u}T) - \nabla^2 T = \gamma_V - \mu T, \tag{3.201}$$

$$C + T = 1 \text{ in } \Omega_\infty, \tag{3.202}$$

$$\frac{\partial C}{\partial r} + \beta C = \frac{\partial T}{\partial r} + \beta (T - 1) = 0 \text{ on } r = R(t), \tag{3.203}$$

$$\frac{dR}{dt} = u(R(t), t), t > 0. \tag{3.204}$$

cells is greater than that of CD8+ T cells, and greater than 1, E_3^0 is globally asymptotically stable. When the relative death rate of CD4+ T cells is less than 1, the relative death rate of CD8+ T cells is greater than that of CD4+ T cells but smaller than the sum of the relative death rate of CD4+ T cells and the maximum enhancement rate of IL-2, we have a positive equilibrium E_4^0. The stability of E_4^0 changes twice.

Two groups of in silico clinical trials were conducted in [95] and each group has 20 protocols. The results of in silico clinical trials show some short-term dynamics of IL-2 immunotherapy. Since different sets of parameter values may represent different tumor conditions or patients, in silico trials may have different outcomes. For example, tumor antigens activate CD4+ T cells. For some tumor conditions, IL-2 administration may not have a significant effect on CD4+ T cells, but for some other tumor conditions, IL-2 administration slows the growth of the CD4+ T cell population.
Short-time administration of IL-2 can always accelerate the increase of the CD8+T cell population, which may be considered as a qualitative confirmation of the increasing proliferation of IL-2 in CD8+ T cells. CD8+ T cells and natural killer cells fight directly against tumor cells. Our in silico trials show this to be the case. When the time for IL-2 administration is longer, the time of the tumor cell population at the low level is longer. When a huge dose of IL-2 is administered, the tumor cell population becomes very low. In other words, IL-2 can control tumor size in a finite period of time. This implies that intermittent administration of IL-2 may be a good strategy for tumor size control. In some trials, IL-2 treatment can reduce the population of tumor cells in the long term. Mathematically, the system converges to the equilibrium E_3 in these trials. When the dose of IL-2 increases, the maximal amplitude of the oscillated tumor cell population arising from a Hopf bifurcation decreases. These implicate that IL-2 influences the tumor in several ways and that individual physical parameters are important for a particular treatment.

3.2.3.2 Analysis of an ODE Virotherapy Model

We are going to analyze the system (3.193) following the work in [262]. First, we non-dimensionalize the system (3.193) by setting

$$\hat{x} = \frac{x}{K}, \hat{y} = \frac{y}{K}, \hat{v} = \frac{v}{K}, \hat{t} = \delta t.$$

The system (3.193) becomes, after dropping all ˆ:

$$\begin{aligned} \frac{dx}{dt} &= rx\left(1 - x - y\right) - axv \\ \frac{dy}{dt} &= axv - y \\ \frac{dv}{dt} &= by - axv - cv, \end{aligned} \tag{3.208}$$

where $a = \frac{\beta K}{\delta}, c = \frac{\gamma}{\delta}, r = \frac{\lambda}{\delta}$.

We define the domain $D = \{(x, y, v) : x \geq 0, y \geq 0, v \geq 0, 0 \leq x + y \leq 1\}$.

Lemma 3.22 *D is a positive invariant domain for the system (3.208).*

Proof. For ($x(0) \geq 0, y(0) \geq 0$, and $v(0) \geq 0$,if the conclusion ($x(t) \geq 0, y(t) \geq 0$, and $v(t) \geq 0$ for $t > 0$ is not true, there must be a time t_1, such that there is at least one component that will be zero first. We check each possible case.
If $x(t_1) = 0$ first, then $x'(t_1) = 0$. From the first equation of (3.208), by the uniqueness of the solution we know $x(t) = 0$ for all $t > t_1$. Then the second equation of (3.208) becomes $y'(t) = -y$. So, $y(t) \geq 0$. since $y(t_1) > 0$. The third equation becomes $v'(t) = by - cv$. Therefore, $v(t) \geq 0$.
If $y(t_1) = 0$ first, then $y'(t_1) = ax(t_1)v(t_1) \geq 0$. So, $y(t) \geq 0$ when $t \geq t_1$ since $x(t) > 0$ and $v(t) > 0$ as assumed.
If $v(t_1) = 0$ first, then $v'(t_1) = by(t_1) \geq 0$. So, after $t_1, v(t) \geq 0$ since $x(t) > 0$ and $y(t) > 0$ as assumed.
If two components are zero simultaneously at t_1, it is easy to check that the third component will be nonnegative when $t > t_1$.
If the three components are zero simultaneously at t_1, then from the uniqueness of the solution, $x(t) = 0, y(t) = 0$, and $v(t) = 0$ for $t > 0$. Therefore, $x(t) \geq 0, y(t) \geq 0$, and $v(t) \geq 0$ for $t \geq 0$. Since the initial value of each component is nonnegative, the solution is non- negative. So, $x'(t) = rx(1-x-y) - axv \leq rx(1-x)$. With $x(0) \leq 1$, by the comparison theorem, we have $x(t) \leq 1$. Notice, $x'(t)+y'(t) = rx(1-x-y)-y \leq rx[1-(x+y)] \leq r(1-(x+y))$. Since $0 \leq x(0) + y(0) \leq 1$, by the comparison theorem, we have $0 \leq x(t) + y(t) \leq 1$ for $t > 0$. ■

We then refer the whole domain D as a global domain.
The system (3.208) always has two equilibrium solutions in the positive invariant domain D, $E_0 = (0, 0, 0)$ and $E_1 = (1, 0, 0)$. When $b > 1 + \frac{c}{a}$, it has three equilibria, E_0, E_1, and a unique positive equilibrium solution E^*

$$E^* = \left(\frac{c}{a(b-1)}, \frac{rc(ab-a-c)}{a(b-1)(ab-a+rc)}, \frac{r(ab-a-c)}{a(ab-a+rc)} \right).$$

Theorem 3.23 *[262] The system (3.208) has three equilibria, $E_0 = (0, 0, 0), E_1 = (1, 0, 0)$, and the positive equilibrium E^*. E_0 is always unstable for all positive values of b. E_1 is globally asymptotically stable when $0 < b < b_{s_1}$, and it is unstable when $b \geq b_{s_1}$. At $b = b_{s_1}$, the positive equilibrium E^* moves into the domain D, a type of transcritical bifurcation occurs with E_1 and E^*. As b increases, while $b_{s_1} < b < b_{s_2}$ and $b \in I_p, E^*$ is locally asymptotically stable; when $b > b_0$ and $b \in I_n, E^*$ is unstable. Hopf bifurcations occur for some $b \geq b_{s_2}$, and these bifurcations give rise to one or three families of periodic solutions. As b becomes large enough, $E^* = (O(\frac{1}{b}), O(\frac{1}{b}), \frac{r}{b})$.*

This theorem is a collections of results of the theorems that will follow. b_{s_1}, b_{s_2}, I_p, and I_n will be defined later.

The Jacobian matrix of the system (3.208) is given by

$$\begin{pmatrix} r-2rx-ry-av & -rx & -ax \\ av & -1 & ax \\ -av & b & -ax-c \end{pmatrix}.$$

Theorem 3.24 *E_0 is unstable for all $b > 0$.*

Proof. At the equilibrium point E_0, the Jacobian matrix is $\begin{pmatrix} -r & 0 & 0 \\ 0 & -1 & 0 \\ 0 & b & -c \end{pmatrix}$.
The eigenvalues are $r, -1$, and $-c$. Since r is positive, E_0 is unstable. ■

For the linearization of the system (3.208) at E_0, the stable invariant subspace is the y-v plane, and the unstable invariant subspace is the x axis. It happens that for the system (3.208), the local stable invariant manifold is in the y-v plane, and the unstable invariant manifold is in the x axis. A possible interpretation is that without viruses and infected tumor cells the tumor will grow from an initial small value around E_0. If all tumor cells are infected, then the tumor will shrink until it disappears into E_0.

Theorem 3.25 *E_1 is globally asymptotically stable when $b < 1 + \frac{c}{a}$; E_1 is unstable $b > 1 + \frac{c}{a}$.*

Proof. At the equilibrium point E_1, the Jacobian matrix is

$$\begin{pmatrix} -r & -r & -a \\ 0 & -1 & a \\ 0 & b & -a-c \end{pmatrix}.$$

The eigenvalues are $\lambda_1 = -r$ and $\lambda_{2,3} = \frac{1}{2}(-(1+a+c) \pm \sqrt{p(1-a-c)^2 + 4ab})$. Hence, when $b < 1 + c/a$, all three eigenvalues are negative. This implies E_1 is locally asymptotically stable. λ_3 is positive when $b > 1 + c/a$, so E_1 is unstable.
To prove that the equilibrium solution E_1 is globally asymptotically stable when $b < 1 + c/a$. Here by the word "globally", we mean the whole positive invariant domain D. We will construct two Lyapunov functions according to different ranges of the parameter b. For convenience, we make a translation of variables, $\bar{x} = 1 - x$, $\bar{y} = y$, and $\bar{v} = v$. After dropping the bars over variables, the system becomes

$$\begin{aligned} \frac{dx}{dt} &= -rx + ry + av + rx^2 - rxy - axv \\ \frac{dy}{dt} &= av - axv - y \\ \frac{dv}{dt} &= by + axv - (a+c)v, \end{aligned} \tag{3.209}$$

while the domain D is translated to

$$D_1 = \{(x, y, v) : 0 \leq x \leq 1, y \geq 0, v \geq 0, 0 \leq x - y \leq 1\}$$

For any initial condition (x_0, y_0, v_0) in the Domain D_1, we know from Lemma 3.20, the solution satisfies $0 \leq x(t) \leq 1, 0 \leq y(t) \leq 1$ and $v(t) \geq 0$. We will construct two Lyapunov functions according to the values of the parameter b to prove $y(t)$ and $v(t)$ approach 0, and then prove $x(t)$ also approaches 0.
When $0 \leq b \leq 1$, we define a Lyapunov function $V_1(x, y, v) = y + v$. It is obvious that $V_1(x, y, v) > 0$, and the orbital derivative $\dot{V}_1(x, y, v) = (b-1)y - cv < 0$.
When $1 \leq b < 1 + c/a$, we define a Lyapunov function $V_2(x, y, v)$ by

$$V_2(x, y, v) = \frac{1}{2}ab(a+c)y^2 + a^2 byv + \frac{1}{2}a^2 v^2.$$

It is easy to see $V_2(x, y, v) > 0$. It can be verified that $\dot{V}_2(x, y, v) < 0$. Therefore, combining these two Lyapunov functions, we have $y(t) \to 0$ and $v(t) \to 0$ as $t \to \infty$ when $b < 1 + c/a$.
Considering the component $x(t)$, we see that

$$\frac{dx}{dt} \leq ry + av - rx.$$

So,

$$0 \leq x(t) \leq ke^{-rt} + e^{-rt} \int_0^t (ry(s) + av(s))e^{rs} ds,$$

which implies $x(t) \to 0$ as $t \to \infty$. ∎

The above theorem has an important biological implication. When the burst size of the oncolytic virus is smaller than $1 + c/a$, the virotherapy always fails. This failure is determined by the replication ability of the oncolytic virus, and it does matter what the initial tumor size, the initial infected portion of the tumor, and the initial amount of injected virus are as long as they are in the domain D. The burst size does not depends on initial conditions. The number $1 + c/a$ is a threshold value for the burst size. We denote it by b_{s_1} as the first threshold. Namely, $b_{s_1} = 1 + c/a$.

Consider the critical case $b = b_{s_1}$. It implies $ab = a + c$. In this case, the linearized system at E_1 has two negative eigenvalues and one zero eigenvalue. In order to determine the stability of the equilibrium solution E_1, we will use the center manifold theorem to reduce the system (3.209) into a center manifold, and study the reduced system.

Theorem 3.26 *E_1 is unstable when $b = b_{s_1} = 1 + c/a$.*

Proof. To reduce the system (3.209) to a center manifold, we first standardize the system, separate it into two parts, the part with zero eigenvalue and the part with negative eigenvalues. The system (3.209) does not have complex eigenvalues in this case. We start with the matrix corresponding to the linear part of the system (3.209), which is $L = \begin{pmatrix} -r & r & a \\ 0 & -1 & a \\ 0 & b & -ab \end{pmatrix}$. It has eigenvalues, $-r, -(1+ab)$ and 0.

The eigenvalue $-r$ has an associated eigenvector $V_1 = (1,0,0)^T$, $-(1+ab)$ has an associated eigenvector $V_2 = (ab-r, 1+ab-r, -b(1+ab-r))^T$, 0 has an associated eigenvector $V_3 = (ar+a, ar, r)^T$. We set a transformation matrix to be $T = (V_1, V_2, V_3)$. Denote $X = (x, y, v)^T$. Then the system (3.209) can be written as $\frac{dX}{dt} = LX + F$, where $F = (rx^2 - rxy - axv, -axv, axv)^T$. Set $X = TY$, then

$$\frac{dY}{dt} = T^{-1}LTY + T^{-1}F,$$

where $T^{-1}LT = \begin{pmatrix} -r & 0 & 0 \\ 0 & -(1+ab) & 0 \\ 0 & 0 & 0 \end{pmatrix}$, and $x = y_1 + (ab-r)y_2 + (ar+a)y_3$, $y = (1+ab-r)y_2 + ary_3$, and $v = -b(1+ab-r)y_2 + ry_3$. Denote $T^{-1}F = (f_1, f_2, f_3)^T$, then we have

$$f_1 = A_{11}y_1^2 + A_{12}y_1y_2 + A_{13}y_1y_3 + A_{22}y_2^2 + A_{23}y_2y_3 + A_{33}y_3^2,$$

$$f_2 = B_{12}y_1y_2 + B_{13}y_1y_3 + B_{22}y_2^2 + B_{23}y_2y_3 + B_{33}y_3^2,$$

$$f_3 = C_{12}y_1y_2 + C_{13}y_1y_3 + C_{22}y_2^2 + C_{23}y_2y_3 + C_{33}y_3^2,$$

where A_{ij}, B_{ij} and C_{ij} are coefficients that can be determined in terms of the parameters.
Then the transformed system can be written as

$$\begin{aligned} \frac{dZ}{dt} &= BZ + (f_1, f_2)^T, \\ \frac{dy_3}{dt} &= Ay_3 + f_3, \end{aligned} \tag{3.210}$$

where $B = \begin{pmatrix} -r & 0 \\ 0 & -(1+ab) \end{pmatrix}$, $A = (0)$, and $Z = (y_1, y_2)$. Then from the Center Manifold Theorem, there is a center manifold given by $Z = h(y_3) = (y_1, y_2)^T = (h_1(y_3), h_2(y_3))$ and it satisfies

$$Bh(y_3) + (f_1(h(y_3), y_3), f2(h(y_3), y_3))^T = Dh(y_3)(Ay_3 + f_3(h(y_3), y_3)).$$

Now using the above equation we reduce the system (3.210) to its center manifold, which is a single equation

$$\frac{dy_3}{dt} = C_{33}y_3^2 + \left(\frac{A_{33}C_{13}}{r} + \frac{B_{33}C_{23}}{1+ab}\right)y_3^3 + \cdots$$

where $C_{33} = \frac{-a^2(a+1)(b-1)}{1+ab} < 0$ since $b = 1 + c/a > 1$. It is easy to see that $y_3 = 0$ is a node. Therefore, for the system (3.209), the origin is unstable. ■

When $b > b_{s_1} = 1 + c/a$, there is a third equilibrium solution $E^* = (\bar{x}, \bar{y}, \bar{v})$ while E_1 is unstable, where $\bar{x} = \frac{c}{a(b-1)}, \bar{y} = \frac{rc(ab-a-c)}{a(b-1)(ab-a+rc)}$, and $\bar{v} = \frac{r(ab-a-c)}{a(ab-a+rc)}$. It is the unique positive equilibrium solution. The Jacobian matrix at this point is

$$\begin{pmatrix} -r\bar{x} & -r\bar{x} & -a\bar{x} \\ a\bar{v} & -1 & a\bar{x} \\ -a\bar{v} & b & -a\bar{x} - c \end{pmatrix} = \begin{pmatrix} -\frac{rc}{a(b-1)} & -\frac{rc}{a(b-1)} & -\frac{c}{b-1} \\ \frac{r(ab-a-c)}{ab-a+rc} & -1 & \frac{c}{b-1} \\ -\frac{r(ab-a-c)}{ab-a+rc} & b & -\frac{bc}{b-1} \end{pmatrix}.$$

The characteristic polynomial is given by

$$p(\lambda) = \lambda^3 + a_1\lambda^2 + a_2\lambda + a_3, \tag{3.211}$$

where $a_1 = \frac{rc+ab-a+abc}{a(b-1)}, a_2 = \frac{rc(bc+b-1)}{a(b-1)^2} + \frac{rc(ab-a-c)(r-a)}{a(b-1)(ab-a+rc)}$, and $a_3 = \frac{rc(ab-a-c)}{a(b-1)}$. By the Routh-Hurwitz Criterion, all roots of the polynomial (3.211) have negative real parts if and only if

$$H_1 = a_1 > 0, H_2 = \begin{vmatrix} a_1 & a_3 \\ 1 & a_2 \end{vmatrix} > 0, H_3 = \begin{vmatrix} a_1 & a_3 & 0 \\ 1 & a_2 & 0 \\ 0 & a_1 & a_3 \end{vmatrix} > 0.$$

Define a function $\phi(b) = \frac{a(b-1)(ab-a+rc)}{ab-a+rc+abc} - \frac{(bc+b-1)(ab-a+rc)}{(b-1)(ab-a-c)}$. Since $b > 1+c/a$, we can conclude that $H_2 > 0$ if and only if $\phi(b) < r - a$, $H_2 < 0$ if and only if $\phi(b) > r - a$, and $H_2 = 0$ if and only if $\phi(b) = r - a$. We will also consider H2 as a function of the parameter burst size b, and denote $H(b) = H_2$. We thus get the following theorem.

Theorem 3.27 *When $\phi(b) < r - a$, the equilibrium solution E^* is locally asymptotically stable.*

Next, we turn our attention to bifurcation analysis. Two types of bifurcations occur in the system (3.208) as the parameter b varies. A transcritical bifurcation at $b = b_{s_1}$ introduces the equilibrium point E^* into the positive invariant domain D. The Hopf bifurcation at some value $b > b_{s_1}$ gives rise to the periodic solutions. In order to analyze these bifurcations, we study the function $H(b)$. The following lemma is proved in [262]:

Lemma 3.28 *The equation $H(b) = 0$ has at least two real roots, one is less than $b_{s_1} = 1 + c/a$, and the another one is greater than b_{s_1}. Furthermore, among all roots that are greater than b_{s_1}, there exists a root denoted by b_0 and a small neighborhood of $b_0, (b_0 - \delta_1, b_0 + \delta_1)$, where $\delta_1 < b_0 - b_{s_1}$, such that $H'(b_0) \neq 0$and $H(b)$ is monotonic in this interval.*

Define $I_p = \{b > b_{s_1}|H(b) > 0\}, I_n = \{b > b_{s_1}|H(b) < 0\}, I_0 = \{b > b_{s_1}|H(b) = 0\}$. From the proof of Lemma 3.8, I_p is not empty, and it is a finite open interval or a union of two finite open intervals. I_n is also not empty, and is an infinite open interval or a union of a finite open interval and an infinite open interval. I_0 is a closed set. I_0 at least has one point, and at most has 3 points. We denote the smallest number in I_0 by b_{s_2}.

Theorem 3.29 *When $b_{s_1} < b < b_{s_2}$, the equilibrium solution E^* is locally asymptotically stable. At this equilibrium point, the tumor load $T(E^*) = \bar{x} + \bar{y} = \frac{c(1+r)}{ab-a+rc} < 1$.*

Proof. From Lemma, $H(b_{s_1}) > 0$. Since $H(b)$ is a continuous function, $H(b)$ is positive until it become zero. So, $H(b) > 0$ for $b_{s_1} < b < b_{s_2}$. Then, all roots of the characteristic polynomial (3.211) have negative real parts by the Routh-Hurwitz Criterion. The verification of the second part is straightforward. ■

Since the tumor load at the equilibrium point E^* is less than 1, this equilibrium point represents a partial success of virotherapy at a modest value of the burst size. This also implies that a permanent reduction of tumor load can be reached.

The following theorem is proved in [262]:

Theorem 3.30 *There exists a neighborhood of b_0, $(b_0 - \delta_0, b_0 + \delta_0)$, such that for each b in this interval the characteristic polynomial $p(\lambda) = \lambda^3 + a_1(b)\lambda^2 + a_2(b)\lambda + a_3(b)$ has a pair of complex conjugate eigenvalues $\lambda(b) = \alpha(b) \pm i\beta(b)$, where $\alpha(b)$ changes sign when it passes through b_0 and $\beta(b) > 0$. Furthermore, when $b = b_0, p(\lambda)$ has a pair of purely imaginary roots and one negative real root, and $\alpha'(b_0) \neq 0$.*

By examining the graph of $H(b)$, there are two cases. In case one where there are three zeros of $H(b)$ that are greater than b_{s_1}, these three zeros are Hopf bifurcation points, and there will be three families of periodic solutions rising from these bifurcation. While in case two where there are one or two zeros of $H(b)$ that are greater than b_{s_1}, but only one zero is Hopf bifurcation point.

Since the exact value of b_0 is not algebraically expressible, the stability, amplitudes, and periods of periodical solutions that occur around b_0 and E^* are difficult to analyze. Numerical simulation are performed in [262] to demonstrate some typical dynamics.

3.2.3.3 Analysis of Combination Treatment Model

We are going to do analysis of combination treatment model one (3.194)–(3.199). The global existence of the model can be obtained in the same fashion as Theorem 3.4 in section 3.1.2.3; we only discuss the asymptotic behavior of the solution as $t \to \infty$.

Let

$$C^* = \frac{K}{2\lambda}\left(\lambda + \gamma_A\delta + \frac{\lambda}{K} - \sqrt{\left(\lambda + \gamma_A\delta + \frac{\lambda}{K}\right)^2 - 4\frac{\lambda}{K}(\lambda + \gamma_A\delta - \gamma_V)}\right), \tag{3.212}$$

$$C^{**} = \frac{K}{2\lambda}\left(\lambda + \gamma_A\delta - \sqrt{(\lambda + \gamma_A\delta)^2 - 4\frac{\lambda}{K}\gamma_A(\delta + 1)}\right). \tag{3.213}$$

Theorem 3.31 *If $C^* < C^{**}$ then $R(t) \to 0$ as $t \to \infty$, while if $C^* > C^{**}$ then $R(t) \to 0$ as $t \to \infty$.*

Proof. Adding Eqs. (3.194) and (3.195), and using (3.196) we have

$$\nabla \cdot \mathbf{u} = h(C), h(C) = \lambda C\left(1 - \frac{C}{K}\right) - \gamma_A - \gamma_A\delta(1 - C). \tag{3.214}$$

Equation (3.194) can be written as

$$\frac{\partial C}{\partial t} + \nabla \cdot (\mathbf{u}C) - \nabla^2 C = f(C), \tag{3.215}$$

where

$$f(C) = Cg(C), g(C) = \lambda C\left(1 - \frac{C}{K}\right) - \gamma_V + \gamma_A\delta(1 - C). \tag{3.216}$$

Note that $g(C)$ has a unique zero in $(0,1)$ at C^* in the light of (3.212), and we consider the ODE system

$$\frac{d\hat{C}}{dt} = f(\hat{C}), \hat{C}(0) = \hat{C}_0; \tag{3.217}$$

where $0 < \hat{C}_0 < 1$. Since $f(C^*) = 0; f(C) > 0$ for $0 < C < C^*$ and $f(C) > 0$ for $C^* < C < 1$, we have $\hat{C}(t) \to C^*$ as $t \to \infty$. By comparison principal, we see that

$$C(r,t) \to C^* \text{ uniformly in } 0 \le r \le R(t) \text{ as } t \to \infty. \tag{3.218}$$

From (3.198), (3.214), and (3.218), we have

$$\frac{1}{R(t)}\frac{dR(t)}{dt} = \frac{1}{R^3(t)}\int_0^{R(t)} h(C(r,t))r^2 dr \to \frac{h(C^*)}{3} \text{ as } t \to \infty.$$

Hence

$$R(t) \to \begin{cases} 0 \text{ if } h(C^*) < 0, \\ \infty \text{ if } h(C^*) > 0. \end{cases} \tag{3.219}$$

From (3.199) and (3.213) we see that $h(C^*) < 0$ if $C^* < C^{**}$ and $h(C^*) > 0$ if $C^* > C^{**}$. So the theorem follows from (3.219). ■

Since Model Two (3.200)–(3.205) is similar to Model One in Section 3.1.1, similar analysis and results such as existence of steady solution can be obtained for (3.200)–(3.205) [121].

3.3 STOCHASTIC MODELS

Cancer progression and treatment response are inherently stochastic due to random mutations in tumor cells, variability in immune cell activation and infiltration, heterogeneous microenvironments and unpredictable therapeutic outcomes. Stochastic models aim to quantify this uncertainty and offer probabilistic predictions useful for designing robust cancer therapies.

Stochastic Models capture random fluctuations in small populations of tumor or immune cells. and reflects rare but critical events, such as immune escape or viral replication failure. They improve prediction of treatment success probabilities and optimal scheduling.

Stochastic Differential Equations (SDEs) models introduce noise terms (e.g., Wiener processes) into ODE models and PDE models. For example, one can add white noise to tumor growth or immune response rates to model uncertainty in tumor growth rates, immune activation, and therapy effectiveness.

Continuous-Time Markov Chains (CTMCs) models cancer and immune cell populations as discrete states evolving over time. They are used to assess extinction probabilities of tumor cells or viruses.

Individual cells/viruses follow probabilistic rules for division, death, infection, or interaction. Agent-Based Models enable detailed modeling of spatial and temporal dynamics under therapy; they are often used for simulating oncolytic virus spread and immune cell trafficking.

3.3.1 Stochastic Model for Virotherapy

In this section, we will present several stochastic models for virotherapy.
Ito SDE models can be derived by applying the modeling procedure in [7,8]. In biochemical applications, the derived SDE system is referred to as the chemical Langevin equation. As in [301], the following SDE model can be derived based on the deterministic model (3.193):

$$\begin{aligned} d\mathbf{X} &= \mathbf{F}(y,v,x)dt + \mathbf{H}(y,v,x)d\mathbf{W}, \\ \mathbf{X}(0) &= (y(0), v(0), x(0))^T, \end{aligned} \tag{3.220}$$

where $\mathbf{X}(t) = (y(t), v(t), x(t))^T, \mathbf{W} = (W_1(t), W_2(t), \cdots W_5(t))^T$ is a vector of five independent Wiener processes; and

$$\mathbf{F} = \left(\beta xv - \delta y, b\delta y - \beta xv - \gamma v, \lambda x\left(1 - \frac{x+y}{K}\right) - \beta xv\right);$$

$$\mathbf{H}(y,v,x) = \begin{pmatrix} \tau_1\sqrt{vx} & \tau_2\sqrt{yx} & -\tau_3\sqrt{y} & 0 & 0 \\ -\tau_1\sqrt{vx} & 0 & -\tau_4\sqrt{y} & \tau_5\sqrt{vx} & 0 \\ -\tau_1\sqrt{vx} & 0 & 0 & 0 & \tau_6\sqrt{x} \end{pmatrix};$$

where $\tau_i, i = 1, 2 \cdots 5$ are positive constants.

On the other hand, in [223], another SDE model is derived based on the deterministic model (3.193). Linear noise to the infected tumor cell population and free virus population are incorporated. that is, $\tau_2 y dW_2$ and $\tau_3 v dW_3$ are added to the second and the third equations of (3.193), respectively. However, for the uninfected tumor cell population, environmental effects are incorporated into per capital growth rate λ. That is, λ is replaced by $\lambda + \tau_1 \frac{dW_1}{dt}$, where $\tau_i, i = 1.2.3$ represent the strength of the noise contributed by each tumor cells. It should be assumed that W_1, W_2, and W_3 are mutually independent Wiener processes. Such, we obtain a system of three Ito stochastic differential equations which is a basic stochastic model for oncolytic viral therapy as follows.

$$\begin{aligned}
\frac{dx}{dt} &= \lambda x \left(1 - \frac{x+y}{K}\right) - \beta x v + \tau_1 x \left(1 - \frac{x+y}{K}\right) dW_1 \\
\frac{dy}{dt} &= \beta x v - \delta y + \tau_2 y dW_2 \\
\frac{dv}{dt} &= b\delta y - \beta x v - \gamma v + \tau_3 v dW_3.
\end{aligned} \tag{3.221}$$

In the deterministic PDE Model One for co-treatment (3.194)–(3.198), we can add linear noise and environmental effects to the infected cancer cell C_i equation and uninfected cancer cell C equation respectively, the following stochastic PDE model can be obtained:

$$\frac{\partial C}{\partial t} + \nabla \cdot (\mathbf{u}C) - \nabla^2 C = \lambda C \left(1 - \frac{C}{K}\right) - \gamma_V C - \gamma_A T C + \tau_1 C T \frac{dW_1}{dt}, \tag{3.222}$$

$$\frac{\partial C_i}{\partial t} + \nabla \cdot (\mathbf{u}C_i) - \nabla^2 C_i = \gamma_V C - \gamma_A (1+\delta) T C_i + \tau_2 T C_i \frac{dW_2}{dt}, \tag{3.223}$$

where T is the density of T cells, we take $T = 1$, and

$$C + C_i = 1 \text{ in } \Omega_\infty, \tag{3.224}$$

$$\frac{\partial C}{\partial r} = \frac{\partial C_i}{\partial r} = 0 \text{ on } r = R(t), \tag{3.225}$$

$$\frac{dR}{dt} = u(R(t), t), t > 0 \tag{3.226}$$

where $\mathbf{u} = u\mathbf{e}_r$.

3.3.2 Stochastic Model for Immunotherapy

Based on the deterministic IL-2 immunotherapy model (3.189), we can incorporate linear noise into the first three equations and environmental effects into the fourth equation. The following system of stochastic ordinary differential equations can be proposed for IL-2 immunotherapy.

$$\begin{aligned}\frac{dI}{dt} &= \beta T_1 - \mu_0 I + s + \tau_1 I dW_1 \\ \frac{dT_1}{dt} &= k_1 C T_1 - \mu_1 T_1 + \tau_2 T_1 dW_2 \\ \frac{dT_2}{dt} &= k_2 C T_2 + \frac{\sigma T_2 I}{g+I} - \mu_2 T_2 + \tau_3 T_2 dW_3 \\ \frac{dC}{dt} &= \lambda C \left(1 - \frac{C}{K}\right) - \alpha T_2 C + \tau_4 C \left(1 - \frac{C}{K}\right) dW_4,\end{aligned} \tag{3.227}$$

in which $\tau_i, i = 1, 2, 3, 4$ represent the strength of the noise contributed by each cells. It should be assumed that W_1, W_2, W_3, and W_4 are mutually independent Wiener processes.

Model one with cancer cell and T cell in section 3.1.1 can be used as a simple example for checkpoint inhibitor therapy since the parameter η can represent a checkpoint inhibitor drug. In that PDE Model One for cancer cells and T cells, we can add noise for η in the cancer cell equation and noise effects for λ_T to the T cell equation respectively, the following stochastic PDE model can be obtained:

$$\frac{\partial C}{\partial t} + \nabla \cdot (\mathbf{u}C) - \nabla^2 C = \lambda_C C \left(1 - \frac{C}{K}\right) - \delta_0 C - \eta T C + \tau_1 C (1 - C) \frac{dW_1}{dt}, \tag{3.228}$$

$$\frac{\partial T}{\partial t} + \nabla \cdot (\mathbf{u}T) - \nabla^2 T = \lambda_T C - \delta_T T + \tau_2 C \frac{dW_2}{dt}, \tag{3.229}$$

where

$$C + T = 1 \text{ in } \Omega_t, \tag{3.230}$$

$$\frac{\partial C}{\partial r} + \beta C = 0, \frac{\partial T}{\partial r} + \beta(T - 1) = 0 \text{ on } r = R(t), \tag{3.231}$$

$$\frac{dR}{dt} = u(R(t), t), t > 0 \tag{3.232}$$

where $\mathbf{u} = u\mathbf{e}_r$, $\beta \geq 0$ is a constant.

3.3.3 Mathematical Analysis and Simulation

3.3.3.1 Analysis of a Stochastic ODE Model for Virotherapy

We are going to analyze the stochastic ODE model (3.221) following the work in [223].

First, we non-dimensionalize the system (3.221) by setting

$$\hat{x} = \frac{x}{K}, \hat{y} = \frac{y}{K}, \hat{v} = \frac{v}{K}, \hat{t} = \delta t.$$

The system (3.221) becomes, after dropping all ˆ from the variables and parameters:

$$\begin{aligned} dx &= [rx\,(1-x-y) - axv]dt + \tau_1 x\,(1-x-y)\,dW_1 \\ dy &= [axv - y]dt + \tau_2 y dW_2 \\ dv &= [by - axv - cv]dt + \tau_3 v dW_3, \end{aligned} \tag{3.233}$$

where $a = \frac{\beta K}{\delta}, c = \frac{\gamma}{\delta}, r = \frac{\lambda}{\delta}$.
In order to apply the results in [149] about asymptotic behaviors of stochastic Kolmogorov systems in non-compact domains, we change variables, set the transformation of variables

$$x = x, y = y, v = yz, or z = v/y,$$

and use Ito's formula, we get

$$dz = (b - axz - cz - axz^2 + z + \tau_2^2 z)dt - \tau_2 z dW2 + \tau_3 z dW3 :$$

(3.233) becomes

$$\begin{aligned} dx &= [rx\,(1-x-y) - axv]dt + \tau_1 x\,(1-x-y)\,dW_1 \\ dy &= [axv - y]dt + \tau_2 y dW_2 \\ dz &= (b - axz - cz - axz^2 + z + \tau_2^2 z)dt - \tau_2 z dW2 + \tau_3 z dW3 : \end{aligned} \tag{3.234}$$

We denote by $u(t) = (x(t); y(t); z(t))$ the solution process of the system (3.234). The drift term and the diffusion term of (3.234) are denoted by

$$f(u) = \begin{pmatrix} rx(1-x-y) - axyz \\ (axz - 1)y \\ b + (1 + \tau_2^2 - ax - c)z - axz^2 \end{pmatrix};$$

and $g(u) = \begin{pmatrix} \tau_1 x(1-x-y) & 0 & 0 \\ 0 & \tau_2 y & 0 \\ 0 & -\tau_2 z & \tau_3 z \end{pmatrix}$.
Assume that we are working on a complete probability space $(\Omega; \mathcal{F}; \{\mathcal{F}_t\}; P)$ with a filtration $\{\mathcal{F}_t\}$ satisfying the usual condition. Let L be the infinitesimal generator of the process u and, for any smooth enough functions $F : \mathbf{R}^3_+ := [0; \infty^3) \to \mathbf{R}$, the generator L acts as

$$LF(u) = F_u \cdot f(u) + \frac{1}{2} trace(g(u)^T F_{uu} g(u));$$

where F_u is the gradient of F and F_{uu} is the Hessian matrix of F. We use P_u or $P_{x;y;z}$ to denote the probability law on Ω when the solution path starts at $u = (x; y; z)$ and E_u or $E_{x;y;z}$ is the expectation corresponding to P_u.

Theorem 3.32 *For any initial value* $(x(0); y(0); z(0)) \in R^3_+ := \{(x; y; z) : x \geq 0; y \geq 0; z \geq 0\}$, *there exists a unique a.s. continuous global solution*

$(x(t); y(t); z(t)), t \geq 0$, that remains in R^3_+ a.s. In particular, if $x(0) = 0$ then $x(t) = 0$ for all $t > 0$ a.s. and if $x(0) > 0$ then $x(t) > 0$ for all $t > 0$ a.s. Similarly, if $y(0) = 0$ then $y(t) = 0$ for all $t > 0$ a.s. and if $y(0) > 0$ then $y(t) > 0$ for all $t > 0$ a.s. Finally, if $z(0) > 0$ then $z(t) > 0$ for all $t > 0$ a.s. Furthermore, the solution $(x(t); y(t); z(t))$ is a strong Markov process that possesses the Feller property.

Proof. We only prove the existence of the global solution, the proof of the positiveness is standard.
Since the drift term $f(u)$ and the diffusion term $g(u)$ are locally Lipschitz continuous, there exists a unique local a.s. continuous solution $u(t)$ up to the explosion time

$$\tau_e = \inf\{t > 0 : \max\{x(t); y(t); z(t)\} = \infty\}.$$

We show that $\tau_e = \infty$ a.s. Consider $V(x; y; z) = x + y + ln(1 + z)$. By Ito's formula, for all $t \in (0; \tau_e)$ we get

$$\begin{aligned} LV(t) &= rx(t)[1 - x(t) - y(t)] - ax(t)y(t)z(t) + ax(t)y(t)z(t) - y(t) \\ &+ \frac{b + (1 + \tau_2^2 - ax(t) - c)z(t) - ax(t)z^2(t)}{1 + z(t)} - \frac{1}{2}(\tau_2^2 + \tau_3^2)\frac{z^2(t)}{(1 + z(t))2} \\ &\leq (b + 1 + \tau_2^2)1_{x+y>1} + (r + b + 1 + \tau_2^2)1_{x+y\leq 1} =: H : \end{aligned}$$

Let $\tau_n := \inf\{t \in [0; \tau_e) : x(t) > nory(t) > norz(t) > n\}$. Clearly, τ_n increases to τ_∞ as $n \to \infty$ where

$$\tau_\infty := \inf\{t2 \in [0; \tau_e) : x(t) = \infty ory(t) = \infty orz(t) = \infty\}.$$

Since $\tau_\infty \leq \tau_e$ a.s., it suffces to prove that $P_{x;y;z}\{\tau_\infty = \infty\} = 1$. Fix $t > 0$, Ito's formula for V implies

$$\begin{aligned} E_{x;y;z}V(t \wedge \tau_n) &:= E_{x;y;z}V(x(t \wedge \tau_n); y(t \wedge \tau_n); z(t \wedge \tau_n)) \\ &= V(x; y; z) + E_{x;y;z}\int_0^{t\wedge\tau_n} LV(x(s); y(s); z(s))ds \\ &\leq K + H(t \wedge \tau_n) \leq K + Ht \end{aligned}$$

where $K := V(x; y; z)$. On the other hand,

$$E_{x;y;z}V(t\wedge\tau_n)\int_{\tau_n<t} V(x(\tau_n); y(\tau_n); z(\tau_n))dP_{x;y;z} \geq (n\wedge ln(1+n))P_{x;y;z}\{\tau_n < t\} :$$

Thus

$$P_{x;y;z}\{\tau_n < t\} \leq \frac{K + Ht}{n \wedge ln(1 + n)} \to 0; \text{ as } n \to \infty.$$

Since $t > 0$ is arbitrary, $P_{x;y;z}\{\tau_\infty < \infty\} = 0$ and hence $\tau_\infty = \infty$ a.s. ■

Next we analyze solutions of the system (3.234) on the boundary ∂R^3_+ firstly. When $x(0) = 0, x(t) = 0$ for all $t \geq 0$ a.s. If $x = 0$ then the system (3.234) becomes

$$dY = -Ydt + \tau_2 Y dW_2$$
$$dZ = [b + (1 + \tau_2^2 - c)Z]dt - \tau_2 Z dW_2 + \tau_3 Z dW_3.$$

The equation for $Y(t)$ implies

$$Y(t) = Y(0)exp\left(-\left(1+\tau_2^2\right)t + \tau_2 W2(t)\right).$$

So $Y(t) \to 0$ a.s. for all $Y(0) = y(0) \geq 0$. Consider the last equation for Z,

$$dZ = [b + (1 + \tau_2^2 - c)Z]dt - \tau_2 Z dW_2 + \tau_3 Z dW_3. \tag{3.235}$$

Fix $\alpha_1 > 0$, consider

$$\begin{aligned} s(Z) &= \int_{\alpha_1}^{Z} exp\left(-\int_{\alpha_1}^{y} \frac{2b - 2(c - 1 - \tau_2^2)u}{(\tau_2^2 + \tau_2^3)u^2} du\right) dy \\ &= C1 \int_{\alpha_1}^{Z} y^{2(c-1-\tau_2^2)/(\tau_2^2+\tau_3^2)} exp\left(\frac{2b}{(\tau_2^2 + \tau_3^2)y}\right) dy \end{aligned}$$

where C_1 is some positive constant. Rewrite the integrand as

$$y^{-2(1+\tau_2^2-c)/(\tau_2^2+\tau_3^2)}\left(1 + \frac{2b}{\tau_2^2 + \tau_3^2}\frac{1}{y} + \frac{1}{2!}\frac{4b^2}{(\tau_2^2 + \tau_3^2)^2}\frac{1}{y^2} + \cdots\right).$$

Since there exists a $k \in \mathcal{Z}_+$ such that $-\frac{2(1+\tau_2^2-c)}{\tau_2^2+\tau_3^2} - k < -1, s(0+) = -\infty$. If $\xi = 2c - 2 - \tau_2^2 + \tau_3^2 < 0$, then $-\frac{2(1+\tau_2^2-c)}{\tau_2^2+\tau_3^2} < -1$, so $s(\infty) < \infty$. By the item 2 of Theorem 3.1 on page 447 in [159], $\lim_{\to\infty} Z(t) = \infty$ a.s. In this case, (3.235) does not have any invariant measure. If $\xi \geq 0$, then $-\frac{2(1+\tau_2^2-c)}{\tau_2^2+\tau_3^2} \geq -1$, this implies that $s(\infty) = \infty$. Then $Z(t)$ oscillates between 0 and 1. Then (3.235) has a unique invariant measure $\pi_1 = \mathrm{IG}\left(-\frac{2(1+\tau_2^2-c)}{\tau_2^2+\tau_3^2} + 1, \frac{2b}{\tau_2^2+\tau_3^2}\right)$, (the inverse gamma distribution with parameters $-\frac{2(1+\tau_2^2-c)}{\tau_2^2+\tau_3^2} + 1$ and $\frac{2b}{\tau_2^2+\tau_3^2}$). When $x(0) > 0, x(t) > 0$ for all $t > 0$ a.s. If $y(0) = 0$, then the second equation of (3.234) implies $y(t) = 0$ for all$t > 0$ a.s. So, when $y = 0$, the equation for x becomes

$$d\tilde{x} = r\tilde{x}(1 - \tilde{x})dt + \tau_1 \tilde{x}(1 - \tilde{x})dW_1. \tag{3.236}$$

Fix $\alpha_2 > 0$, we compute

$$s(\tilde{x}) = \int_{\alpha_2}^{\tilde{x}} exp\left(-\int_{\alpha_2}^{y} \frac{2ru(1-u)}{\tau_1^2 u^2 (1-u)2} du\right) dy = C_2 \int_{\alpha_2}^{\tilde{x}} \left(\frac{1}{y} - 1\right)^{2r/\tau_1^2} dy;$$

where C_2 is some positive constant. Clearly, $s(1_-) < \infty$. Since $\lim_{y\to 0_+}(\frac{1}{y} - 1)^{2r/\tau_1^2} = \infty$, for any $M > 0$, there exists a $0 < \delta_0 < \alpha_2$ so that, if $0 < y < \alpha_2$, then $(\frac{1}{y} - 1)^{2r/\tau_1^2} \geq \frac{M}{\delta C_2}$. But we have

$$\begin{aligned} s(0_+) &= -C_2 \int_{\alpha_2}^{0} \left(\frac{1}{y} - 1\right)^{2r/\tau_1^2} dy \\ &\leq -C_2 \int_{\delta}^{0} \left(\frac{1}{y} - 1\right)^{2r/\tau_1^2} dy \leq -M \end{aligned}$$

Letting $M \to \infty$, it gives $s(0+) = -\infty$. This means that $\lim_{t\to\infty} \tilde{x}(t) = 1$ a.s. for any $\tilde{x}(0) = x(0) > 0$.
When $x = 1$ and $y = 0$, the last equation for z becomes

$$d\tilde{z} = [b + (1 + \tau_2^2 - a - c)\tilde{z} - a\tilde{z}^2]dt - \tau_2 \tilde{z} dW_2 + \tau_3 \tilde{z} dW_3. \tag{3.237}$$

Fix $\alpha > 0$, consider

$$\begin{aligned} s(Z) &= \int_{\alpha}^{Z} exp\left(-\int_{\alpha}^{y} \frac{2b + 2(1 + \tau_2^2 - a - c)u - 2au^2}{(\tau_2^2 + \tau_2^3)u^2} du\right) dy \\ &= C_3 \int_{\alpha}^{Z} y^{2(c-1-\tau_2^2)/(\tau_2^2+\tau_3^2)} exp\left(\frac{2b}{(\tau_2^2 + \tau_3^2)} \frac{1}{y} + \frac{2a}{(\tau_2^2 + \tau_3^2)}\right) dy \end{aligned}$$

where C_3 is some positive constant. Write the integrand as

$$\begin{aligned} y^{-2(1+\tau_2^2-c)/(\tau_2^2+\tau_3^2)} \Bigg\{ 1 &+ \frac{2b}{\tau_2^2 + \tau_3^2} \frac{1}{y} + \frac{2b}{\tau_2^2 + \tau_3^2} y + \\ &\frac{1}{2!} \left(\frac{4b^2}{(\tau_2^2 + \tau_3^2)^2} \frac{1}{y2} + \frac{8ab}{\tau_2^2 + \tau_3^2} + \frac{4a^2}{\tau_2^2 + \tau_3^2} y^2 \right) + \cdots \Bigg\}. \end{aligned}$$

Since there exists a $k_1, k_2 \in \mathcal{Z}_+$ such that $-\frac{2(1+\tau_2^2-c)}{\tau_2^2+\tau_3^2} - k_1 < -1$, and $-\frac{2(1+\tau_2^2-c)}{\tau_2^2+\tau_3^2} - k_2 > -1$. Hence $s(0+) = -\infty$ and $s(\infty) = \infty$. So $\tilde{z}(t)$ oscillates between 0 and 1, and thus (3.236) has a unique invariant measure $\pi_2 \sim$ GIG $(\theta; \chi; \phi)$, which is the generalized inverse Gaussian distribution with parameters $\theta \in R, \chi > 0$, and $\phi > 0$ (see [165]), whose density takes the form

$$p(\tilde{z}) = \frac{(a/b)^{\theta/2}}{2K_\theta(4\sqrt{ab}/(\tau_2^2 + \tau_3^2))} \tilde{z}^{\theta-1} \exp\left(-\frac{1}{2}(\chi\tilde{z}^{-1} + \phi\tilde{z})\right), \tilde{z} \in (0, \infty).$$

Where $\theta := \frac{2(1+\tau_2^2-a-c)}{\tau_2^2+\tau_3^2} - 1, \chi := \frac{4b}{\tau_2^2+\tau_3^2}$, and $\phi := \frac{4a}{\tau_2^2+\tau_3^2}$; $K_\theta(\cdot)$ is the modified Bessel function of the third kind with index θ. By law of large numbers,

$$\lim_{t\to\infty} \frac{1}{t} \int_0^t \tilde{z}(s)ds = \int_0^\infty \tilde{z}\pi_2(d\tilde{z}) = R_\theta(w)\sqrt{b/a},$$

where $R_\theta(w) := \frac{K_{\theta+1}(w)}{K_\theta(w)}$ and $w := 4\sqrt{ab}/(\tau_2^2 + \tau_3^2))$.
In summary, on the boundary ∂R^3_+

- If $\xi = 2c-2-\tau_2^2+\tau_3^2 < 0$, then the system (3.234) has only one invariant measure $\mu_2 := \delta_1^* \times \delta_0^* \times \pi_2$.
- If $\xi = 2c - 2 - \tau_2^2 + \tau_3^2 \geq 0$, then the system (3.234) has two invariant measure $\mu_1 := \delta_0^* \times \delta_0^* \times \pi_1$ and μ_2.

Note that

$$\int_{\partial R^3} \left(axz - 1 - \frac{\tau_2^2}{2} \right) d\mu_1 = -1 - \frac{\tau_2^2}{2} < 0,$$

$$\int_{\partial R^3} \left(axz - 1 - \frac{\tau_2^2}{2} \right) d\mu_2 = \sqrt{ab} R_\theta(w) - \frac{\tau_2^2}{2}.$$

We define a combined parameter as the threshold

$$\lambda := \sqrt{ab} R_\theta(w) - \frac{\tau_2^2}{2}.$$

Theorem 3.33 *[223] Assume that the initial values $u = (x; y; z)$ are in $R^{3;o}_+ := \{(x; y; z) : x > 0; y > 0; z > 0\}$ such that $x + y \leq 1$. The complete classification of solutions of the system (3.234) is as follows. Case 1. When $\xi < 0$, there is only one ergodic invariant measure μ_2 for solutions of (3.234) on the boundary ∂R^3_+.*

- *If $\lambda < 0$ then $x(t)$ converges to 1 a.s., $y(t)$ converges to 0 a.s., and $z(t)$ converges a.s. to π_2 weakly.*
- *If $\lambda > 0$ then the solution $u(t)$ is strongly stochastically persistent in the sense that the solution converges to its unique invariant probability measureμ_3 supported by $R^{3;o}_+$.*

Case 2. When $\xi > 0$, there are two ergodic invariant measures μ_1 and μ_2 for solutions of (3.234) on the boundary ∂R^3_+.

- *If $\lambda < 0$ and $\tau_1 < \sqrt{2r}$, then $x(t)$ converges to 1 a.s., $y(t)$ converges to 0 a.s., and $z(t)$ converges a.s. to μ_2 weakly.*
- *If $\lambda < 0$ and $\tau_1 > \sqrt{2r}$, then solutions starting near the interior of supp(μ_2) will tend to stay close and concentrate on supp(μ_1).*
- *If $\lambda > 0$ and $\lambda_1 < \sqrt{2r}$, then the solution $u(t)$ is strongly stochastically persistent.*
- *If $\lambda > 0$ and $\lambda_1 > \sqrt{2r}$, then $x(t)$ and $y(t)$ both converge a.s. to 0.*

Proof. The idea of the proof is to apply Theorems 1.1 and 1.3 in [149] to the system (3.234), we omit the details here. ■

Proposition 3.34 *The deterministic part of the system (3.234)(see also (3.208) in section 3.2.3.2) has three possible nonnegative equilibrium solutions,* $E_1 = (0; 0; b/(c-1)), E_2 = (1; 0; \frac{1}{2a}((1-a-c) + \sqrt{(1-a-c)^2 + 4ab})$, *and* $E_3 = (\frac{1}{a\bar{z}}; \frac{r(1-a/\bar{z})}{r+a\bar{z}}; \bar{z})$ *where* $\bar{z} = \frac{b-1}{c}$. *The ergodic invariant measures* μ_1 *and* μ_2 *correspond to* E_1 *and* E_2*, respectively, in the sense that the means of the distributions of* μ_1 *and* μ_2 *approaches* E_1 *and* E_2*, respectively, when* $(\tau_1; \tau_2; \tau_3)$ *approaches (0; 0; 0).*

From the transformation of variables, the information about the system (3.233) can be obtained. We write them as the interpretation of our main theorem. We will give some medical interpretation of these results and compare with our study in section 3.2.3.2.

Interpretation 1. *Consider the non-dimensionalized uninfected tumor cell population* $x(t)$*, infected tumor cell population* $y(t)$*, and free virus population* $v(t)$ *start in* $R_+^{3;o} := \{(x; y; z) : x > 0; y > 0; v > 0\}$ *such that* $x + y \leq 1$*, which corresponds to the system (3.234). Then, according to the thresholds* ξ *and* λ*, we can describe how each population will evolve as follows.*
Case 1. When $\xi < 0$*, the tumor cannot be eradicated completely a.s.*

- *If* $\lambda < 0$ *then* $(x(t); y(t); v(t))$ *converges to* $\bar{\mu}_2 = \delta_1^* \times \delta_0^* \times \delta_0^*$ *a.s.*

- *If* $\lambda > 0$ *then* $(x(t); y(t); v(t))$ *is strongly stochastically coexistence in the sense that* $(x(t); y(t); v(t))$ *converges to a unique invariant probability measure* $\bar{\mu}_3$ *supported by* $R_+^{3;o}$.

Case 2. When $\xi \geq 0$*, there is some possibilities to eradicate the tumor by oncolytic viruses.*

- *If* $\lambda < 0$*, and* $\tau_1 < \sqrt{2r}$*, then* $(x(t); y(t); v(t))$ *converges to* $\bar{\mu}_2 = \delta_1^* \times \delta_0^* \times \delta_0^*$ *a.s.*

- *If* $\lambda > 0$*, and* $\tau_1 < \sqrt{2r}$*, then the solution* $(x(t); y(t); v(t))$ *is strongly stochastically coexistence.*

- *If* $\lambda > 0$*, and* $\tau_1 > \sqrt{2r}$*, then* $(x(t); y(t); v(t))$ *converges to* $\bar{\mu}_1 = \delta_0^* \times \delta_0^* \times \delta_0^*$ *a.s.*

Using the transformation of variables or directly deduce, we have a similar proposition to Proposition 3.32.

Proposition 3.35 *The deterministic part of the system (3.234) has three equilibrium solutions,* $Q_1 = (0; 0; 0), Q_2 = (1; 0; 0)$*, and* $Q_3 = (\frac{1}{a\bar{z}}; \frac{r(1-a/\bar{z})}{r+a\bar{z}}; \frac{r(1-a/\bar{z})}{a+r/\bar{z}})$. *The system (3.234) has three ergodic invariant probability measures* $\bar{\mu}_1 = \delta_1^* \times \delta_0^* \times \delta_0^*, \bar{\mu}_2 = \delta_1^* \times \delta_0^* \times \delta_0^*$ *and* $\bar{\mu}_3$*, which correspond to* Q_1, Q_2, Q_3*, respectively.*

In section 3.2.3.2, we obtained asymptotic properties of the deterministic part of the system (3.234). There are three equilibrium solutions Q_1, Q_2, and Q_3. Q_1 is always unstable for any positive values of parameters. Q_2 is globally asymptotically stable when the virus burst size b is smaller a threshold value b_{s_1}, while it is unstable if b is greater than b_{s_1}. There is a second threshold value of the viral burst size bs2, and under the second threshold value and other conditions, Q_3 is locally asymptotically stable. The system undergoes Hopf bifurcations with three families of periodic solutions when the virus burst size passes the second threshold value b_{s_2}. It is interesting that Q_3 can be approximated by $(O(1/b); O(1/b); r/a)$ when the viral burst size b is very big. After incorporating environmental noise and stochastic effects into the system, there are three invariant probability measures in which solutions will approach them under various conditions. We have two combined parameters ξ and λ to describe asymptotical properties of solutions to the systems (3.233) or (3.234) as in Theorem 3.31. However, we would like to understand these results from the original system or how environmental noise and stochastic effects change the dynamical behaviors of the original system (3.208). Then, we need to understand how these two combined parameters connect to original parameters and their biological meanings. We have a proposition about the parameter λ.

Proposition 3.36 *The parameter $\lambda = \sqrt{ab}R_\theta(w) - 1 - \tau_2^2/2$ is an increasing function of the virus burst size b. Also consider λ is a function of noise intensities τ_2 and τ_3, and set $\bar{\lambda} := \lim_{(\tau_2;\tau_3)\to(0;0)} \lambda$. Then $\bar{\lambda} = 0$ if and only if $b = b_{s_1} = 1 + c/a$, $\bar{\lambda} < 0$ if and only if $b < b_{s_1}$, and $\bar{\lambda} > 0$ if and only if $b > b_{s_1}$; $\bar{\lambda}$ also is a increasing function of b.*

The parameter ξ combines infected tumor cell lysis rate δ, virus degradation rate γ , and their stochastic variation τ_2 and τ_3, which describes possibilities if the tumor can be eradicated. More specifically, $\xi = 2c - 2 - \tau_2^2 + \tau_3^2 = \frac{2T_\delta}{T_\gamma} - 2 - \tau_2^2 + \tau_3^2$, where T_δ is the average life time of infected tumor cells, and T_{gamma} is the average life time of free viruses in tumor tissue. $\xi < 0$ means $\frac{T_\delta}{T_\gamma} + \frac{\tau_3^2}{2} < \tau_2^2/2 + 1$. We may interpret that, if the ratio between the life time of infected tumor cells to the life time of free viruses is small and stochastic effects of viruses also is small comparing with stochastic effects of infected tumor cells, it is impossible to eradicate the tumor for viral therapy. However, in this situation, the viral therapy may partly success which depends on λ, or implicitly the outcome of the virotherapy depends on the virus burst size b. As in the deterministic model (3.208), if b is smaller than the threshold b_{s_1} which corresponds to $\lambda < 0$ (it is deduced from continuity of λ as a function of b, τ_2, and τ_3), then the infected tumor cell population and virus population will disappear, and only tumor cell population is left a.s., or the system approaches the invariant probability measure $\bar{\mu}_2 = \delta_1^* \times \delta_0^* \times \delta_0^*$. If b is greater than the threshold b_{s_1} which corresponds to $\lambda > 0$, three populations will coexist, or the system approaches the invariant probability measure $\bar{\mu}_3$, in which we may say viral therapy achieve some partial success. When $\xi > 0$ which means $\frac{T_\delta}{T_\gamma} + \frac{\tau_3^2}{2} > \tau_2^2/2 + 1$. We may interpret that, if the ratio between the life time of infected tumor cells to the life time of free viruses is big and stochastic effects of viruses also is big comparing with stochastic effects of infected tumor cells, there is some possibilities to eradicate the tumor by viral therapy. In this case, there is a third threshold value for stochastic variations of tumor cell growth τ_1 that comes to play some roles. This value is $2r = 2\frac{\rho}{\delta}$, scaled tumor cell growth rate. When b is smaller than the threshold b_{s_1} which corresponds to $\lambda < 0$, the noise intensity τ_1 or tumor cell variance τ_2 is smaller than the double of the scaled tumor cell growth rate, then the viral treatment will completely fail. When b is greater than the threshold bs1 which corresponds to $\lambda > 0$, and the noise intensity $\tau_1^2/2$ is not strong or smaller than scaled tumor cell growth rate, the system eventually will have three populations coexist, where the viral therapy reaches partial success. However, unlike in the corresponding deterministic model (3.208), when b is greater than the threshold b_{s_1} which corresponds to $\lambda > 0$, and the noise intensity $\tau_1^2/2$ is strong or greater than scaled tumor cell growth rate, the viral therapy will eradicate the tumor. A medical implication could be that viral therapy can success without too big virus burst size.

APPENDIX A

A Review of Dynamical Systems

The theory of dynamical systems studies how systems evolve over time according to deterministic rules. In continuous time, such systems are often modeled by ordinary differential equations (ODEs). In the appendix, we review some key concepts and results in the theory of dynamic systems [12, 52, 138, 170, 175, 199, 251, 281].

A.1 LINEAR SYSTEM

Let A be a $n \times n$ matrix, consider the following linear system

$$\dot{\mathbf{x}} = A\mathbf{x}, \quad \mathbf{x} = \mathbf{x}_0,$$

where $\mathbf{x}, \mathbf{x}_0 \in \mathbb{R}^n$.

Let $\sigma(A)$ denote the spectrum of A. Define:

$$\begin{aligned}
\sigma_s &= \{\lambda \in \sigma(A) : \Re(\lambda) < 0\}, \\
\sigma_u &= \{\lambda \in \sigma(A) : \Re(\lambda) > 0\}, \\
\sigma_c &= \{\lambda \in \sigma(A) : \Re(\lambda) = 0\}.
\end{aligned}$$

Corresponding invariant subspaces:

$$\mathbb{R}^n = E^s \oplus E^u \oplus E^c.$$

The linear flow e^{At} satisfies exponential decay on E^s and exponential growth on E^u.

A two-dimensional linear system can be written as

$$\dot{x} = a_{11}x + a_{12}y, \quad \dot{y} = a_{21}x + a_{22}y,$$

DOI: 10.1201/9781003376675-A

or in matrix form,

$$\dot{\mathbf{x}} = A\mathbf{x}, \quad A = \begin{pmatrix} a_{11} & a_{12} \\ a_{21} & a_{22} \end{pmatrix}, \quad \mathbf{x} = \begin{pmatrix} x \\ y \end{pmatrix}.$$

The eigenvalues λ_1, λ_2 of A determine the local dynamics. They satisfy

$$\lambda^2 - (\operatorname{tr} A)\lambda + \det A = 0,$$

where $\operatorname{tr} A = T = a_{11} + a_{22}$ and $\det A = D = a_{11}a_{22} - a_{12}a_{21}$.

Classification via Trace–Determinant Plane

Type	Conditions	Behavior
Saddle	$D < 0$	Unstable
Stable node	$D > 0, T < 0, T^2 > 4D$	Asymptotically stable
Unstable node	$D > 0, T > 0, T^2 > 4D$	Unstable
Stable focus	$D > 0, T < 0, T^2 < 4D$	Spiral in
Unstable focus	$D > 0, T > 0, T^2 < 4D$	Spiral out
Center	$T = 0, D > 0$	Closed orbits

A.2 NONLINEAR SYSTEM

Consider a smooth autonomous system:

$$\dot{x} = f(x), \quad f \in C^r(\mathbb{R}^n, \mathbb{R}^n), \ r \geq 1, \tag{A.1}$$

where an equilibrium point x_0 satisfies $f(x_0) = 0$.

A.2.1 Linearization and Spectral Decomposition

Let $A = Df(x_0)$ denote the Jacobian at the equilibrium. Linearizing about x_0 yields

$$\dot{y} = Ay, \qquad y = x - x_0.$$

Linearization predicts local behavior but cannot capture global nonlinear phenomena such as limit cycles.

A.2.2 Invariant Sets and Flows

Flow Map The flow $\Phi_t(x_0)$ is defined by

$$\frac{d}{dt}\Phi_t(x_0) = f(\Phi_t(x_0)), \quad \Phi_0(x_0) = x_0.$$

Invariant Set A subset $S \subset \mathbb{R}^n$ is *invariant* if

$$x_0 \in S \implies \Phi_t(x_0) \in S, \quad \forall t \in \mathbb{R}.$$

Typical examples: equilibria, periodic orbits, and manifolds.

A.2.3 Stable, Unstable, and Center Manifolds

Stable and Unstable Manifolds

Definition A.1 *Let x_0 be a hyperbolic equilibrium. The* local stable *and* local unstable manifolds *are defined as:*

$$W^s_{\text{loc}}(x_0) = \{x : \Phi_t(x) \to x_0 \ \text{as}\ t \to +\infty\},$$
$$W^u_{\text{loc}}(x_0) = \{x : \Phi_t(x) \to x_0 \ \text{as}\ t \to -\infty\}.$$

Theorem A.1 (Local Stable Manifold Theorem) *If x_0 is hyperbolic, there exist C^r submanifolds $W^s_{\text{loc}}(x_0)$ and $W^u_{\text{loc}}(x_0)$ such that*

$$T_{x_0} W^s_{\text{loc}} = E^s, \quad T_{x_0} W^u_{\text{loc}} = E^u,$$

and they are invariant under the flow:

$$\Phi_t(W^s_{\text{loc}}) \subset W^s_{\text{loc}}, \quad \Phi_t(W^u_{\text{loc}}) \subset W^u_{\text{loc}}.$$

Moreover, on W^s_{loc},

$$\|\Phi_t(x) - x_0\| \le Ce^{-\alpha t}, \ t > 0.$$

Center Manifold

Definition A.2 *A C^r submanifold $W^c(x_0)$ is a* center manifold *if*

(i) $T_{x_0} W^c = E^c$,

(ii) it is locally invariant: $x(0) \in W^c_{\text{loc}} \Rightarrow \Phi_t(x(0)) \in W^c_{\text{loc}}$ for small t.

Theorem A.2 (Center Manifold Theorem) *If $Df(x_0)$ has eigenvalues with zero real part, there exists a locally invariant C^r manifold W^c_{loc} tangent to E^c at x_0. The reduced flow on W^c_{loc} governs local dynamics and determines stability or bifurcation.*

In particular, if we consider the system

$$\dot{x} = Ax + f(x, y), \quad \dot{y} = By + g(x, y), \tag{A.2}$$

where $x \in \mathbb{R}^c$, $y \in \mathbb{R}^s$, A has eigenvalues with zero real parts (center directions), and B has eigenvalues with negative real parts (stable directions). Assume f and g are sufficiently smooth and vanish at the origin along with their first derivatives.

Theorem (Center Manifold Theorem). There exists a locally invariant manifold W^c of dimension c, called the *center manifold*, that can be expressed as

$$W^c = \{(x, y) \in \mathbb{R}^{c+s} \mid y = h(x), \ h(0) = 0, \ Dh(0) = 0\}.$$

The reduced dynamics on W^c is governed by

$$\dot{x} = Ax + f(x, h(x)).$$

Moreover, the stability and bifurcation behavior of the full system near the origin are determined by the reduced system on the center manifold.

We are going to see how the center manifold theorem can be applied in bifurcation analysis.

A.2.4 Lyapunov's Direct Method

Geometric invariant manifolds describe the structure of motion; Lyapunov's method provides analytical criteria for stability.

Definition A.3 (Lyapunov Function) *A continuously differentiable function $V : \mathbb{R}^n \to \mathbb{R}$ is a* Lyapunov function *for $\dot{x} = f(x)$ at an equilibrium x_0 if*

$$V(x_0) = 0, \quad V(x) > 0 \text{ for } x \neq x_0,$$

and the derivative along trajectories,

$$\dot{V}(x) = \nabla V(x) \cdot f(x),$$

is negative semidefinite (or negative definite) near x_0.

Theorem A.3 (Lyapunov Stability Theorem) *Let x_0 be an equilibrium of $\dot{x} = f(x)$, and let V be a Lyapunov function in a neighborhood D of x_0.*

(i) If $\dot{V}(x) \leq 0$ in D, then x_0 is stable.

(ii) If $\dot{V}(x) < 0$ in $D \setminus \{x_0\}$, then x_0 is asymptotically stable.

(iii) If $\dot{V}(x) > 0$ in $D \setminus \{x_0\}$, then x_0 is unstable.

This theorem establishes sufficient conditions for stability without solving the differential equations explicitly.

A.2.5 LaSalle's Invariance Principle

Lyapunov's theorem ensures asymptotic stability when $\dot{V}(x)$ is negative definite. If $\dot{V}(x)$ is only negative semidefinite, we need an extended result to describe asymptotic convergence.

Theorem A.4 (LaSalle's Invariance Theorem) *Let $\dot{x} = f(x)$ with f continuous, and let $V : \mathbb{R}^n \to \mathbb{R}$ be continuously differentiable such that $\dot{V}(x) \leq 0$ in a compact, positively invariant set Ω. Let*

$$E = \{x \in \Omega : \dot{V}(x) = 0\}.$$

Then every trajectory starting in Ω approaches the largest invariant set $M \subset E$ as $t \to \infty$:

$$\lim_{t \to \infty} \operatorname{dist}(\Phi_t(x_0), M) = 0.$$

Corollary. If E contains only the equilibrium x_0, then x_0 is asymptotically stable.

Remarks.

- LaSalle's theorem generalizes Lyapunov's method by relaxing the need for strict negativity of $\dot{V}$.
- It connects the analytic notion of invariance (via $\dot{V} = 0$) to the geometric invariant sets of the flow.
- The equilibrium's basin of attraction corresponds to the stable manifold when the system is smooth.

A.2.6 Relationship Between Invariant Manifolds and Lyapunov Theory

- The *stable manifold* coincides locally with the set of points where a Lyapunov function decreases monotonically.
- The *invariant set* in LaSalle's theorem can often be identified as a center or stable manifold.
- Lyapunov functions can be used to verify the existence or smoothness of invariant manifolds (e.g., through energy-like integrals).
- For dissipative systems, the asymptotic dynamics are confined to compact invariant sets (attractors), which may be manifolds or more complex invariant structures.

A.3 PHASE PLANE ANALYSIS

The *phase plane* is the geometric representation of trajectories $(x(t), y(t))$ in $\mathbb{R}^2$. Important tools include:

- **Nullclines:** Curves where $\dot{x} = 0$ or $\dot{y} = 0$. Their intersections give equilibrium points.
- **Direction field:** A graphical indication of trajectory slopes.
- **Invariant sets:** Regions where trajectories remain confined.

Phase plane analysis reveals qualitative features such as oscillations, convergence, and divergence even without analytic solutions.

A.4 LIMIT CYCLE

A *limit cycle* is a closed trajectory that is isolated, meaning nearby trajectories are not closed. If $\mathbf{x}(t)$ is a periodic solution with minimal period $T > 0$, then

$$\mathbf{x}(t + T) = \mathbf{x}(t).$$

A limit cycle Γ is *stable* if nearby trajectories spiral toward it, and *unstable* if they spiral away.
Poincaré–Bendixson Theorem: If a bounded trajectory in the plane remains in a compact region that contains no equilibrium points, then it approaches a periodic orbit (limit cycle).
This theorem provides a powerful existence result for 2D systems.

Example: The Van der Pol Oscillator The Van der Pol equation

$$\ddot{x} - \mu(1 - x^2)\dot{x} + x = 0$$

can be rewritten as

$$\dot{x} = y, \quad \dot{y} = \mu(1 - x^2)y - x.$$

For $\mu > 0$, the origin is an unstable focus, but the system exhibits a stable limit cycle.

A.5 BIFURCATIONS

Bifurcation theory studies qualitative changes in the behavior of dynamical systems as parameters vary. We summarizes the fundamental concepts, types, analytical and numerical methods, and typical examples of bifurcations in continuous and discrete systems. Applications across physics, biology, and engineering are also highlighted.

Consider a parameter-dependent dynamical system

$$\dot{x} = f(x, \mu), \tag{A.3}$$

where $x \in \mathbb{R}^n$ and $\mu \in \mathbb{R}$ is a control parameter. A **bifurcation** occurs at a critical parameter value $\mu = \mu_c$ where the qualitative structure of trajectories changes. These changes can involve the creation, annihilation, or stability exchange of equilibria or periodic orbits.

Bifurcation theory provides tools to connect local stability (through eigenvalue analysis) with global dynamical behavior, explaining transitions to oscillations, patterns, or chaos.

A.5.1 Classification of Bifurcations

Bifurcations can be broadly categorized as *local* or *global*, depending on whether they can be detected by analyzing the linearization near an equilibrium.

Local Bifurcations: Local bifurcations occur when eigenvalues of the Jacobian $D_x f(x^*, \mu)$ cross the imaginary axis.
1. **Saddle-Node (Fold) Bifurcation** Two equilibria collide and annihilate:

$$\dot{x} = \mu - x^2. \tag{A.4}$$

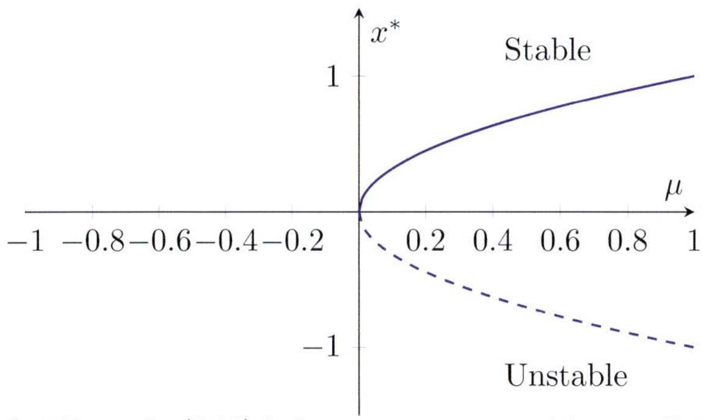

Figure A.1 Saddle-node (fold) bifurcation: two equilibria collide and annihilate at $\mu = 0$.

2. **Transcritical Bifurcation** Two equilibria exchange stability:

$$\dot{x} = \mu x - x^2. \tag{A.5}$$

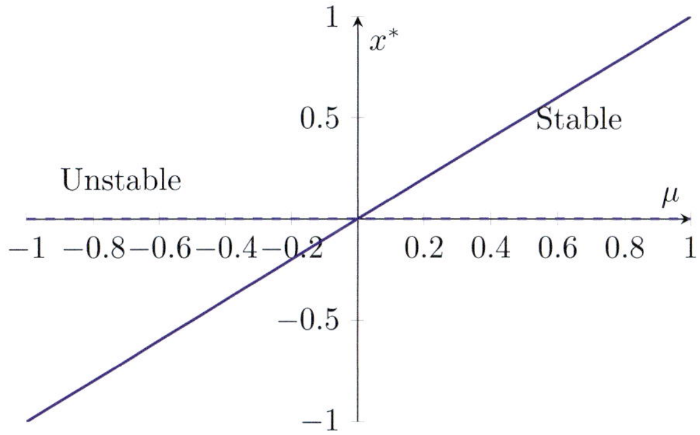

Figure A.2 Transcritical bifurcation: two equilibria exchange stability at $\mu = 0$.

3. **Pitchfork Bifurcation** A symmetric equilibrium gives rise to two new equilibria:

$$\dot{x} = \mu x - x^3. \tag{A.6}$$

4. **Hopf Bifurcation** A pair of complex conjugate eigenvalues cross the imaginary axis, giving rise to a limit cycle:

$$\begin{cases} \dot{x} = \mu x - y - x(x^2 + y^2), \\ \dot{y} = x + \mu y - y(x^2 + y^2). \end{cases} \tag{A.7}$$

Global Bifurcations: Global bifurcations involve topological changes in trajectories far from equilibria.

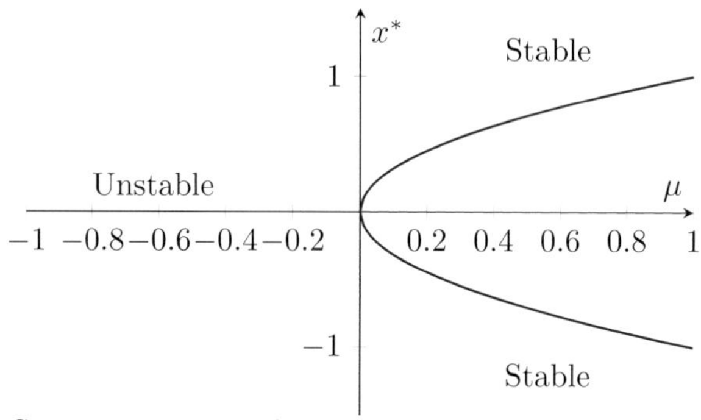

Figure A.3 Supercritical pitchfork bifurcation: a symmetric pair of stable equilibria emerge from an unstable one.

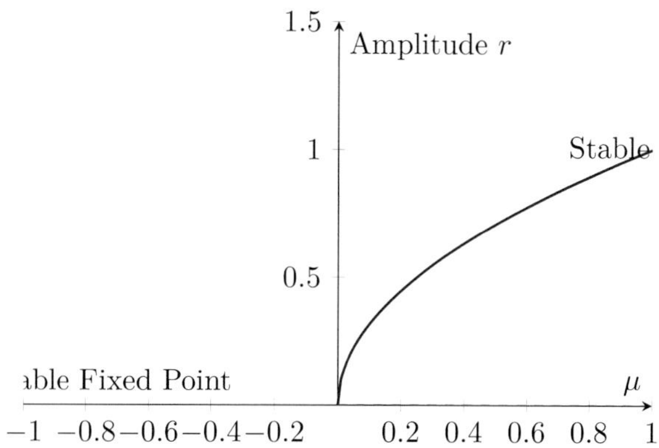

Figure A.4 Supercritical Hopf bifurcation: stable oscillations emerge as μ increases through zero.

- **Homoclinic Bifurcation:** A trajectory connects a saddle point to itself.
- **Heteroclinic Bifurcation:** A trajectory connects two different saddle points.
- **Period-Doubling (Flip) Bifurcation:** A periodic orbit doubles its period, potentially leading to chaos.

A.5.2 Applications of Center Manifold Theorem in Bifurcation Analysis

The center manifold theorem allows reduction of multi-dimensional systems to their essential one- or two-dimensional dynamics:

- **Saddle-node, pitchfork, and transcritical bifurcations** reduce to one-dimensional normal forms, e.g. $\dot{x} = \mu - x^2$ or $\dot{x} = \mu x - x^3$.

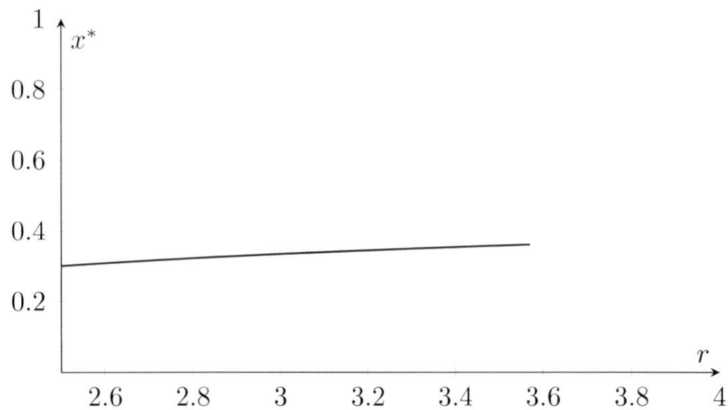

Figure A.5 Schematic of the period-doubling route to chaos in the logistic map.

- **Hopf bifurcation** reduces to a two-dimensional system representing oscillatory modes, leading to the normal form

$$\dot{r} = \mu r - \beta r^3, \qquad \dot{\theta} = \omega + O(r^2),$$

where r and θ are amplitude and phase variables.

Hence, even in high-dimensional systems, the essential bifurcation behavior can be captured in low dimensions via center manifold reduction.

Geometric Interpretation:

The center manifold acts as a *slow manifold* where the dynamics unfold after fast modes decay. Near equilibrium, trajectories are rapidly attracted to W^c, after which the slower bifurcation dynamics dominate.

Example: explicit center manifold reduction

We illustrate the center manifold reduction with a prototypical two-dimensional system in which one direction is *center* (eigenvalue zero at the bifurcation) and the other is *stable* (strictly negative eigenvalue). Consider

$$\begin{aligned} \dot{x} &= \mu x - x^3 + a\,xy, \\ \dot{y} &= -\lambda y + b\,x^2, \end{aligned} \tag{A.8}$$

where $x, y \in \mathbb{R}$, μ is the bifurcation parameter, and $\lambda > 0$ (so the y-direction is stable for μ near 0). The nonlinear terms are chosen to provide typical coupling terms; a, b are constants.

Step 1: Linearization and spectral splitting At the origin the Jacobian is

$$J(0,0) = \begin{pmatrix} \mu & 0 \\ 0 & -\lambda \end{pmatrix}.$$

At the bifurcation value $\mu = 0$ the eigenvalues are 0 (center) and $-\lambda$ (stable).

The center manifold is one-dimensional and can be written locally as

$$W^c = \{(x, y) : y = h(x),\ h(0) = 0,\ h'(0) = 0\}.$$

Step 2: Ansatz for the center manifold Seek h as a power series in x. Consistency with $h(0) = h'(0) = 0$ gives

$$h(x) = \alpha x^2 + \beta x^3 + O(x^4). \tag{A.9}$$

Step 3: Invariance equation Invariance of W^c implies that trajectories starting on the manifold stay on it. Differentiating $y = h(x)$ along trajectories gives

$$\dot{y} = h'(x)\dot{x}.$$

Using (A.8) we substitute $\dot{y}$ and $\dot{x}$:

$$-\lambda h(x) + bx^2 \;=\; h'(x)\big(\mu x - x^3 + axh(x)\big).$$

This functional equation is solved order-by-order in x.

Step 4: Match coefficients to determine α Compute left and right sides to $O(x^2)$. From (A.9):

$$\text{LHS} = -\lambda(\alpha x^2 + \beta x^3) + bx^2 + O(x^4) = (-\lambda\alpha + b)x^2 + (-\lambda\beta)x^3 + O(x^4).$$

Differentiate h: $h'(x) = 2\alpha x + 3\beta x^2 + O(x^3)$. Then

$$\text{RHS} = (2\alpha x + 3\beta x^2)\big(\mu x - x^3 + ax(\alpha x^2) + O(x^4)\big).$$

To leading orders,

$$\text{RHS} = 2\alpha\mu x^2 + O(x^3).$$

Equating the x^2-coefficients on both sides:

$$2\alpha\mu = -\lambda\alpha + b.$$

Solving for α yields

$$\alpha(\,2\mu + \lambda\,) = b \qquad \Longrightarrow \qquad \alpha = \frac{b}{2\mu + \lambda}. \tag{A.10}$$

Near the bifurcation $\mu \approx 0$ we may use the leading-order approximation

$$\alpha = \frac{b}{\lambda} + O(\mu).$$

Step 5: Reduced equation on the center manifold The reduced dynamics on W^c is

$$\dot{x} = \mu x - x^3 + axh(x).$$

Substitute $h(x) = \alpha x^2 + O(x^3)$:

$$\dot{x} = \mu x - x^3 + a\alpha x^3 + O(x^4) = \mu x - \big(1 - a\alpha\big)x^3 + O(x^4).$$

Hence, the leading-order normal form is

$$\dot{x} = \mu x - c\,x^3 + O(x^4), \qquad c \;=\; 1 - a\alpha. \tag{A.11}$$

Using (A.10) at leading order (set $\mu = 0$ in, α if desired), we often take

$$c \approx 1 - \frac{ab}{\lambda}.$$

Interpretation - If $c > 0$ the reduced equation $\dot{x} = \mu x - cx^3$ is the canonical form of a *supercritical pitchfork / transcritical style* bifurcation (stable nonzero equilibria appear for $\mu > 0$). - If $c < 0$ the cubic term has the opposite sign and may indicate a *subcritical* bifurcation (unstable branches) or require higher-order terms to decide the scenario.

Thus the center manifold reduction has transformed the original two-dimensional problem (A.8) into the one-dimensional normal form (A.11), with the effective nonlinear coefficient c expressed explicitly in terms of the original coupling constants a, b, λ.

Remark on higher-order terms One can continue the matching to determine β and $O(x^4)$ corrections for higher accuracy; the algebra is the same but lengthier. For many qualitative conclusions the cubic truncation suffices.

A.5.3 Bifurcation of Limit Cycles

Hopf Bifurcation

A *Hopf bifurcation* occurs when a fixed point changes stability and a small amplitude limit cycle emerges or disappears. Consider a system depending on a parameter μ:

$$\dot{x} = f(x, y, \mu), \quad \dot{y} = g(x, y, \mu).$$

At the bifurcation value $\mu = \mu_c$, a pair of complex conjugate eigenvalues of the Jacobian cross the imaginary axis:

$$\lambda_{1,2}(\mu_c) = \pm i\omega_0, \qquad \frac{d}{d\mu}\,\mathrm{Re}(\lambda_{1,2})\Big|_{\mu=\mu_c} \neq 0.$$

This transition causes the equilibrium to lose stability, giving rise to periodic oscillations.

Normal Form

The canonical form near a Hopf bifurcation is

$$\dot{z} = (\mu + i\omega_0)z - |z|^2 z,$$

where $z = x + iy$. For $\mu < 0$, the origin is a stable focus; for $\mu > 0$, it becomes unstable and a stable limit cycle of radius $\sqrt{\mu}$ emerges.

APPENDIX B

A Review of Parabolic Partial Differential Equations

In this appendix, we review some concepts and results in the theory of parabolic partial differential equations [9, 99, 105, 188, 191, 218, 300].

B.1 PARABOLIC EQUATIONS

Parabolic partial differential equations (PDEs) describe diffusion-type processes in time-dependent systems, such as heat conduction, population dynamics, and stochastic diffusion. The classical prototype is the *heat equation*

$$u_t - \Delta u = f(x,t), \quad (x,t) \in \Omega \times (0,T], \tag{B.1}$$

subject to appropriate boundary and initial conditions.

Let $\Omega \subset \mathbb{R}^n$ be a bounded domain with smooth boundary $\partial\Omega$. Consider the linear parabolic equation

$$u_t - a_{ij}(x,t)D_{ij}u - b_i(x,t)D_i u - c(x,t)u = f(x,t), \tag{B.2}$$

with $a_{ij} = a_{ji}$ and the uniform ellipticity condition

$$\lambda|\xi|^2 \leq a_{ij}(x,t)\xi_i\xi_j \leq \Lambda|\xi|^2, \quad \forall \xi \in \mathbb{R}^n. \tag{B.3}$$

Weak Maximum Principle: Suppose u satisfies

$$u_t - a_{ij}D_{ij}u - b_i D_i u - cu \leq 0 \quad \text{in } \Omega_T = \Omega \times (0,T],$$

with $u \leq 0$ on the parabolic boundary $\partial_p\Omega_T$. Then

$$u(x,t) \leq 0 \quad \text{for all } (x,t) \in \Omega_T.$$

DOI: 10.1201/9781003376675-B

This expresses that the solution cannot exceed its boundary maximum. The proof uses the parabolic comparison principle and barrier arguments.

Strong Maximum Principle: If $u_t - \mathcal{L}u \leq 0$ and u attains a nonnegative maximum at an interior point, then u is constant.

This generalizes the elliptic strong maximum principle to the parabolic setting.

Schauder Estimates: Schauder estimates quantify the smoothness of solutions in Hölder spaces. If u solves

$$u_t - a_{ij}(x,t)D_{ij}u = f(x,t) \quad \text{in } Q_T = \Omega \times (0,T],$$

and $a_{ij}, f \in C^{\alpha,\alpha/2}(\overline{Q_T})$, then

$$\|u\|_{C^{2+\alpha,1+\alpha/2}(\overline{Q_T})} \leq C\left(\|f\|_{C^{\alpha,\alpha/2}(\overline{Q_T})} + \|u\|_{C^0(\overline{Q_T})}\right),$$

where C depends on the ellipticity constants, α, and Ω.

Interpolation inequalities and Identities :

For any smooth function v, we have the following interpolation inequality [188]:

$$|v|_{C^{\alpha,\frac{\alpha}{2}}_{r,t}} \leq |v|^{\frac{\alpha}{1+\beta}}_{C^{1+\beta,\frac{1+\beta}{2}}_{r,t}} \quad \| v \|^{\frac{1+\beta-\alpha}{1+\beta}}_{L^\infty}, \text{ for } \beta > 0.$$

For L^p and Sobolev spaces, interpolation results bridge regularity spaces. For example, for parabolic Sobolev spaces $W^{2,1}_p(Q_T)$,

$$\left(L^p(Q_T), W^{2,1}_p(Q_T)\right)_{\theta,p} = B^{2\theta,\theta}_{p,p}(Q_T),$$

where $(\cdot,\cdot)_{\theta,p}$ denotes real interpolation, and $B^{2\theta,\theta}_{p,p}$ are Besov spaces. Interpolation provides a framework for time-space regularity of weak solutions.

B.2 EXISTENCE AND UNIQUENESS RESULTS

Theorem B.1 ***Classical Solutions***: *If a_{ij}, f are smooth and Ω has a smooth boundary, there exists a unique classical solution $u \in C^{2+\alpha,1+\alpha/2}(\overline{Q_T})$ satisfying* (B.2).

This follows from the Schauder theory.

Theorem B.2 ***Weak Solutions***: *For less regular data, define*

$$V = \{u \in L^2(0,T; H^1_0(\Omega)) : u_t \in L^2(0,T; H^{-1}(\Omega))\}.$$

Then there exists a unique $u \in V$ *satisfying*

$$\langle u_t, \phi \rangle + \int_\Omega a_{ij} D_i u D_j \phi \, dx = \int_\Omega f \phi \, dx, \quad \forall \phi \in H_0^1(\Omega),$$

with $u(0) = u_0$.

This result follows from the Lax–Milgram theorem and energy estimates.

B.3 SEMIGROUP THEORY

Definition B.1 *A semigroup* $S(t)$ *on a Banach space* $\mathcal{B}$ *is a family of bounded linear operators* $\{S(t)\}_{t \geq 0}$ *with the properties that* $S(t) \circ S(s) = S(t+s)$ *for any* $s, t \geq 0$ *and that* $S(0) = Id$. *A semigroup is furthermore, called "strongly continuous" if the map* $(x, t) \to S(t)x$ *is strongly continuous. A strongly continuous semigroup is also sometimes called a* C_0*-semigroup.*

Definition B.2 *The generator* L *of a* C_0*-semigroup is given by*

$$Lx = \lim_{t \to 0} t^{-1}(S(t)x - x),$$

on the set $D(L)$ *of all elements* $x \in \mathcal{B}$ *such that this limit exists (in the sense of strong convergence in* $\mathcal{B}$*).*

Theorem B.3 *(Hille-Yosida) A closed densely defined operator* L *on the Banach space* $\mathcal{B}$ *is the generator of a* C_0*-semigroup* $S(t)$ *with* $\|S(t)\| \leq Me^{at}$ *if and only if all* λ *with* $\Re\lambda > a$ *lie in its resolvent set and the bound* $\|R_\lambda^n\| \leq M(\Re\lambda - a)^{-n}$ *holds there for every* $n \geq 1$.

B.3.1 Sectorial Operators

An operator A on a Banach space X is called **sectorial** if there exists $\theta \in (0, \pi)$ such that the spectrum $\sigma(A)$ is contained in the sector

$$\Sigma_\theta = \{\lambda \in \mathbb{C} : |\arg \lambda| \leq \theta\},$$

and for all λ outside Σ_θ,

$$\|(\lambda I - A)^{-1}\| \leq \frac{C}{|\lambda|}.$$

Sectorial operators generate analytic semigroups.

B.3.2 Analytic Semigroup Definition

A strongly continuous semigroup $\{T(t)\}_{t \geq 0}$ on X is called **analytic** if there exists $\theta > 0$ such that $T(z)$ is holomorphic for all z in the sector

$$S_\theta = \{z \in \mathbb{C} : |\arg z| < \theta\},$$

and $\|T(z)\| \leq Me^{\omega \Re z}$ for some $M, \omega > 0$.

A sectorial operator A on X generates an analytic semigroup e^{At}. Analytic semigroups satisfy stronger regularity and decay properties than general C_0-semigroups.

B.3.3 Generation of Analytic Semigroups by Elliptic Operators

Let A be a uniformly elliptic operator defined by

$$Au = \nabla \cdot (a(x)\nabla u),$$

with $D(A) = H^2(\Omega) \cap H_0^1(\Omega)$. Then with Dirichlet boundary conditions, $-A$ generates an analytic semigroup on $L^p(\Omega)$ for $1 < p < \infty$. In particular, the Laplacian Δ with $D(\Delta) = H^2(\Omega) \cap H_0^1(\Omega)$ satisfies

$$\|e^{t\Delta}\|_{L^p \to L^p} \leq 1, \quad \|\Delta e^{t\Delta}\|_{L^p \to L^p} \leq \frac{C}{t}.$$

This implies that $e^{t\Delta}$ is analytic in t and exponentially stable.

B.3.4 Fractional Powers and Interpolation Spaces

For a sectorial operator A, define fractional powers via the Balakrishnan integral:

$$A^{-\alpha} = \frac{1}{\Gamma(\alpha)} \int_0^\infty t^{\alpha-1} e^{-tA}\, dt, \quad \alpha > 0.$$

The domains $D(A^\alpha)$ form a continuous interpolation scale:

$$[X, D(A)]_\theta = D(A^\theta),$$

which connects functional analysis with PDE regularity theory. For elliptic A, we have $D(A^{1/2}) = H_0^1(\Omega)$.

B.3.5 Mild and Strong Solutions

Let A on X be a sectorial operator, $u_0 \in X, f(t) \in L^1([0,T], X)$. The abstract Cauchy problem

$$u'(t) + Au(t) = f(t), \quad u(0) = u_0,$$

has a unique mild solution

$$u(t) = e^{-tA}u_0 + \int_0^t e^{-(t-s)A} f(s)\, ds,$$

which becomes a strong solution if $u_0 \in D(A)$ and $f \in L^\infty(0, T; X)$.

B.3.6 Analyticity and Regularization

Analytic semigroups immediately regularize data:

$$\|A^k e^{-tA} u_0\|_X \le C_k t^{-k} \|u_0\|_X.$$

In PDE language, even rough initial data $u_0 \in L^2(\Omega)$ becomes smooth for $t > 0$. This property underpins short-time regularity and smoothing for nonlinear parabolic systems.

For $u'(t) + Au(t) = f(t)$, analytic semigroup theory gives

$$u(t) = e^{-tA} u_0 + \int_0^t e^{-(t-s)A} f(s)\, ds,$$

and the mapping $f \mapsto u$ is bounded from $L^p(0,T;X)$ to $W^{1,p}(0,T;X) \cap L^p(0,T;D(A))$.

B.3.7 Applications

Analytic semigroup methods unify:

- linear and nonlinear parabolic PDEs,
- quasilinear and semi-linear diffusion equations,
- existence, uniqueness, and regularity proofs,
- long-time stability and invariant manifold theory.

They also underpin abstract results like the Crandall–Liggett theorem and Henry's geometric theory for semi-linear parabolic equations.

APPENDIX C

A Review of Stochastic Differential Equations

In this appendix, we review some concepts and results in probability theory, stochastic differential equations, and stochastic partial differential equations [32, 91, 167, 171, 189, 195, 208, 273].

C.1 FOUNDATIONS

C.1.1 Basic Notations of Probability Theory

Sample Space (Ω): The set of all possible outcomes of a random experiment:

$$\Omega = \{\omega_1, \omega_2, \dots\}$$

Event ($A, B, \dots$): A subset of the sample space, $A \subseteq \Omega$.

- The empty set $\emptyset$ represents an impossible event.
- The whole space Ω represents a certain event.

A **σ-algebra** $\mathcal{F}$ on Ω is a collection of subsets of Ω such that:

1. $\Omega \in \mathcal{F}$
2. If $A \in \mathcal{F}$, then $A^c \in \mathcal{F}$
3. If $A_1, A_2, A_3, \dots \in \mathcal{F}$, then $\bigcup_{i=1}^{\infty} A_i \in \mathcal{F}$

This ensures closure under complements and countable unions.

A **probability measure** P is a function

$$P : \mathcal{F} \to [0, 1]$$

that satisfies Kolmogorov's axioms:

DOI: 10.1201/9781003376675-C

1. $P(A) \geq 0$ for all $A \in \mathcal{F}$
2. $P(\Omega) = 1$
3. (Countable additivity) If $A_i \cap A_j = \emptyset$ for $i \neq j$, then

$$P\left(\bigcup_{i=1}^{\infty} A_i\right) = \sum_{i=1}^{\infty} P(A_i)$$

The triplet $(\Omega, \mathcal{F}, P)$ is called a **probability space**.
For events A, B with $P(B) > 0$,

$$P(A|B) = \frac{P(A \cap B)}{P(B)}.$$

Product rule:

$$P(A \cap B) = P(A|B)P(B).$$

Two events A and B are **independent** if

$$P(A \cap B) = P(A)P(B).$$

A collection of events $\{A_i\}$ is **mutually independent** if this holds for all finite subsets.

Tightness of Probability Measures

A sequence (or family) of probability measures (μ_n) on $\mathbb{R}^d$ is said to be *tight* if

$$\forall \varepsilon > 0,\ \exists \text{ compact set } K_\varepsilon \subset \mathbb{R}^d \text{ such that } \mu_n(K_\varepsilon) \geq 1 - \varepsilon, \quad \forall n.$$

In other words, most of the probability mass of μ_n is contained in some compact set uniformly in n.

Importance: Tightness ensures relative compactness in the space of probability measures endowed with the weak topology (by Prokhorov's theorem). It guarantees that from any tight sequence, one can extract a weakly convergent subsequence.

A **random variable (RV)** is a measurable function

$$X : \Omega \to \mathbb{R}$$

meaning that for every real x,

$$\{\omega : X(\omega) \leq x\} \in \mathcal{F}.$$

The **cumulative distribution function (CDF)** of X is

$$F_X(x) = P(X \leq x).$$

Properties:

- F_X is non-decreasing.
- $\lim_{x\to-\infty} F_X(x) = 0$, $\lim_{x\to\infty} F_X(x) = 1$.
- F_X is right-continuous.

Probability Mass and Density Functions:
Discrete case:

$$P(X = x_i) = p(x_i), \quad \sum_i p(x_i) = 1.$$

Continuous case:

$$f(x) \geq 0, \quad \int_{-\infty}^{\infty} f(x)dx = 1, \quad P(a \leq X \leq b) = \int_a^b f(x)dx.$$

Expectation:

$$E[X] = \begin{cases} \sum_i x_i p(x_i), & \text{discrete,} \\ \int_{-\infty}^{\infty} x f(x)\, dx, & \text{continuous.} \end{cases}$$

Variance:

$$\mathrm{Var}(X) = E[(X - E[X])^2] = E[X^2] - (E[X])^2.$$

Covariance:

$$\mathrm{Cov}(X, Y) = E[(X - E[X])(Y - E[Y])].$$

Correlation:

$$\rho_{XY} = \frac{\mathrm{Cov}(X, Y)}{\sqrt{\mathrm{Var}(X)\mathrm{Var}(Y)}}.$$

Let $(X_n)_{n\geq 1}$ be a sequence of random variables on a probability space $(\Omega, \mathcal{F}, \mathbb{P})$, and let X be another random variable.

Almost Sure Convergence: We say that X_n converges *almost surely* (a.s.) to X if

$$X_n \xrightarrow{a.s.} X \quad \text{if and only if} \quad \mathbb{P}\big(\lim_{n\to\infty} X_n = X\big) = 1.$$

That is, for almost every $\omega \in \Omega$, $X_n(\omega) \to X(\omega)$.

Convergence in Probability: We say that X_n converges *in probability* to X if

$$X_n \xrightarrow{\mathbb{P}} X \quad \text{if and only if} \quad \forall \varepsilon > 0, \ \lim_{n\to\infty} \mathbb{P}(|X_n - X| > \varepsilon) = 0.$$

Intuitively, the probability that X_n deviates from X by more than ε vanishes as $n \to \infty$.

Convergence in Distribution: We say that X_n converges *in distribution* (or weakly) to X if

$$X_n \xrightarrow{d} X \quad \text{if and only if} \quad \lim_{n\to\infty} F_{X_n}(x) = F_X(x)$$

for all continuity points x of the distribution function F_X of X. Equivalently, for every bounded and continuous function $f : \mathbb{R} \to \mathbb{R}$,

$$\lim_{n\to\infty} \mathbb{E}[f(X_n)] = \mathbb{E}[f(X)].$$

Relations Between Convergences:

The following implications hold:

$$X_n \xrightarrow{a.s.} X \implies X_n \xrightarrow{\mathbb{P}} X \implies X_n \xrightarrow{d} X.$$

However, the converse implications generally do not hold.

Key Theorems and Results:

Theorem C.1 *Law of Total Probability If $\{B_i\}$ is a partition of Ω, then*

$$P(A) = \sum_i P(A|B_i)P(B_i).$$

Theorem C.2 *Bayes' Theorem*

$$P(B_j|A) = \frac{P(A|B_j)P(B_j)}{\sum_i P(A|B_i)P(B_i)}.$$

Theorem C.3 *Chebyshev's Inequality*

$$P(|X - E[X]| \geq k\sigma) \leq \frac{1}{k^2}.$$

Let (X_n) be i.i.d. random variables with finite mean $\mu = \mathbb{E}[X_1]$. Define the sample average:

$$\bar{X}_n = \frac{1}{n}\sum_{i=1}^{n} X_i.$$

Theorem C.4 *Weak Law of Large Numbers(WLLN) If $\mathbb{E}[|X_1|] < \infty$, then*

$$\bar{X}_n \xrightarrow{\mathbb{P}} \mu.$$

That is, for all $\varepsilon > 0$,

$$\lim_{n\to\infty} \mathbb{P}(|\bar{X}_n - \mu| > \varepsilon) = 0.$$

Proof (via Chebyshev's inequality): *If* $\mathrm{Var}(X_1) = \sigma^2 < \infty$, *then*

$$\mathbb{P}(|\bar{X}_n - \mu| > \varepsilon) \le \frac{\mathrm{Var}(\bar{X}_n)}{\varepsilon^2} = \frac{\sigma^2}{n\varepsilon^2} \to 0.$$

Theorem C.5 *Strong Law of Large Numbers (SLLN)*
If $\mathbb{E}[|X_1|] < \infty$, *then*

$$\bar{X}_n \xrightarrow{a.s.} \mu.$$

That is, with probability one, the sample mean converges to the true mean.
Kolmogorov's version: *If* (X_n) *are independent with* $\mathbb{E}[X_n] = 0$ *and*

$$\sum_{n=1}^{\infty} \frac{\mathrm{Var}(X_n)}{n^2} < \infty,$$

then $\frac{1}{n}\sum_{i=1}^{n} X_i \to 0$ *almost surely.*

Theorem C.6 *Central Limit Theorem (CLT)*
Let (X_n) *be i.i.d. random variables with mean* μ *and variance* $\sigma^2 > 0$. *Define*

$$S_n = \sum_{i=1}^{n} X_i, \qquad Z_n = \frac{S_n - n\mu}{\sigma\sqrt{n}}.$$

Then

$$Z_n \xrightarrow{d} Z \sim \mathcal{N}(0, 1).$$

That is, the normalized sum of i.i.d. random variables converges in distribution to the standard normal law.

Lindeberg–Feller CLT: If (X_n) are independent with $\mathbb{E}[X_n] = 0$, variances σ_n^2, and $s_n^2 = \sum_{i=1}^{n} \sigma_i^2$, and the Lindeberg condition holds:

$$\forall \varepsilon > 0, \quad \frac{1}{s_n^2} \sum_{i=1}^{n} \mathbb{E}\big[X_i^2 \mathbf{1}_{\{|X_i| > \varepsilon s_n\}}\big] \to 0,$$

then

$$\frac{1}{s_n} \sum_{i=1}^{n} X_i \xrightarrow{d} \mathcal{N}(0, 1).$$

Lyapunov CLT: If for some $\delta > 0$,

$$\frac{1}{s_n^{2+\delta}} \sum_{i=1}^{n} \mathbb{E}[|X_i|^{2+\delta}] \to 0,$$

then the same convergence in distribution to $\mathcal{N}(0, 1)$ holds.

Connection Between LLN and CLT:

Theorem	Type of Convergence	Scaling	Limit
Law of Large Numbers	In probability / a.s.	$1/n$	Deterministic (μ)
Central Limit Theorem	In distribution	$1/\sqrt{n}$	Random (Normal law)

Conditional Expectation: Let $X \in L^1(\Omega, R)$ be a random variable. Let $g \subset F$ is a sub-σ-algibra of F so (ω, g) is a measurable space. By Radon-Nikodym Thm, there exists a on such Y, almost surely unique, such that

$$\int_G Y(w)dP(w) = \int_G X(w)dP(w) \text{ for all } G \in g$$

and Y is an integrable g measurable random variable. Y is called the conditional expectation of X under the condition g, and we write $Y = E(x|g)$. If g is the $\delta - algebra$ generate by a random variable Y, we write $E(X|g) = E(X]Y)$.

Property of conditional expectation:

1. If X is $g - measurable, then E(X|g) = X$
2. $E(aX + bY|g) = aE(X|g) + bE(Y|g), a, b \in R$
3. X is $g - measurable \Rightarrow E(XY|g) = XE(Y|g)$
4. If $\delta(X), g$ are independent $\Rightarrow E(X|g) = 0$
5. $g_1 \subset g_2 \subset F \Rightarrow E(E(X|g_2)|g_1) = E(X|g_1)$

C.1.2 Stochastic Process

A **stochastic process** is a family of random variables

$$\{X_t : t \in T\}$$

defined on a probability space $(\Omega, \mathcal{F}, \mathbb{P})$, where T is an index set (often $T = \mathbb{N}$ or $T = [0, \infty)$). For each $\omega \in \Omega$, the map $t \mapsto X_t(\omega)$ is called a *sample path* or *realization* of the process.

Examples:

- Discrete-time process: X_n for $n \in \mathbb{N}$.
- Continuous-time process: X_t for $t \geq 0$.

A **filtration** $(\mathcal{F}_t)_{t \in T}$ is an increasing family of sub-σ-algebras of $\mathcal{F}$:

$$\mathcal{F}_s \subseteq \mathcal{F}_t \subseteq \mathcal{F}, \quad \text{for all } s \leq t.$$

It represents the evolution of information over time. A stochastic process (X_t) is said to be **adapted** to $(\mathcal{F}_t)$ if

$$X_t \text{ is } \mathcal{F}_t\text{-measurable for all } t.$$

Let $\{X_t\}_{t \geq 0}$ be on R^d-valued stochastic process. It is said to be continuous (resp, right continuous, left continuous) on $t \geq 0$ if for almost all $\omega \in \Omega$, $X_t(\omega)$ is continuous (right continuous, or left continuous) on $t \geq 0$. It is said to be cadlag, if it is right continuous and for almost all $\omega \in \Omega$ the left limit $\lim_{s \to t} X_s(\omega)$ exists and is finite for all $t \geq 0$).
$\{X_t\}$ is $\{F_t\}$-adapted if for every t,X_t is F_t-measurable.
$\{X_t\}$ is said to be progressive by measurable or progressive if for every $T > 0$, $\{X_t\}_{0 \leq t \leq T}$ regarded as a function from $[O, T] \times \Omega$ to R^d is $B([O, T]) \times F_T$-measurable, where $B([O, T])$ is the family of all Borel subsets of $[O, T]$.

Let $(\Omega, \mathcal{F}, (\mathcal{F}_t)_{t \geq 0}, \mathbb{P})$ be a filtered probability space, and (X_t) an integrable stochastic process adapted to $(\mathcal{F}_t)$. (X_t) is a **martingale** if

$$\mathbb{E}[|X_t|] < \infty, \quad \text{and} \quad \mathbb{E}[X_t \mid \mathcal{F}_s] = X_s, \quad \forall s \leq t.$$

(X_t) is a **supermartingale** if

$$\mathbb{E}[X_t \mid \mathcal{F}_s] \leq X_s, \quad \forall s \leq t.$$

(X_t) is a **submartingale** if

$$\mathbb{E}[X_t \mid \mathcal{F}_s] \geq X_s, \quad \forall s \leq t.$$

A stochastic process $X = \{X_t\}_{t \geq 0}$ is called square integrable if $E|X_t^2| < \infty$ for all $t \geq 0$.

If $\{X_t\}_{t \geq 0}$ is square integrable continuous martingale, then there exists a unique continuous integrable adapted increasing process denoted by $\{< M, M >_t\}$ such that $\{M_t^2 - < M, M >_t\}$ is a continuous martingale vanishing at $t = 0$. $\{< M, M >_t\}$ is called the quadratic variation of M. Let $\{N_t\}_t \geq 0$ be another square integrable continuous martingale; we define: $< M, N >_t = \frac{1}{2}(< M+N, M+N >_t - < M, M >_t - < N, N >_t)$ and call $\{< M, N >_t\}$ the joint quadratic variation of M and N. It is useful to know that $\{< M, N >_t\}$ is the unique continuous integrable adapted process of finite variation such that $\{M_t N_t - < M, N >_t\}$ is a continuous martingale vanishing at $t = 0$.

A random variable $\tau : \Omega \to (0, \infty)$ is called a $\mathcal{F}_t$ - stopping time (or stopping time) if $\{w; \tau(w) \leq t\} \in \mathcal{F}_t$ for $\forall t > 0$.

A right continuous adapted process $M = \{M_t\}_t \geq 0$ is called a local martingale if there exists a non-decreasing sequence $\{\tau_k\}_k \geq$ of stopping times with $\tau_k \to \infty$ as such that $\{M_{\tau_k \wedge t} - M\}_t \geq 0$ is a martiangle.

Doob's Martingale Convergence Theorem : If (X_t) is a nonnegative supermartingale, then there exists an a.s. finite limit:

$$X_t \xrightarrow{a.s.} X_\infty \quad \text{as } t \to \infty.$$

Doob's Optional Sampling Theorem:
Let (X_t) be a martingale, and $\tau_1 \leq \tau_2$ be bounded stopping times. Then

$$\mathbb{E}[X_{\tau_2} \mid \mathcal{F}_{\tau_1}] = X_{\tau_1}.$$

In particular,

$$\mathbb{E}[X_{\tau_2}] = \mathbb{E}[X_{\tau_1}].$$

Extensions: If the martingale is uniformly integrable, this result holds even for unbounded stopping times provided τ_1 and τ_2 are finite almost surely.
Brownian motions:
Let (Ω, F, P) be a probability space with filtration $\{F_t\}_{t>0}$. A one-dimensional Brownian motion is a real-valued continuous $\{F_t\}$-adapted process $\{B_t\}_{t\geq 0}$ with the following properties:

1. $B_t = 0$ as $t = 0$
2. for $0 \leq s < t < \infty$, the increment $B_t - B_s$ is normally distributed with mean 0 and variance $t - s$.
3. for $0 \leq s < t < \infty, B_t - B_s$ is independent of F_s.
4. **Continuity:** The sample paths $t \mapsto B_t(\omega)$ are continuous almost surely.

Properties of Brownian motion:

- $\{B_t\}$ is a continuous square integrable martingale, and its quadratic variation $< B, B >_t = t$ for all $t \geq 0$
- For almost every $w \in \Omega$, the Brownian sample path $B(w)$ is nowhere differentiable.
- For almost every $w \in \Omega, B(w)$ is locally Holder continuous with exponent δ if $\delta \in (0, \frac{1}{2})$. But $B(w)$ is not Holder continuous with $\delta > \frac{1}{2}$.
- **Law of the Iterated Logarithm (LIL):**

$$\limsup_{t\to\infty} \frac{B_t}{\sqrt{2t \log\log t}} = 1, \liminf_{t\to\infty} \frac{B_t}{\sqrt{2t \log\log t}} = -1; \quad \text{a.s.}$$

and

$$\limsup_{t\to 0^+} \frac{B_t}{\sqrt{2t \log\log(1/t)}} = 1, \liminf_{t\to 0^+} \frac{B_t}{\sqrt{2t \log\log(1/t)}} = -1. \quad \text{a.s.}$$

A d-dimensional process $\{B_t = (B_t^1, \cdots, B_t^d)\}_{t\geq 0}$ is called a d-dimensional Brownian motion if $\{B_t^i\}$ a one-dimensional Brownian motion and $\{B_t^1\} \cdots \{B_t^d\}$ are independent.

A d-dimensional Brownian motion is a d-dimensional continuous martingle with the joint quadratic variation $< B^i, B^j >_t = \delta_{ij} t$ for $1 \leq i, j \leq d$ and

$$\delta_{ij} = \begin{cases} 0 & i \neq j \\ 1 & i = 1 \end{cases}$$

C.1.3 Stochastic Integrals

Denote by $M^2([a,b]; R)$ the space of all real-valued measurable $\{F_t\}$-adapted process $f = \{f(t)\}_{a \leq t \leq b}$ such that $||f||_{ab}^2 = E\int_a^b |f(t)|^2 dt < \infty$.

A real valued stochastic process $g = \{g(t)\}_{a \leq t \leq b}$ is called a simple (or step) process if there exists a partition $a = t_0 < t_1 < \cdots < t_k = b$ of $[a, b]$ and bounded random variables ξ_i, $0 \leq i \leq k-1$, such that ξ_i is F_{ti}-measurable and $g(t) = \xi_0 I_{[t_0, t_1]} + \Sigma_{i=1}^{t-1} \xi_i I_{[t_i, t_{i+1}]}(t)$. Denote by $M_0([a,b], R)$ the family of all such processes.

Let $g \in M_0([a,b], R)$, define $\int_a^b g(t) dB_t = \Sigma_{i=0}^{k-1} \xi_i (B_{t_{i+t}} - B_{t_i})$.

Let $f \in M^2([a,b], R)$. The Ito integral of f is defined by $\int_a^b f(t) dB_t = \lim_{n\to\infty} \int_a^b g_n(t) dB_t$ in $L^2(\Omega, R)$, where $\{g_n\}$ is a sequence of simple process such that $\lim_{n\to\infty} E\int_a^b |f(t) - g_n(t)|^2 dt = 0$.

Properties of Ito Integral:

1. $\int_a^b f(t) dB_t$ is F_b-measurable
2. $E\int_a^b f(t) dB_t = 0$
3. $E|\int_a^b f(t) dB_t|^2 = E\int_a^b |f(t)|^2 dt$

Ito's Formula:

Let $\{B_t\}_{t\geq 0}$ be a one-dimensional Brownian motion on (Ω, F, P), with filtration $\{F_t\}$.

Let $L^1\{R_+; R^d\}$ denote the family of all R^d-valued measurable $\{F_k\}$-adapted process $f = \{f(t)\}_{t\geq 0}$ such that $\int_0^T |f(t)| dt < \infty$ for every $T > 0$.

A one dimensional Ito process $x(t)$ is a continuous adapted process on $t \geq 0$ of the form

$$x(t) = x(0) + \int_0^t f(s) ds + \int_0^t g(s) dB_s,$$

where $f \in L^1(R_t, R)$, $g \in L^2(R_t, R)$.

We shall say that $x(t)$ has **stochastic differential** $dx(t)$ given by $dx(t) = f(t)dt + g(t)dB_t$.

Theorem C.7 *(The one-dimensional Ito formula) Let $x(t)$ be an Ito process with $dx(t) = f(t)dt + g(t)dB_t$ and $V \in C^{2,1}(RxR_t, R)$, then $V(x((t), t)$ is again an Ito process with*

$$\partial V(x(t), t) = [V_t(X(t), t) + V_x(x(t), t)f(t) + \frac{1}{2}V_{xx}(x(t), t)g^2(t)]dt \\ + V_x(x(t), t)g(t)dB_t.$$

Let $B(t) = (B_1(t), \cdots, B_m(t))^T, t \geq 0$ be an m-dimensional Brownian motion on (Ω, F, P) with filtration $\{F_t\}_{t\geq 0}$.

A d-dimensional Ito process $x(t) = (x_1(t), \cdots, x_d(t)^T$ on $t \geq 0$ is given by

$$x(t) = x(0) + \int_0^t f(s)ds + \int_0^t g(s)dB(s)$$

for $f(t) \in L^1(R+; R^d), g(t) \in L^2(R+, R^{d\times m})$ and we denote $dx(t) = f(t)dt + g(t)dB(t)$.

Let $C^{2,1}(R^d \times R_t; R)$ denote the family of all real valued functions $V(x, t)$ on $R^d \times R_t$ such that they are continuously twice differentiable in x and one differentiable in t. We set $V_t = \frac{\partial V}{\partial t}$, $V_x = (\frac{\partial V}{\partial x_1}, \cdots, \frac{\partial V}{\partial x_d})$, and

$$V_{xx} = \left(\frac{\partial^2 V}{\partial x_i, \partial x_j i}\right)_{d\times d} = \begin{pmatrix} \frac{\partial^2 v}{\partial x_i, \partial x_1}, \cdots, \frac{\partial^2 v}{\partial x, \partial x_d} \\ \frac{\partial^2 v}{\partial x_d, \partial x_1}, \cdots, \frac{\partial^2 v}{\partial X_d \partial x_d} \end{pmatrix}.$$

Theorem C.8 *(The multi-dimensional Ito formula) If $dx(t) = f(t)dt + g(t)dB(t), f \in L^1(R^+, R^d), g \in L^2(R^+, R^{d\times m})$. Let $V \in C^{2,1}(R^d \times R_t, R)$, then $V(x(t), t)$ is an Ito process and*

$$dV(x(t), t) = V_t(x(t), t) + V_x(x(t), t)f(t) \\ + \frac{1}{2}trace[g^T(t)V_{xx}(x(t), t)g(t)]\}dt + V_x(x(t), t)g(t)dB(t).$$

Now we formally introduce $dtdt = 0, dB_idt = 0, dB_idB_i = dt, dB_idB_j = 0$ for $i \neq j$. Then $dx_i(t)dx_i(t) = \Sigma_{k=1}^m g_{ik}(t)g_{ik}(t)dt$ and the Ito formula becomes

$$dV(x(t), t) = V_t(x(t), t)dt + V_x(x(t), t)dx(t) + \frac{1}{2}dx^T(t)V_{xx}(x(t), t)dx(t).$$

Theorem C.9 *(Integration by parts) Let $x(t)$ be one-dimensional Ito process with $dx(t) = f(t)dt + g(t)dB(t)$ when $f \in L^1(R^+, R), g(t) \in$*

$L^1(R^+, R^{1\times m}), B(t)$ is m-dimensional Brownian motion. Let $g(t), t \geq 0$ be a real-valued continuous adapted process of finite variation. Then $d[x(t)y(t)] = y(t)dx(t) + x(t)dy(t)$. i.e

$$x(t)y(t) = \int_0^t y(s)[f(s)ds + g(s)dB(s)] + \int_0^t x(s)dy(s).$$

C.2 STOCHASTIC DIFFERENTIAL EQUATIONS

A standard d-dimensional Ito SDE has the following form:

$$dX_t = b(t, X_t)\,dt + \sigma(t, X_t)\,dW_t, \quad X_0 = x_0,$$

where $b: [0, T] \times \mathbb{R}^d \to \mathbb{R}^d$ is the drift coefficient, $\sigma: [0, T] \times \mathbb{R}^d \to \mathbb{R}^{d\times m}$ is the diffusion coefficient, and W_t is an m-dimensional Wiener process.

If X_t is adapted to the filtration generated by W_t, and satisfies the SDE almost surely, then X_t is a **strong solution**. If there exists a filtered probability space and Wiener process W_t such that the SDE holds in distribution, then X_t is a **weak solution**. If two solutions on the same probability space with same W_t and X_0 are indistinguishable, then the solution is **pathwise unique**. If the distribution of X_t is unique, even if the underlying space differs, then the solution is **unique in law**.

C.2.1 Existence and Uniqueness

Let $b(t, x)$ and $\sigma(t, x)$ satisfy: (1) Lipschitz condition: For every $R > 0$, there exists $L_R > 0$ such that

$$\|b(t, x) - b(t, y)\| + \|\sigma(t, x) - \sigma(t, y)\| \leq L_R\|x - y\|, \quad \forall \|x\|, \|y\| \leq R.$$

(2) Linear growth condition: There exists $K > 0$ such that

$$\|b(t, x)\|^2 + \|\sigma(t, x)\|^2 \leq K(1 + \|x\|^2).$$

Theorem C.10 *If b, σ satisfy the Lipschitz and linear growth conditions, then for every initial value $X_0 = x_0$, there exists a unique strong solution X_t on $[0, T]$ such that*

$$\mathbb{E}\left[\sup_{0\leq t\leq T} \|X_t\|^2\right] < \infty.$$

Theorem C.11 *Pathwise Uniqueness and Yamada–Watanabe Theorem: If weak existence and pathwise uniqueness hold, then a unique strong solution exists.*

Remark C.12 *When the coefficients are not Lipschitz, solutions may still exist under weaker assumptions:*
1. **Monotonicity condition:**

$$(x - y)^\top(b(x) - b(y)) + \|\sigma(x) - \sigma(y)\|^2 \leq K\|x - y\|^2.$$

2. **One-sided Lipschitz** *and* **coercivity** *conditions are often used (see Mao, 2007).*

C.2.2 Invariant Measures

Consider the SDE on $\mathbb{R}^n$:

$$dX_t = b(X_t)\,dt + \sigma(X_t)\,dW_t,$$

where $b : \mathbb{R}^n \to \mathbb{R}^n$ is the drift, $\sigma : \mathbb{R}^n \to \mathbb{R}^{n\times m}$ the diffusion coefficient, and W_t an m-dimensional Wiener process. Let P_t denote the associated Markov semigroup:

$$(P_t f)(x) = \mathbb{E}[f(X_t^x)].$$

C.2.2.1 *Definition*

A probability measure μ on $\mathbb{R}^n$ is *invariant* if

$$\int_{\mathbb{R}^n} (P_t f)(x)\,\mu(dx) = \int_{\mathbb{R}^n} f(x)\,\mu(dx), \quad \forall t \geq 0,\ f \in C_b(\mathbb{R}^n).$$

Equivalently, if $X_0 \sim \mu$, then $X_t \sim \mu$ for all t.

C.2.2.2 *Fokker–Planck Equation*

Let ρ_t be the density of X_t. Then

$$\frac{\partial \rho_t}{\partial t} = L^* \rho_t,$$

where L is the generator

$$Lf = b \cdot \nabla f + \tfrac{1}{2}(\sigma\sigma^\top) : \nabla^2 f,$$

and L^* is its formal adjoint. An invariant density ρ satisfies $L^*\rho = 0$.

C.2.2.3 *Existence and Uniqueness*

Existence follows from the Krylov–Bogolyubov theorem under tightness. Uniqueness is ensured by ergodicity, which holds if the process is irreducible, strongly Feller, and recurrent, or if b is dissipative and $\sigma\sigma^\top$ is uniformly elliptic. See [32].

C.2.2.4 *Gradient Systems*

For a gradient SDE

$$dX_t = -\nabla V(X_t)\,dt + \sqrt{2\beta^{-1}}\,dW_t,$$

the invariant measure is the Gibbs measure

$$\mu(dx) = Z^{-1} e^{-\beta V(x)}\, dx,$$

where $Z = \int_{\mathbb{R}^n} e^{-\beta V(x)}\, dx$.

C.2.2.5 Ergodicity

If the process is ergodic, then for $f \in L^1(\mu)$,

$$\lim_{T\to\infty} \frac{1}{T} \int_0^T f(X_t)\, dt = \int f(x)\, \mu(dx), \qquad \text{a.s.}$$

and the law of X_t converges to μ as $t \to \infty$.

C.3 GAUSSIAN MEASURES, CYLINDRICAL WIENER PROCESS, AND ITO INTEGRAL IN HILBERT SPACES

Notation and Setting

Let $(H, \langle\cdot,\cdot\rangle_H, \|\cdot\|_H)$ be a separable real Hilbert space. The Borel σ-algebra on H is denoted by $B(H)$. The spaces of bounded, trace-class, and Hilbert–Schmidt operators on H are respectively, $\mathcal{L}(H)$, $\mathcal{L}_1(H)$, and $\mathcal{L}_2(H)$.

C.3.1 Gaussian Measures on Hilbert Spaces

A Borel probability measure μ on H is Gaussian if for every $h \in H$, the real random variable $\langle X, h\rangle_H$ (with X distributed according to μ) is Gaussian. Such a measure is completely determined by its mean $m \in H$ and covariance operator Q:

$$m = \int_H x\, \mu(dx), \qquad Qh = \int_H \langle x - m, h\rangle_H (x - m)\, \mu(dx).$$

Covariance Operator

The covariance operator Q is self-adjoint, positive semidefinite, and trace-class if and only if $\int_H \|x\|_H^2\, \mu(dx) = \mathrm{Tr}(Q) < \infty$. In an orthonormal basis (e_n) with eigenvalues (λ_n) of Q, we can write

$$X = \sum_{n=1}^{\infty} \sqrt{\lambda_n} \xi_n e_n, \qquad \xi_n \overset{iid}{\sim} N(0,1).$$

Cameron–Martin Space

The Cameron–Martin space associated with μ is

$$H_\mu = Q^{1/2}(H),$$

with inner product $\langle Q^{1/2}u, Q^{1/2}v\rangle_{H_\mu} = \langle u, v\rangle_H$. The Cameron–Martin formula states that for $h \in H_\mu$,

$$\frac{d\mu_h}{d\mu}(x) = \exp\left(\langle x, h\rangle_{H_\mu} - \tfrac{1}{2}\|h\|^2_{H_\mu}\right),$$

where $\mu_h(\Gamma) = \mu(\Gamma - h)$, $\Gamma \in B(H)$.

Fernique's Theorem:

There exists $\alpha > 0$ such that

$$\int_H e^{\alpha\|x\|^2_H}\, d\mu(x) < \infty.$$

C.3.2 Cylindrical Wiener Processes

A family $W = \{W_t\}_{t\geq 0}$ is a cylindrical Wiener process on H if for each $h \in H$, the process $W_t(h)$ is a real Brownian motion with variance $t\|h\|^2_H$ and W_t is linear in h. For finite $\{h_i\}$, the joint process $(W_t(h_1), \dots, W_t(h_n))$ is a standard Gaussian vector with covariance $t[\langle h_i, h_j\rangle_H]$.

Series Representation

For an orthonormal basis (e_n) and independent Brownian motions (β_n),

$$W_t^{\mathrm{cyl}} = \sum_{n=1}^{\infty} \beta_n(t) e_n$$

is a cylindrical Wiener process. The series does not converge in H when H is infinite-dimensional.

Q-Wiener Process

Given a trace-class $Q \in \mathcal{L}(H)$, the process

$$W_t^Q = \sum_{n=1}^{\infty} \sqrt{\lambda_n}\beta_n(t) e_n$$

is an H-valued Q-Wiener process, satisfying $\mathbb{E}\|W_t^Q\|^2_H = t\,\mathrm{Tr}(Q)$.

C.3.3 Ito Integral in Hilbert Spaces

Let U, H be separable Hilbert spaces and W^Q a Q-Wiener process on U. We wish to define

$$\int_0^T \Phi(s)\, dW_s^Q,$$

where $\Phi(s) : U \to H$ is progressively measurable.

Integrability Condition

The integral exists if

$$\mathbb{E}\int_0^T \|\Phi(s)Q^{1/2}\|^2_{\mathcal{L}_2(U,H)}\, ds < \infty.$$

Series Definition

Let (e_n) be an orthonormal basis of U diagonalizing Q with eigenvalues (λ_n), and (β_n) independent Brownian motions:

$$\int_0^T \Phi(s)\, dW_s^Q := \sum_{n=1}^{\infty}\int_0^T \Phi(s)(\sqrt{\lambda_n}e_n)\, d\beta_n(s).$$

The series converges in $L^2(\Omega; H)$.

Ito Isometry

$$\mathbb{E}\left\|\int_0^T \Phi(s)\, dW_s^Q\right\|_H^2 = \mathbb{E}\int_0^T \|\Phi(s)Q^{1/2}\|^2_{\mathcal{L}_2(U,H)}\, ds.$$

Ito Formula

For an Itô process

$$X_t = X_0 + \int_0^t A_s\, ds + \int_0^t \Phi_s\, dW_s^Q,$$

and a twice Fréchet-differentiable $F : H \to \mathbb{R}$,

$$F(X_t) = F(X_0) + \int_0^t DF(X_s)[A_s]ds + \int_0^t DF(X_s)[\Phi_s dW_s^Q] + \frac{1}{2}\int_0^t \mathrm{Tr}\big(D^2F(X_s)(\Phi_s Q^{1/2})(\Phi_s Q^{1/2})^*\big)ds.$$

C.4 STOCHASTIC PARTIAL DIFFERENTIAL EQUATIONS

Stochastic partial differential equations (SPDEs) generalize deterministic PDEs by including random perturbations, often modeled by Wiener processes or space–time white noise. They describe diverse phenomena in physics, biology, and finance where randomness plays a structural role, such as heat conduction with random sources or stochastic reaction–diffusion systems.

A typical abstract form of an SPDE on a Hilbert space H is

$$dX_t = (AX_t + B(X_t))\, dt + G(X_t)\, dW_t, \quad X_0 = x_0 \in H, \tag{C.1}$$

where

- A is the generator of a C_0-semigroup $S(t)$ on H (typically representing diffusion or dissipation),
- $B : H \to H$ and $G : H \to \mathcal{L}_2(U, H)$ are the drift and diffusion coefficients,
- W_t is a cylindrical Wiener process on another Hilbert space U.

The main questions of interest are:

1. Does a solution X_t exist (in a suitable sense)?
2. Is the solution unique (pathwise or in law)?
3. How regular are the trajectories?

C.4.1 Solution Frameworks

Different frameworks have been developed to treat SPDEs depending on the nature of the noise and the regularity of coefficients.

C.4.1.1 *Mild Solutions: Semigroup Approach (Da Prato–Zabczyk [91])*

Let A generate a C_0-semigroup $(S(t))_{t\geq 0}$ on H. A *mild solution* to (C.1) satisfies

$$X_t = S(t)x_0 + \int_0^t S(t-s)B(X_s)\,ds + \int_0^t S(t-s)G(X_s)\,dW_s. \tag{C.2}$$

If B and G are globally Lipschitz and satisfy linear growth bounds, standard Picard iteration arguments yield existence and uniqueness of a mild solution $X \in L^2(\Omega; C([0,T]; H))$.

Theorem (Da Prato & Zabczyk [91]). Assume A generates a C_0-semigroup $S(t)$ on H, and B, G are globally Lipschitz and of linear growth. Then, for every $x_0 \in L^2(\Omega; H)$, there exists a unique mild solution to (C.1), satisfying

$$\mathbb{E}\left[\sup_{t\in[0,T]} \|X_t\|_H^2\right] < \infty.$$

C.4.1.2 *Variational (Monotone) Solutions [189]*

For nonlinear SPDEs with monotone operators, e.g. stochastic p-Laplacian equations, Lipschitz conditions fail. The variational method considers a Gelfand triple

$$V \hookrightarrow H \hookrightarrow V^*,$$

and interprets the equation weakly as

$$\langle dX_t, \phi\rangle = \langle A(X_t), \phi\rangle\, dt + \langle G(X_t)\, dW_t, \phi\rangle, \tag{C.3}$$

for test functions $\phi \in V$. Existence and uniqueness follow from Minty–Browder monotonicity and compactness arguments.

Theorem (Pardoux type [216]). If $A : V \to V^*$ is hemicontinuous, coercive, and monotone, and $G : V \to \mathcal{L}_2(U, H)$ satisfies appropriate Lipschitz and growth conditions, then there exists a unique variational solution

$$X \in L^2(\Omega; L^2(0, T; V)) \cap L^2(\Omega; C([0, T]; H)).$$

C.4.1.3 Walsh Random-Field Formulation [273]

For space–time white noise $\dot{W}(t, x)$, the equation

$$\partial_t u = \mathcal{L}u + F(u) + \dot{W}(t, x)$$

is ill-defined in classical sense. Walsh (1986) developed a stochastic integral with respect to the *martingale measures*, allowing the definition of random-field solutions:

$$u(t, x) = (G_t * u_0)(x) + \int_0^t \int_{\mathbb{R}^d} G_{t-s}(x - y) F(u(s, y))\, dy\, ds + \int_0^t \int_{\mathbb{R}^d} G_{t-s}(x - y) M(ds, dy),$$

where G_t is the heat kernel and M is a martingale measure associated with $\dot{W}$.

Existence and uniqueness of such solutions hold for Lipschitz F provided the *Dalang condition* on the noise's spectral measure is satisfied.

Dalang Condition [87]: Let μ be the spectral measure of the spatial covariance of $\dot{W}$. Then the stochastic convolution is well-defined iff

$$\int_{\mathbb{R}^d} \frac{1}{1 + |\xi|^2}\, \mu(d\xi) < \infty.$$

This restricts the allowable spatial dimension and correlation of the noise.

C.4.1.4 Extensions and Modern Developments

Regular SPDEs: When noise and nonlinearities are sufficiently regular, classical theory ensures X_t has continuous paths in H and inherits semigroup smoothing.

Singular SPDEs and Renormalization:

Equations such as the KPZ equation or the Φ^4_3 model are *singular*: products of distributions arising from space–time white noise are undefined. Recent breakthroughs include:

- Hairer's *theory of regularity structures* [144], which gives a general fixed-point and renormalization framework for singular SPDEs.
- Paracontrolled distributions and renormalization group approaches that provide alternative solution frameworks.

C.4.2 Invariant Measures for Stochastic Partial Differential Equations (SPDEs)

Invariant measures are fundamental tools in the study of the long-time behavior of stochastic partial differential equations (SPDEs). They describe the steady-state distributions toward which the system converges under its stochastic dynamics.

Formally, given an SPDE of the form

$$dX_t = (AX_t + F(X_t))\,dt + B(X_t)\,dW_t, \tag{C.4}$$

where A is typically an unbounded linear operator generating a C_0-semigroup on a separable Hilbert space H, F is a nonlinear drift, B is the noise coefficient, and W_t is a cylindrical Wiener process, the associated Markov semigroup $(P_t)_{t\geq 0}$ acts on bounded measurable functions $\varphi : H \to \mathbb{R}$ by

$$P_t\varphi(x) = \mathbb{E}[\varphi(X_t^x)].$$

C.4.2.1 *Definition and Basic Properties*

Definition C.1 (Invariant Measure) *A Borel probability measure μ on H is called an* invariant measure *for (P_t) if*

$$\int_H P_t\varphi(x)\,\mu(dx) = \int_H \varphi(x)\,\mu(dx), \qquad \forall\varphi \in \mathcal{B}_b(H),\ t \geq 0.$$

Equivalently, $P_t^*\mu = \mu$.

Definition C.2 (Stationarity and Ergodicity) *A process $(X_t)_{t\in\mathbb{R}}$ is* stationary *if all finite-dimensional distributions are time-shift invariant, with law μ. The invariant measure μ is* ergodic *if for any bounded measurable φ,*

$$\lim_{T\to\infty} \frac{1}{T}\int_0^T \varphi(X_t)\,dt = \int_H \varphi(x)\,\mu(dx) \quad a.s.$$

C.4.2.2 Existence and Uniqueness Theorems

Existence via Krylov–Bogoliubov

Theorem C.13 (Krylov–Bogoliubov) *If for some $x \in H$ the family of measures*

$$\mu_T := \frac{1}{T} \int_0^T P_t(x, \cdot)\, dt$$

is tight, then there exists a subsequence μ_{T_n} converging weakly to a measure μ, and μ is invariant for (P_t).

In SPDEs, tightness is typically established by energy or Lyapunov-type estimates combined with compact embeddings between Sobolev spaces.

Uniqueness and Ergodicity

Uniqueness of invariant measures and ergodicity are often obtained through one or more of the following criteria:

- **Strong Feller property + irreducibility**: implies uniqueness of the invariant measure.
- **Harris theorem**: If there exists a Lyapunov function $V : H \to [0, \infty)$ and a small set $\mathcal{C} \subset H$ such that

  $$P_t V(x) \leq \lambda V(x) + b, \qquad x \in H,$$

  and a minorization condition holds on $\mathcal{C}$, then (P_t) is geometrically ergodic.
- **Coupling methods**: Construct coupled solutions (X_t^x, X_t^y) such that $\mathbb{P}(X_t^x = X_t^y) \to 1$ as $t \to \infty$.

C.4.2.3 Linear SPDEs and Gaussian Invariant Measures

Consider the linear stochastic evolution equation

$$dX_t = AX_t\, dt + B\, dW_t.$$

If A generates an exponentially stable semigroup and B is bounded (or Hilbert–Schmidt), then there exists a unique Gaussian invariant measure $\mathcal{N}(0, Q_\infty)$ where the covariance operator Q_∞ satisfies the Lyapunov equation

$$AQ_\infty + Q_\infty A^* + BB^* = 0.$$

If $Ae_k = \lambda_k e_k$ and $Be_k = b_k e_k$, then the modal variances are

$$\mathbb{E}|\langle X_t, e_k \rangle|^2 = \frac{b_k^2}{-2\lambda_k}.$$

C.4.2.4 Example: Stochastic Heat Equation

The 1D stochastic heat equation with Dirichlet boundary conditions

$$\partial_t u = \partial_{xx} u + \sigma dW(t, x)$$

on $[0, 1]$ can be expanded in the eigenbasis $e_k(x) = \sqrt{2}\sin(k\pi x)$:

$$dX_k = -\lambda_k X_k \, dt + \sigma_k \, d\beta_k(t), \quad \lambda_k = (k\pi)^2.$$

Each mode is an Ornstein–Uhlenbeck process with invariant variance

$$q_k = \frac{\sigma_k^2}{2\lambda_k}.$$

Bibliography

[1] G. Abi Younes, N. El Khatib, V. Volpert, A free boundary mathematical model of atherosclerosis, Appl. Anal. 103(1) (2024), 240-262.

[2] E. Ackerman, J.W. Rosevear, W.F. McGuckin, A mathematical model of the glucose tolerance test, Phys. Med. Biol. 9 (2) (1964), 203.

[3] E. Ackerman, L.C. Gatewood, J.W. Rosevear, G.D. Molnar, Model studies of blood-glucose regulation, Bull. Math. Biophys. 27 (1965), S21.

[4] J. Adam and N. Bellomo, Editors, A Survey of Models on timor Immune Systems Dynamics, Birkhliuser, Boston, (1996).

[5] A. Aldakhil, Stationary solution and its linear stability in a cancer model, Master's Thesis, *Morgan State University*, (2021).

[6] A. Aldakhil, Analysis and Simulation of a Free Boundary Problem Modeling2 Tumor Evolution, PhD Dissertation, Morgan State University, 2025.

[7] E. Allen, Modeling with Ito Stochatic Differential Equations. Springer; Dordrecht, The Netherlands: 2007.

[8] L.J.S. Allen, An Introduction to Stochastic Processes with Applications to Biology. 2. CRC Press; Boca Raton, London, New York: 2010.

[9] H. Amann, *Linear and Quasilinear Parabolic Problems*, Birkhäuser, 1995.

[10] A. Poznyak, A.V. Grechko, P. Poggio, V.A. Myasoedova, V. Alfieri, and A.N. Orekhov. The Diabetes Mellitus Atherosclerosis Connection: The Role of Lipid and Glucose Metabolism and Chronic Inflammation, Int. J. Mol. Sci. 21 (2020), 1835.

[11] N.A. Averinos, and P. Neofytou, Mathematical Modeling and Simulation of Atherosclerosis Formation and Progress: A Review. Annals of Biomedical Engineering, 47 (8) (2019), 1764-1785.

[12] V.I. Arnold, *Ordinary Differential Equations*, MIT Press, 1992.

[13] Z. Bajzer, T. Carr, K. Josic, S.J. Russel, and D. Dingli, Modeling of cancer virotherapy with recombinant measles viruses, J. Theoretical Biology, 252 (2008), 109-122.

[14] A. Basu, C. Dalla Man, R. Basu, G. Toffolo, C. Cobelli, and R.A. Rizza, Effects of type 2 diabetes on insulin secretion, insulin action, glucose effectiveness, and postprandial glucose metabolism, Diabetes Care 32 (2009), 866.

[15] B.V. Bazaliy, and A. Friedman, A free boundary problem for an elliptic-parabolic system: Application to a model of tumor growth. Commun. Partial Diff. Eqns 28 (2003), 517-560.

[16] B.V. Bazaliy, and A. Friedman, Global existence and asymptotic stability for an elliptic parabolic free boundary problem: an application to a model of tumor growth. Indiana Math. J 52 (2003), 1265-1304.

[17] J.A. Beckman, M.A. Creager, and P. Libby, Diabetes and Atherosclerosis, JAMA, 287 (19) (2002).

[18] P. Bekima, and X. Xie, Well-posedness of a Stochastic Model for Glucose, Insulin, β-Cell Mass Kinetics, preprint, 2024.

[19] N. Bellomo, and L. Preziosi, Modeling and mathematical problems related to tumor evolution and its interaction with the immune system. Math. Comput. Modeling 32 (2000), 413-542.

[20] R.N. Bergman, Origins and History of the Minimal Model of Glucose Regulation. Front. Endocrinol. 11 (2021), 583016.

[21] R.N. Bergman, and C. Cobelli, Minimal modeling/partition analysis and the estimation of insulin sensitivity, Fed. Proc. 39 (1980), 110.

[22] R.N. Bergman, Y.Z. Ider, C.R. Bowden, and C. Cobelli, Quantitative estimation of insulin sensitivity, Am. J. Physiol. 236 (1979), E667.

[23] R.N. Bergman, The minimal model: yesterday, today and tomorrow., in: R.N. Bergman, J.C. Lovejoy (Eds.), The Minimal Model Approach and Determination of Glucose Tolerance, LSU Press, 1997, pp. 3–50.

[24] R.N. Bergman, The minimal model of glucose regulation: a biography, in: J. Novotny, M. Green, R. Boston (Eds.), Mathematical Modeling in Nutrition and Health, Kluwer Academic/Plenum, 2001.

[25] R. Bertram, J. Previte, A. Sherman, T.A. Kinard, and L.S. Satin, The phantom burster model for pancreatic β-cells, Biophys. J. 79 (2000), 2880-2892.

[26] R. Bertram, and J. Rubin, Multi-timescale systems and fast-slow analysis, Math. Biosci. 287 (2017), 105-121.

[27] R. Bertram , I. Marinelli, P.A. Fletcher, L.S. Satin, and A.S. Sherman, Deconstructing the integrated oscillator model for pancreatic β-cells, Math. Biosci. 365 (2023), 109085.

[28] R. Bertram, L.S. Satin, and A.S. Sherman, Closing in on the mechanisms of pulsatile insulin secretion, Diabetes 67 (2018), 351–359.

[29] R. Bertram, L. Satin, M. Zhang, P. Smolen, and A. Sherman, Calcium and glycolisis mediate multiple bursting modes in pancreatic islets, Biophys. J. 87 (2004), 3074.

[30] R. Bertram, and A. Sherman, A calcium-based phantom bursting model for pancreatic islets, Bull. Math. Biol. 66 (2004), 1313.

[31] A. Bertuzzi, S. Salinari, and G. Mingrone, Insulin granule trafficking in b-cells: mathematical model of glucose-induced insulin secretion, Am. J. Physiol. Endocrinol. Metab. 293 (2007), E396.

[32] V. Bogachev, N. Krylov, M. Röckner, and S.V. Shaposhnikov, Fokker-Planck-Kolmogorov Equations, Mathematical Surveys and Monographs, volume 207, 2015, American Mathematical Society.

[33] V.W. Bolie, Coefficients of normal blood glucose regulation, J. Appl. Physiol. 16 (1961), 783.

[34] A. Boutayeb, and A. Chetouani, A critical review of mathematical models and data used in diabetology, BioMedical Engineering OnLine 5 (2006), 43.

[35] A. Boutayeb, and M.E.N. Lamlili, Computational Mathematics and Modeling for Diabetes. Industrial and Applied Mathematics, 2025.

[36] E.M. Bradshaw, K. Raddassi, W. Elyaman et al., Monocytes from patients with type 1 diabetes spontaneously secrete proinflammatory cytokines inducing Th17 cells, Journal of Immunology, 183 (7) (2009), 4432-4439.

[37] E. Breda, M.K. Cavaghan, G. Toffolo, K.S. Polonsky, and C. Cobelli, Oral glucose tolerance test minimal model indexes of beta-cell function and insulin sensitivity. Diabetes 50 (2001), 150-158.

[38] P.L. Brubaker, E.L. Ohayon, L.M. D'Alessandro, and K.H. Norwich, A mathematical model of the oral glucose tolerance test illustrating the effects of the incretins, Ann. Biomed. Eng. 35 (2007), 1286.

[39] M.A. Bulelzai, and J.L.A. Dubbeldam, A mathematical model of plaque formation. Journal of Theoretical Biology, 309 (2012), 1-10.

[40] H.M. Byrne, The importance of intercellular adhesion in the development of carcinomas. IMA Journal of Mathematics Applied in Medicine & Biology 14 (1997), 305-323.

[41] H.M. Byrne, A weakly nonlinear analysis of a model of avascular solid tumour growth. J Math Biol. 39 (1999), 59-89.

[42] H.M. Byrne and M.A.J. Chaplain, Growth of nonnecrotic tumor in the presence and absence of inhibitor, Math.Bioscience, 130 (1995), 151-181.

[43] H.M. Byrne, and M.A. Chaplain, Modeling the role of cell-cell adhesion in the growth and development of carcinomas. Mathematical and Computer Modeling 24 (1996), 1-7.

[44] H.M. Byrne and M.A.J. Chaplain, Free boundary value problems associated with the growth and development of multicellular spheroids. Eur. J. Appl. Math 8 (1997), 639-658.

[45] H.M. Byrne, T. Alarcn, M.R. Owen, S.W. Webb, and P.K. Maini, Modeling aspects of cancer dynamics: A review. Phi. Trans. R. Soc. A 364 (2006), 1563-1578.

[46] H.M. Byrne and P. Matthews, Asymmetric growth of models of avascular solid tumors: exploiting symmetries. IMA J. Math. Appl. Med. Biol 19 (2002), 129.

[47] R. Caballero, M.A. Martinez, and E. Peña, "Fully coupled hybrid in-silico modeling of atherosclerosis: A multi-scale framework integrating CFD, transport phenomena and agent-based modeling." Frontiers in Bioengineering and Biotechnology, 13 (2025), 1549104.

[48] V. Calvez, A. Ebde, N. Meunier, and A. Raoult, Mathematical Modeling of the atherosclerotic plaque formation. CEMRACS 2008 - Modeling and Numerical Simulation of Complex Fluids 28 (2009), 1-12.

[49] V. Calvez and A. Ebde, Mathematical modeling of the atherosclerotic plaque formation. ESAIM Proc. CEMRACS 2008 - Model. Numer. Simul. Complex Fluids (2010), 1-16.

[50] K.L. Chambers, M. Myerscough, M.G. Watson, and H.M. Byrne. "Blood Lipoproteins Shape the Phenotype and Lipid Content of Early Atherosclerotic Lesion Macrophages: A Dual-Structured Mathematical Model". Bulletin of Mathematical Biology, 86 (2024), 112.

[51] C.G. Caro, J.M. Fitz-Gerald, and R.C. Schroter, Atheroma and arterial wall shear. The Lancet, 297 (1971), 464-466.

[52] J. Carr, *Applications of Centre Manifold Theory*, Springer, 1981.

[53] V. Carvalho, D. Pinho, R.A. Lima, J. Teixeira, and S. Teixeira. "Blood Flow Modeling in Coronary Arteries: A Review". Fluids (2021), 6020053.

[54] A. Caumo, R.N. Bergman, C. Cobelli, Insulin sensitivity from meal tolerance tests in normal subjects: a minimal model index, J. Clin. Endocrinol. Metab. 85 (2000), 4396.

[55] U. Chakravarthy, R.G. Hayes, A.W. Stitt, E. McAuley, and D.B. Archer. Constitutive nitric oxide synthase expression in retinal vascular endothelial cells is suppressed by high glucose and advanced glycation end products. Diabetes. 47 (1998), 945-952.

[56] M.A.J. Chaplain, Avascular growth, angiogenesis and vascular growth in solid tumors: The mathematical Modeling of stages of tumor development, Modeling and Simulation Problems on firnor-Immune System Dynamics, Special Issue of Mathl. Comput. Modeling 23 (6) (1996), 47–87.

[57] M.A.J. Chaplain, Special Issue on Mathematical Models for the Growth, Development and Treatment of Tumours, Math. Models Meth. Appt. Sci. 9 (1999).

[58] M.A.J. Chaplain, Pattern formation in cancer. In: Chaplain M.A.J., et al., editors. On Growth and Form: Spatio-Temporal Pattern Formation in Biology. Wiley; New York: 2000.

[59] M.A.J. Chaplain, M. Ganesh, and I.G. Graham, Spatio-temporal pattern formation on spherical surfaces: numerical simulation and application to solid tumour growth. J. Math. Biol 42 (2001), 387-423.

[60] T. Chavakis, A. Bierhaus, P.P. Nawroth, RAGE (receptor for advanced glycation end products): a central player in the inflammatory response. Microbes Infect. 6 (2004), 1219-1225.

[61] T.R. Chay and J. Keizer, Minimal model for membrane oscillations in the pancreatic β-cell. Biophys. J. 42 (1983), 181–190.

[62] X. Chen, and A. Friedman, A free boundary problem for an elliptic-hyperbolic system: an application to tumor growth, SIAM J. Math. Anal. 35 (4) (2003), 974-986.

[63] Y.D. Chen, S. Wang, and A. Sherman, Identifying the targets of the 751 amplifying pathway for insulin secretion in pancreatic beta-cells by kinetic modeling of granule exocytosis. Biophys J. 95 (2008), 2226-2241.

[64] G.P. Chen, X.Q. Zhang, T. Wu, L. Li, J. Han, and C.Q. Du, Alteration of mevalonate pathway in proliferated vascular smooth muscle from diabetic mice: possible role in high-glucose-induced atherogenic process, Journal of Diabetes Research, 2015 (379287) (2015), 11.

[65] C. Chothia, The nature of the accessible and buried surfaces in proteins. J Mol Biol. 105 (1976), 1-12.

[66] C.-S. Chou and A. Friedman, Introduction to Mathematical Biology modeling, Analysis, and Simulations, Springer International Publishing Switzerland, 2016.

[67] M. Cilla, E. Pena, and M.A. Martinez, Mathematical modeling of atheroma plaque formation and development in coronary arteries. J.R. Soc. Interface 11 (2013), 20130866.

[68] C.A. Cobbold, J.A. Sherratt, and S.R.J. Maxwell, Lipoprotein oxidation and its significance for atherosclerosis: a mathematical approach. Bull. Math. Biol. 64 (2002), 65-95.

[69] C. Cobelli, C. Dalla Man, G. Toffolo, R. Basu, A. Vella, and R. Rizza, The oral minimal model method. Diabetes 63 (2014), 1203-1213.

[70] C. Cobelli, G.M. Toffolo, C. Dalla Man, M. Campioni, P. Denti, A. Caumo, P. Butler, and R. Rizza, Assessment of beta cell function in humans, simultaneously with insulin sensitivity and hepatic extraction, from intravenous and oral glucose test, Am. J. Physiol. Endocrinol. Metab. 293 (2007), E1.

[71] A. Corti, C. Chiastra, M. Colombo, M. Garbey, F. Migliavacca, and S. Casarin. "A fully coupled computational fluid dynamics - agent-based model of atherosclerotic plaque development: Multiscale modeling framework and parameter sensitivity analysis". Computers in biology and medicine, 118 (2020), 103623.

[72] V. Cristini, H.B. Frieboes, X. Li, J.S. Lowengrub, P. Macklin, S. Sanga, S.M. Wise, and X. Zheng, Nonlinear modeling and simulation of tumor growth. In: Bellomo, N., editor. Modeling and Simulation in Science, Engineering and Technology. Birkhauser; Boston: 2008.

[73] V. Cristini, J.S. Lowengrub, Q. Nie, Nonlinear simulation of tumor growth. J. Math. Biol 46 (2003), 191-224.

[74] S. Cui, Analysis of a mathematical model for the growth of tumors under the action of external inhibitors. J. Math. Biol 44 (2002), 395-426. [PubMed: 12021982]

[75] S. Cui, Analysis of a free boundary problem modeling tumor growth. Acta Math. Sin 21 (2005), 1071-1082.

[76] S. Cui. Well-posedness of a multidimensional free boundary problem Modeling the growth of nonnecrotic tumors, J. Functional Analysis 245 (2007), 1-18.

[77] S. Cui, Asymptotic stability of the stationary solution for a hyperbolic free boundary problem modeling tumor growth. SIAM J. Math. Anal 40 (2008), 1692-1724.

[78] S. Cui, Asymptotic stability of the stationary solution for a parabolic-hyperbolic free boundary problem modeling tumor growth, SIAM J. Math. Anal. 45 (5)(2013), 2870-2893.

[79] S. Cui, Linearized stability for a multi-dimensional free boundary problem Modeling two-phase tumour growth, Nonlinearity 27 (5)(2014), 1045-1079.

[80] S. Cui, and J. Escher, Asymptotic behaviour of solutions of a multidimensional moving boundary problem modeling tumor growth. Commun. Partial Diff. Eqns 33 (2008), 636-655.

[81] S. Cui and J. Escher, Well-posedness and stability of a multi-dimensional tumor growth model. Arch. Ration. Mech. Anal 191 (2009), 173-193.

[82] S. Cui and A. Friedman, Analysis of a mathematical model of the effect of inhibitors on the growth of tumors. Math. Biosci 164 (2000), 103-137.

[83] S. Cui and A. Friedman, A free boundary problem for a singular system of differential equations: an application to a model of tumor growth. Trans. Am. Math. Soc 255 (2003), 3537-3590.

[84] S. Cui and A. Friedman, Formation of necrotic cores in the growth of tumors: analytic results. Acta Mat. Sci 26 (2006), 781-796.

[85] S. Cui and X. Wei, Global existence for a parabolic-hyperbolic free boundary problem Modeling tumor growth. Acta Math. Appl. Sin 21 (2005), 597-614.

[86] S. Cui and Y. Zhuang, Bifurcation solutions of a free boundary problem modeling tumor growth with angiogenesis J. Math. Anal. Appl. 468 (2018), no. 1, 391-405.

[87] R.C. Dalang, Extending the martingale measure stochastic integral with applications to spatially homogeneous SPDEs. *Electronic Journal of Probability*, 4 (1999), 1-29.

[88] C. Dalla Man, A. Caumo, and C. Cobelli, The oral glucose minimal model: estimation of insulin sensitivity from a meal test. IEEE Trans Biomed Eng 49: 419-429, 2002.

[89] C. Dalla Man, A. Caumo, R. Basu, R. Rizza, G. Toffolo, C. Cobelli, Minimal model estimation of glucose absorption and insulin sensitivity from oral test: validation with a tracer method, Am. J. Physiol. Endocrinol. Metab. 287 (2004) E637.

[90] C. Dalla Man, K.E. Yarasheski, A. Caumo, H. Robertson, G. Toffolo, K.S. Polonsky, C. Cobelli, Insulin sensitivity by oral glucose minimal models: validation against clamp, Am. J. Physiol. Endocrinol. Metab. 289 (2005) E954.

[91] G. Da Prato and J. Zabczyk, Stochastic equations in infinite dimensions, Cambridge University Press, 1992.

[92] A. De Gaetano, and O. Arino, Mathematical Modeling of the intravenous glucose tolerance test, J. Math. Biol. 40 (2000), 136.

[93] A. De Gaetano, T. Hardy, B. Beck, E. Abu-Raddad, P. Palumbo, J. Bue-Valleskey, and N. Prksen, Mathematical models of diabetes progression, Am. J. Physiol. Endocrinol. Metab. 295 (6) (2008), E1462.

[94] D. Dingli, M.D. Cascino, K. Josic, S.J. Russell, and Z. Bajzer, Mathematical modeling of cancer radiovirotherapy, Math. Biosci., 199 (2006), 55-78.

[95] M. Dixon, T.A. Phan, J.C. Dallon, and J.P. Tian, Mathematical model for IL-2-based cancer immunotherapy, Math Biosci. 372 (2024), 109187.

[96] G. Douglas, and K.M. Channon. The pathogenesis of atherosclerosis. Medicine (Baltimore) 42 (2014), 480-484.

[97] G. Bard Ermentrout, David H. Terman, Mathematical Foundations of Neuroscience, Springer New York, 2010.

[98] J. Escher, Classical solutions to a moving boundary problem for an elliptic-parabolic system, Interface Free Bound. 6 (2004), 175-193.

[99] L.C. Evans, *Partial Differential Equations*, 2nd ed., AMS, 2010.

[100] P. Ferroni, S. Basili, A. Falco, and G. Dav, Platelet activation in type 2 diabetes mellitus, Journal of Thrombosis and Haemostasis, 2 (8) (2004), 1282-1291.

[101] N. Filipovic, et al. Multi-physics Modeling of atherosclerosis. Computational Methods in Applied Mechanics and Engineering, 200(33-36) (2011), 2954-2966.

[102] N. Filipovic, Z. Teng, M. Radovic, I. Saveljic, D. Fotiadis, and O. Parodi, Computer simulation of three-dimensional plaque formation and progression in the carotid artery. Med. Biol. Eng. Comput. 51:607-616, 2013.

[103] P.-W. Fok. Mathematical model of intimal thickening in atherosclerosis: Vessel stenosis as a free boundary problem. Journal of Theoretical Biology 314 (2012) 23-33.

[104] P.W. Fok, K.R. Sanft, and T. Chou, Reaction-diffusion model of atherogenesis. Journal of Theoretical Biology, 264(2) (2010), 253-263.

[105] A. Friedman, Partial differential equations of parabolic type, Prentice Hall, Inc.,Englewood Cliffs, N.J., 1964.

[106] A. Friedman, A hierarchy of cancer models and their mathematical challenges. Discrete Cont. Dyn. Syst. Ser. B4 (2004), 147-159.

[107] A. Friedman, A free boundary problem for a coupled system of elliptic, hyperbolic and stokes equations. Int. Free Bound 8 (2006), 247-261.

[108] A. Friedman, Free boundary problems in biology, Phil. Trans. R. Soc. A, 373 (2015), 20140386.

[109] A. Friedman, Free boundary problems arising in biology, Discrete & Continuous Dynamical Systems - B, 23 (2018), 193-202.

[110] A. Friedman, Mathematical biology: Modeling and Analysis, CBMS Regional Conference Series in Mathematics, Number 127, 2018.

[111] A. Friedman, and W. Hao, A mathematical model of atherosclerosis with reverse cholesterol transport and associated risk factors. Bull. Math. Biol. 77 (2015), 758-781.

[112] A. Friedman, W. Hao, and B. Hu, A free boundary problem for steady small plaques in the artery and their stability, J. Differential Equations 259(2015), 1227-1255.

[113] A. Friedman, W. Hao, and K.-Y. Lam, A cancer model with nonlocal free boundary dynamics, Journal of Mathematical Biology 85 (2022), 46.

[114] A. Friedman, B. Hu, Asymptotic stability for a free boundary problem arising in a tumor model. J. Diff. Eqns 227 (2005), 598-639.

[115] A. Friedman, B. Hu, Bifurcation from stability to instability for a free boundary problem arising in a tumor model. Arch. Ration. Mech. Anal 180 (2006), 293-330.

[116] A. Friedman, B. Hu, Bifurcation from stability to instability for a free boundary problem modeling tumor growth by stokes equation. J. Math. Anal. Appl 327 (2007), 643-664.

[117] A. Friedman, B. Hu, Stability and instability of Liapunov-Schmidt and Hopf bifurcation for a free boundary problem arising in a tumor model. Trans. Am. Math. Soc 360 (2008), 5291-5342.

[118] A. Friedman, and C.-Y. Kao, Mathematical Modeling of Biological Processes, Springer International Publishing Switzerland, 2014.

[119] A. Friedmen, C.-Y. Kao, and R. Leander, On the dynamics of radially symmetric granulomas. J Math Anal Appl 412 (2) (2014), 776-791.

[120] A. Friedman and X. Lai, Combination therapy for cancer with oncolytic virus and checkpoint inhibitor: A mathematical model, PLoS ONE, 13 (2018), e0192449.

[121] A. Friedman and X. Lai, Free boundary problems associated with cancer treatment by combination therapy, Discrete & Continuous Dynamical Systems - A, 39 (2019), 6825-6842.

[122] A. Friedman and K.-Y. Lam, On the stability of steady states in a granuloma model, J. Differential Equations 256 (2014), 3743-3769.

[123] A. Friedman and K.-Y. Lam, Analysis of a free-boundary tumor model with angiogenesis, J. Differential Equations 259 (12) (2015), 7636-7661.

[124] A. Friedman and F. Reitich, Analysis of a mathematical model for the growth of tumors. J. Math. Biol 38 (1999), 262-284.

[125] A. Friedman and F. Reitich, On the existence of spatially patterned dormant malignancies in a model for the growth of non-necrotic vascular tumors. Math. Models Methods Appl. Sci 11 (2001), 601-625.

[126] A. Friedman and F. Reitich, Symmetry-breaking bifurcation of analytic solutions to free boundary problems: an application to a model of tumor growth. Trans. Am. Math. Soc 353 (2001), 1587-1634.

[127] A. Friedman, J.P. Tian, G. Fulci, E.A. Chiocca, and J. Wang, Glioma virotherapy: Effects of innate immune suppression and increased viral replication capacity, Cancer Research, 66 (2006), 2314-2319.

[128] M.H. Friedman, C.B. Bargeron, D. Duncan, and G.M. Hutchins, Effect of arterial compliance and non-Newtonian rheology on correlation between wall shear stress and intimal thickness. Atherosclerosis, 120(1-2) (1996), 1-8.

[129] U. Gayaki, S. Daronde, A. Tale, and A. Barhate, "A Review of Machine Learning Algorithms in Diabetes Management". 2025 4th International Conference on Sentiment Analysis and Deep Learning (ICSADL) (2025), 766-771.

[130] L.C. Gatewood, E. Ackerman, J.W. Rosevear, G.D. Molnar, Test of a mathematical model of the blood-glucose regulatory system, Comput. Biomed. Res. 2 (1968), 1.

[131] N. Ghaffari Laleh, C.M.L. Loeffler, J. Grajek, K. Stakova, A.T. Pearson, H.S. Muti, et al., Classical mathematical models for prediction of response to chemotherapy and immunotherapy. PLoS Comput Biol 18 (2) (2022), e1009822.

[132] I. Gessaghi, C. Chiastra, F. Migliavacca, and G. Dubini, Influence of wall shear stress patterns on plaque progression in coronary arteries: a patient-specific computational study. Biomechanics and Modeling in Mechanobiology, 14(4) (2015), 703-718.

[133] G.S. Getz, and C.A. Reardon, Animal models of Atherosclerosis. Arterioscler Thromb VascBiol. 32 (2012), 1104-1115.

[134] D.V. Giang, Y. Lenbury, A. De Gaetano, and P. Palumbo, Delay model of glucose-insulin systems: global stability and oscillated solutions conditional on delays, J. Math. Anal. Appl. 343 (2) (2008) 996.

[135] H.P. Greenspan, Models for the growth of a solid tumor by diffusion, Studies in appl. math. 53 (1972), 317-340.

[136] H.P. Greenspan, On the growth and stability of cell cultures and solid tumors. J. Theor. Biol 56 (1976), 229-242.

[137] G.M. Grodsky, A threshold distribution hypothesis for packet storage of insulin and its mathematical modeling. J Clin Invest 51 (1972), 2047-2059.

[138] J. Guckenheimer and P. Holmes, *Nonlinear Oscillations, Dynamical Systems, and Bifurcations of Vector Fields*, Springer, 1983.

[139] T. Gui, A. Shimokado, Y. Sun, T. Akasaka, and Y. Muragaki, Diverse Roles of Macrophages in Atherosclerosis: From Inflammatory Biology to Biomarker Discovery. Mediators of Inflammation 2012 (2012), ID693083.

[140] J. Ha, S.T. Chung, M. Springer, J.Y. Kim, P. Chen, A. Chhabra, M.G. Cree, C. Diniz Behn, A.E. Sumner, S.A. Arslanian, and A.S. Sherman, Estimating insulin sensitivity and β-cell function from the oral glucose tolerance test: validation of a new insulin sensitivity and secretion (ISS) model. Am J Physiol Endocrinol Metab 326 (2024), E454-E471.

[141] J. Ha, L.S. Satin, and A.S. Sherman, A Mathematical Model of the Pathogenesis, Prevention, and Reversal of Type 2 Diabetes. Endocrinology 157 (2016), 624-635.

[142] J. Ha and A. Sherman, Type 2 diabetes: one disease, many pathways. Am J Physiol Endocrinol Metab 319 (2020), E410-E426.

[143] S. Hadebe, B. Ndlovu, and K. Maguraushe, "Managing Diabetes Using Machine Learning and Digital Twins". Indonesian Journal of Innovation and Applied Sciences (IJIAS) (2025). https://doi.org/10.47540/ijias.v5i2.1981.

[144] M. Hairer, A theory of regularity structures. *Inventiones Mathematicae*, 198(2) (2014), 269-504.

[145] S. Hamasaki, T. Kobori, Y. Yamazaki, A. Kitaura, A. Niwa, T. Nishinaka, M. Nishibori, S. Mori, S. Nakao, and H. Takahashi, Effects of scavenger receptors-1 class A stimulation on macrophage morphology and highly modified advanced glycation end product-protein phagocytosis. Sci. Rep. 2018, 8, 5901.

[146] E. Hanzawa, Classical solutions of the Stefan problem. Tohoku Math. J. (1981), 297-335.

[147] W. Hao, and A. Friedman, The LDL-HDL profile determines the risk of atherosclerosis: a mathematical model. PLoS ONE 9 (2014), 1-15.

[148] J.R. Harrington, The Role of MCP-1 in Atherosclerosis. Stem Cells 18 (2000), 65-66.

[149] A. Hening and H.D. Nguyen, Coexistence and extinction for stochastic Kolmogorov systems, Ann. Appl. Probab., 28 (2018), 1893-1942.

[150] M.M. Hennes, Insulin resistant lypolisis in abdominally obese hypertensive individuals. Hypertension. 29 (1996), 120-126.

[151] A.G. Hoekstra, B. Chopard, D. Coster, and A. Lutz, Multiscale Modeling of atherosclerosis: computational challenges and opportunities. Interface Focus, 8(6) (2018), 20180016.

[152] C.Y. Hsu, S. Chien, and C.C. Wu, Wall shear stress and plaque development: insights from computational fluid dynamics models. Journal of the Royal Society Interface, 18(178) (2021), 20200803.

[153] Y. Huang and B. Hu, Symmetry-breaking longitude bifurcations for a free boundary problem modeling small plaques in three dimensions, Journal of Mathematical Biology, 85 (2022), Paper No. 58, 44 pp.

[154] Y. Huang and B. Hu, Symmetry-breaking combined latitude-longitude bifurcations for a free boundary problem modeling small plaques, Discrete Contin. Dyn. Syst. Ser. B 29 (10) (2024), 4120-4149.

[155] Y. Huang, Z. Zhang, and B. Hu, Bifurcation for a free-boundary tumor model with angiogenesis, Nonlinear Anal. Real World Appl. 35 (2017), 483-502.

[156] Y. Huang, Z. Zhang, and B. Hu, Bifurcation from stability to instability for a free boundary tumor model with angiogenesis Discrete Contin. Dyn. Syst. 39 (5) (2019), 2473-2510.

[157] V. Lissoni, G. Luraghi, M. Stefanati, J.F.R. Matas, and F. Migliavacca, "Computational methods used to investigate atherosclerosis progression in coronary arteries: structural FEA, CFD or FSI". Computer methods and programs in biomedicine, 270 (2025): 108959.

[158] N. Ikeda, and S. Watanabe, A Comparison Theorem for Solutions of Stochastic Differential Equations and its Applications. Osaka Journal of Mathematics, 14 (1977), 619-633.

[159] N. Ikeda, and S. Watanabe, Stochastic Differential Equations and Diffusion Processes, 2nd edition, North-Holland Publishing Co., Amsterdam, 1989.

[160] T. Imanishi, et al., Patient-specific computational modeling of coronary artery disease progression using serial imaging. European Heart Journal - Cardiovascular Imaging, 20(7) (2019), 781-789.

[161] T. Inoguchi, P. Li, et al., High glucose level and free fatty acid stimulate reactive oxygen species production through protein kinase C-dependent activation of NAD(P)H oxsidase in cultured vascular cells. Diabetes. 49 (2000), 1939-1945.

[162] J. Janin and C. Chothia, Role of Hydrophobicity in the Binding of Coenzymes. Biochemistry 17 (1978), 2943-2948.

[163] M.T. Johnstone, S.J. Creager, K.M. Scales, et al., Impaired endothelium-dependent vasodilation in patients with insulin-dependent diabetes mellitus. Circulation, 88 (1993), 2510-2516.

[164] L.A. Johnson, H.S. Kim, M.J. Knudson, C.T. Nipp, X. Yi, and N. Maeda, "Diabetic atherosclerosis in APOE*4 mice: synergy between lipoprotein metabolism and vascular inflammation," Journal of Lipid Research, 54(2) (2013), 386-396.

[165] B. Jorgensen, Statistical Property of the Generalized Inverse Gaussian Distribution, Springer-Verlag New York, 1982.

[166] J.E. Kanter, F. Kramer, S. Barnhart, et al., Diabetes promotes an inflammatory macrophage phenotype and atherosclerosis through acyl-CoA synthetase 1, Proceedings of the National Academy of Sciences of the United States of America, 109 (12) (2012), E715-E724.

[167] I. Karatzas and S. Shreve, Brownian Motion and Stochastic Calculus, Springer, 1991.

[168] R. Kaur, M. Kaur, and J. Singh, Endothelial dysfunction and platelet hyperactivity in type 2 diabetes mellitus: molecular insights and therapeutic strategies, Cardiovasc Diabetol 17 (2018), 121.

[169] M. Khakpour, and K. Vafai. Critical assessment of arterial transport models. Int. J. Heat Mass Transf. 51 (2008), 807–822.

[170] H.K. Khalil, *Nonlinear Systems*, 3rd Edition, Prentice Hall, 2002.

[171] R. Khasminskii, Stochastic Stability of Differential Equations, Springer, 2012.

[172] N. El Khatib, S. GZenieys, B. Kazmierczak, and V. Volpert, Reaction-diffusion model of atherosclerosis development. Journal of mathematical biology, 65 (2) (2012), 349-374.

[173] P.B. Khokhar, C. Gravino, and F. Palomba, "Advances in artificial intelligence for diabetes prediction: insights from a systematic literature review". Artificial intelligence in medicine, 164 (2025), 103132. https://doi.org/10.1016/j.artmed.2025.103132.

[174] D.N. Ku, D.P. Giddens, C.K. Zarins, and S. Glagov, Pulsatile flow and atherosclerosis in the human carotid bifurcation. Arteriosclerosis, 5(3) (1985), 293-302.

[175] Y.A. Kuznetsov, *Elements of Applied Bifurcation Theory*, Springer, 3rd ed., 2013.

[176] O.A. Ladyzhenskaya and N.N. Uraltseva, *Linear and quasilinear elliptic equations*, Academic press, New York, 1968.

[177] X. Lai and A. Friedman, Combination therapy of cancer with cancer vaccine and immune checkpoint inhibitor: A mathematical model, PLoS ONE, 12 (2017), e0178479.

[178] X. Lai and A. Friedman, How to schedule VEGF and PD-1 inhibitors in combination cancer therapy? BMC Syst Biol 13(1) (2019), 30.

[179] E. Lee, and D. Terman, Uniqueness and Stability of Periodic Bursting Solutions, Journal of Differential Equations 158 (1999), 48-78.

[180] S. Lee, et al., AI-assisted multiscale Modeling for plaque progression and rupture risk prediction. Nature Biomedical Engineering, 8(1) (2024), 45-58.

[181] H. Li, S. Hou, X. Wei, Analysis of a free boundary tumor model with time-dependent in the presence of inhibitors Discrete Contin. Dyn. Syst. Ser. B 29 (9) (2024), 3887-3907.

[182] J. Li, Y. Kuang, B. Li, Analysis of IVGTT glucose-insulin interaction models with time delay, Discrete Contin. Dyn. Syst. Ser. B. 1 (1) (2001) 103.

[183] J. Li, Y. Kuang, Analysis of a model of the glucose-insulin regulatory system with two delays, SIAM J. Appl. Math. 67 (3) (2007) 757.

[184] J. Li, Y. Kuang, C.C. Mason, Modeling the glucose-insulin regulatory system and ultradian insulin secretory oscillations with two explicit time delays, J. Theor. Biol. 242 (2006) 722.

[185] J. Li, M. Wang, A. De Gaetano, P. Palumbo, S. Panunzi, The range of time delay and the global stability of the equilibrium for an IVGTT model, Math. Biosci. 235 (2012) 128.

[186] X. Li, V. Cristini, Q. Nie, J.S. Lowengrub, Nonlinear three-dimensional simulation of solid tumor growth. Discrete Dyn. Contin. Dyn. Syst. B7 (2007), 581-604.

[187] Z. Li, Z. Qiao, and T. Tang, *Numerical Solution of Differential Equations: Introduction to Finite Difference and Finite Element Methods*, Cambridge University Press, 2017.

[188] G.M. Lieberman, Second Order Parabolic Differential Equations, World Scientific Publishing Co., 1996.

[189] W. Liu, and M. Rochner, Stochastic partial differential equations: an introduction, Springer, 2015.

[190] J.S. Lowengrub, H.B. Frieboes, F. Jin, Y.-L. Chuang, X. Li, P. Macklin, S.M. Wise, and V. Cristini, Nonlinear Modeling of cancer: bridging the gap between cells and tumours, Nonlinearity. 23(1) (2010), R1-R9.

[191] A. Lunardy, Analytic semigroups and optimal regularity in parabolic problems. Birkhĺauser, (1995).

[192] A.J. Lusis, Atherosclerosis. Nature 407 (2000), 233-241.

[193] G.E. Mahlbachera, K.C. Reihmera, and H.B. Frieboesa, Mathematical Modeling of Tumor-Immune Cell Interactions, J Theor Biol. 21(469) (2019), 47-60.

[194] A. Makroglou, J. Li, and Y. Kuang, Mathematical models and software tools for the glucose-insulin regulatory system and diabetes: an overview, Applied Numerical Mathematics 56 (2006) 559-573.

[195] X. Mao, Stochastic Differential Equations and Applications, 2nd Edition, Woodhead Publishing, 2011.

[196] E. Di Marco, S.P. Gray, K. Kennedy, et al., NOX4-derived reactive oxygen species limit fibrosis and inhibit proliferation of vascular smooth muscle cells in diabetic atherosclerosis, Free Radical Biology & Medicine, 97 (2016), 556-567.

[197] A. Mari, G. Pacini, E. Murphy, B. Ludvik, and J.J. Nolan, A model-based method for assessing insulin sensitivity from the oral glucose tolerance test. Diabetes Care 24 (2001), 539-548.

[198] A. Mari, A. Tura, A. Gastaldelli, and E. Ferrannini, Assessing insulin secretion by modeling in multiple-meal tests: role of potentiation, Diabetes 51 (2002), S221.

[199] J.E. Marsden and M. McCracken, *The Hopf Bifurcation and Its Applications*, Springer, 1976.

[200] C. McKay, S. McKee, N. Mottram, T. Mulholland, and S. Wilson, Towards a model of atherosclerosis. Strathclyde Mathematics Research Report, 2005.

[201] J.P. McKenna, J. Ha, M.J. Merrins, L.S. Satin, A. Sherman, R. Bertram, Ca^{2+} effects on ATP production and consumption have regulatory roles on oscillatory islet activity, Biophys. J. 110 (2016), 733–742.

[202] M. McLaurin, Analysis and simulation of mathematical models of the intravenous glucose tolerance test, Master Project, Morgan State University, 2023.

[203] M.J. Merrins, A.R.V. Dyke, A.K. Mapp, M.A. Rizzo, and L.S. Satin, Direct measurements of oscillatory glycolysis in pancreatic islet β-cells using novel FRET biosensors for pyruvate kinase M2 activity, J. Biol. Chem. 288 (2013), 33312–33322.

[204] P.A. Modesti, A. Fortini, G.F. Gensini, D. Vanni, D. Prisco, and R. Abbate, Human prostacyclin platelet receptors in diabetes mellitus, Thrombosis Research, 63(5) (1991), 541-548.

[205] S. Mundi, M. Massaro, E. Scoditti, M.A. Carluccio, V.W.M. Van Hinsbergh, M.L. Iruela-Arispe, and R. De Caterina, Endothelial permeability, LDL deposition, and cardiovascular risk factors: a review. ESC Cardiovascular Research. 114 (2018), 35-52.

[206] E. Muscelli, A. Mari, A. Natali, B.D. Astiarraga, S. Camastra, S. Frascerra, J.J. Holst, E. Ferrannini, Impact of incretin hormones on b-cell function in subjects with normal or impaired glucose tolerance, Am. J. Physiol. Endocrinol. Metab. 291 (2006), E1144.

[207] E. Muscelli, A. Mari, A. Casolaro, S. Camastra, G. Seghieri, A. Gastaldelli, J.J. Holst, and E. Ferrannini, Separate impact of obesity and glucose tolerance on the incretin effect in normal subjects and type 2 diabetic patients, Diabetes 57 (2008), 1340.

[208] B. Oksendal, Stochastic Differential Equations: An Introduction with Applications, 6th ed., Springer, 2013.

[209] F.W.J. Olver, Asymptotics and special functions, Academic press, New York, 1974.

[210] G. Orasanu and J. Plutzky, The pathologic continuum of diabetic vascular disease, Journal of the American College of Cardiology, 53 (Supplement 5) (2009), S35-S42.

[211] P. Palumbo, S. Ditlevsen, A. Bertuzzi, and A. De Gaetano, Mathematical modeling of the glucose-insulin system: A review, Mathematical Biosciences 244 (2013), 69-81.

[212] P. Palumbo, and A. De Gaetano, An islet population model for the endocrine pancreas, J. Math. Biol. 61 (2) (2010), 171.

[213] P. Palumbo, S. Panunzi, A. De Gaetano, Qualitative behavior of a family of delay-differential models of the glucose-insulin system, Discrete Contin. Dyn. Syst. Ser. B. 7 (2) (2007), 399.

[214] A.V. Panfilov, H. Dierckx, V. Volpert. (INVITED) Reaction-diffusion waves in cardiovascular diseases. Physica D. 399 (2019), 1-34.

[215] S. Panunzi, P. Palumbo, and A. De Gaetano, A discrete single delay model for the intra-venous glucose tolerance test, Theor. Biol. Med. Model. 4 (2007).

[216] E. Pardoux, Equations aux dérivées partielles stochastiques non linéaires monotones. *These de doctorat, Université Paris-Sud*, 1975.

[217] A. Parton, V. McGilligan, M. O'Kane, F.R. Baldrick, and S. Watterson, Computational Modeling of atherosclerosis. Briefings in Bioinformatics, 17(4) (2016), 562-575.

[218] A. Pazy, *Semigroups of Linear Operators and Applications to Partial Differential Equations*, Springer, 1983.

[219] M.G. Pedersen, R. Bertram, and A. Sherman, Intra- and inter-islet synchronization of metabolically driven insulin secretion, Biophys. J. 89 (2005), 107.

[220] M.G. Pedersen, A. Corradin, G.M. Toffolo, and C. Cobelli, A subcellular model of glucose-stimulated pancreatic insulin secretion, Phil. Trans. R. Soc. A 366 (2008), 3525.

[221] M.G. Pedersen, and A. Sherman, Newcomer insulin secretory granules as a highly calcium-sensitive pool, Proc. Natl. Acad. Sci. USA 106 (2009) 7432.

[222] M.G. Pedersen, G.M. Toffolo, and C. Cobelli, Cellular modeling: insight into oral minimal models of insulin secretion, Am. J. Physiol. Endocrinol. Metab. 298 (2010), E597.

[223] T.A. Phan, and J.P. Tian, Basic stochastic model for tumor virotherapy, MBE, 17(4) (2020), 4271-4294.

[224] T.A. Phan, and J.P. Tian,, Hopf bifurcation without parameters in deterministic and stochastic modeling of cancer virotherapy, part I, J Math Anal Appl, 514(1) (2022), 126278.

[225] U. Picchini, A. De Gaetano, S. Panunzi, S. Ditlevsen, G. Mingrone, A mathematical model of the euglycemic hyperinsulinemic clamp, Theor. Biol. Med. Model. 2 (2005), 44.

[226] U. Picchini, S. Ditlevsen, and A. De Gaetano, Modeling the euglycemic hyperinsulinemic clamp by stochastic differential equations, J. Math. Biol. 53 (5) (2006), 771.

[227] U. Picchini, S. Ditlevsen, and A. De Gaetano, Maximum likelihood estimation of a time-inhomogeneous stochastic differential model of glucose dynamics, Math. Med. Biol. 25 (2008), 141.

[228] G.M. Pieper, P. Langenstroer, and W. Siebeneich, Diabetic induced endothelial dysfunction in rat aorta: role of hydroxyl radicals, Cardiovascular Research, 34(1) (1997), 145-156.

[229] A. Quehenberger, P. Bierhaus, and C. Fasching, et al., Endothelin 1 transcription is controlled by nuclear factor-kappaB in AGE-stimulated cultured endothelial cells. Diabetes. 49 (2000), 1561-1570.

[230] E.W. Raines, and R. Ross, Smooth muscle cells and the pathogenesis of the lesions of atherosclerosis. Br Heart J. 69 (1993), 30-37.

[231] T.J. Reape, and P. Groot, Chemokines and atherosclerosis. Atherosclerosis 147 (1999), 213-225.

[232] J. Rinzel, A formal classification of bursting mechanisms in excitable systems, in: E. Teramoto, M. Yamaguti (Eds.), Mathematical Topics in Population Biol- ogy, Morphogenesis and Neurosciences, in: Lecture Notes in Biomathematics, vol. 71, Springer, Berlin, 1987, pp. 267–281.

[233] G.B. Rinzel, Ermentrout, Analysis of neural excitability and oscillations, in: C. Koch, I. Segev (Eds.), Methods in Neuronal Modeling: From Synapses to Networks, Vol. 2, MIT Press, Cambridge, 1998, pp. 251-292.

[234] V.C. Rispoli, et al., A mechanistic computational model for predicting the effect of lipid-lowering therapy on atherosclerosis progression. PLOS Computational Biology, 18(4) (2022), e1010027.

[235] R.P. Robertson, Chronic Oxidative Stress as a Central Mechanism for Glucose Toxicity in Pancreatic Islet Beta Cells in Diabetes. J Biol Chem 279 (2004), 42351-42354.

[236] P. Rorsman, and E. Renstrom, Insulin granule dynamics in pancreatic beta cells. Diabetologia 46 (2003), 1029-45.

[237] P. Rorsman, and M. Braun, Regulation of insulin secretion in human pancreatic islets. Annu Rev Physiol 75 (2013), 155-79.

[238] R. Ross, J. Masuda, E.W. Raines, A.M. Gown, S. Katsuda, et al., Localization of PDGF-B protein in macrophages in all phases of atherogenesis. Science 248 (1990), 1009-1012.

[239] A.M. Schmidt, S. Du Yan, J.L. Wautier, and D. Stern, Activation of receptor for advanced glycation end products: a mechanism for chronic vascular dysfunction in diabetic vasculopathy and atherosclerosis. Circ Res. 84 (1999), 489-497.

[240] Y. Setty, S. Ramaswamy, and K.A. Rejniak, Multiscale and hybrid modeling frameworks of tumor and atherosclerotic plaque microenvironments. Current Opinion in Biomedical Engineering, 13 (2020), 148-157.

[241] H. Shen, X. Wei, Linear stability analysis for the free boundary problem modeling and tumor growth with angiogenesis in the presence of inhibitors, J. Differential Equations 364 (2023), 244-295.

[242] X.Shi, Q. Zheng, J. Li, and X. Zhou, Analysis of a stochastic IVGTT glucose-insulin model with time delay. *AIMS, Mathematical Biosciences and Engineering*, (2020), 2310-2340.

[243] T. Silva, A. Sequeira, R. Santos, and J. Tiago. Mathematical modeling of atherosclerotic plaque formation coupled with a non-Newtonian model of blood flow. Conf. Pap. Math. (2013) (2013), 1-14.

[244] C. Simonetto, T.V. Azizova, Z. Barjaktarovic, J. Bauersachs, P. Jacob, J.C. Kaiser, et al., A mechanistic model for atherosclerosis and its application to the cohort of Mayak workers. PLoS ONE 12(4) (2017), e0175386.

[245] C. Simonetto, S. Rospleszcz, M. Heier, C. Meisinger, A. Peters, and J. Kaiser, "Simulating the dynamics of atherosclerosis to the incidence of myocardial infarction, applied to the KORA population". Statistics in Medicine, 40 (2021), 3299-3312.

[246] R. Singh, S. Devi, and R. Gollen, Role of free radical in atherosclerosis, diabetes and dyslipidaemia: larger-than-life. Diabetes Metab Res Rev 31 (2015), 113-126.

[247] P. Smolen, A model for glycolytic oscillations based on skeletal muscle phosphofructokinase kinetics, J. Theoret. Biol. 174 (1995), 137–148.

[248] M. Soleimani, B. Dashtbozorg, M. Mirkhalaf, and S. Mirkhalaf. "A multiphysics-based artificial neural networks model for atherosclerosis." Heliyon, 9 (2023), e17902.

[249] A. Soro-Paavonen, A.M. Watson, J. Li, K. Paavonen, A. Koitka, A.C. Calkin, D. Barit, M.T. Coughlan, B.G. Drew, G.I. Lancaster, et al., Receptor for advanced glycation end products (RAGE) deficiency attenuates the development of atherosclerosis in diabetes. Diabetes, 57 (2008), 2461-2469.

[250] W.D. Stanbro, Modeling the interaction of peroxynitrite with low-density lipoproteins. II: reaction/diffusion model of peroxynitrite in low-density lipoprotein particles. J. Theor. Biol. 205 (2000), 465-471.

[251] S.H. Strogatz, *Nonlinear Dynamics and Chaos: With Applications to Physics, Biology, Chemistry, and Engineering*, CRC Press, 2018.

[252] H. Sun, X. Zhang, and L. Zhao, et al., Attenuation of atherosclerotic lesions in diabetic apolipoprotein E-deficient mice using gene silencing of macrophage migration inhibitory factor, Journal of Cellular and Molecular Medicine, 19(4) (2015), 836-849.

[253] X. Sun and B. Hu, Mathematical modeling and computational prediction of cancer drug resistance, Briefings in Bioinformatics, 19(6) (2018), 1382-1399.

[254] K.R. Swanson, C. Bridge, J.D. Murray, E.C. Alvord, Jr., Virtual and real brain tumors: using mathematical modeling to quantify glioma growth and invasion. J. Neuro. Sci 216 (2003), 1-10.

[255] K.R. Swanson, R.C. Rostomily, E.C. Alvord Jr., A mathematical modeling tool for predicting the survival of individual patients following resection of glioblastoma: a proof of principle. Br. J. Cancer 98 (2008), 113-119.

[256] Y. Tao and M. Chen, An elliptic-hyperbolic free boundary problem Modeling cancer therapy. Nonlinearity 19 (2006), 419-440.

[257] Y. Tao and Q. Guo, The competitive dynamics between tumor cells, a replicationcompetent virus and an immune response. J. Math. Biol 51 (2005), 37-74. [PubMed: 15772825]

[258] Y. Tao, N. Yoshida, and Q. Guo, Nonlinear analysis of a model of vascular tumour growth and treatment. Nonlinearity 17 (2004), 867-895.

[259] D. Terman, Chaotic spikes arising horn a model for bursting in excitable membranes, SIAM J. A/y/. MU//I. 51 (1991), 1418-1450.

[260] D. Terman, The transition from bursting to continuous spiking in excitable membrane models, J. Nonheor Sci. 2 (1992), I35-182.

[261] M.P. Thon, R.H. Selzer, S. Sinha, and J.J. Saucerman, A computational model of plaque composition in atherosclerosis. PLoS Computational Biology, 13(8) (2017), e1005640.

[262] J.P. Tian, the replicability of oncolytic virus: defining conditions in tumor virotherapy, Mathematical biosciences, and engineering 8(3) (2011).

[263] J. Tian, Y. Liu, Y. Liu, K. Chen, and S. Lyu, Cellular and Molecular Mechanisms of Diabetic Atherosclerosis: Herbal Medicines as a Potential Therapeutic Approach, Oxidative Medicine and Cellular Longevity, Volume 2017, Article ID 9080869, 16 pages.

[264] G. Toffolo, R.N. Bergman, D.T. Finegood, C.R. Bowden, C. Cobelli, Quantitative estimation of beta cells sensitivity to glucose in the intact organism: a minimal model of insulin kinetics in dog, Diabetes 29 (1980), 979.

[265] B. Topp, K. Promislow, G. Devries, R.M. Miuraa, and D.T. Finegood, A Model of b-Cell Mass, Insulin, and Glucose Kinetics: Pathways to Diabetes. J. Theor. Biol. 206 (2000), 605-619.

[266] G. Tomaso, V. Daz-Zuccarini, and C. Pichardo-Almarza. A multiscale model of atherosclerotic plaque formation at its early stage. IEEE Trans. Biomed. Eng. 58 (2011), 3460-3463.

[267] B. Trachet, et al., From animal models to patient-specific computational models of atherosclerosis. Annals of Biomedical Engineering, 49(1) (2021), 22-39.

[268] K. Tsaneva-Atanasova, C.L. Zimliki, R. Bertram, A. Sherman, Diffusion of calcium and metabolites in pancreatic islets: killing oscillations with a pitchfork, Biophys. J. 90 (2006), 3434.

[269] A.G. van der Giessen, et al., Multimodal data integration in computational models of atherosclerosis. Frontiers in Physiology, 14 (2023), 1123450.

[270] I.A. van den Oever, H.G. Raterman, M.T. Nurmohamed, and S. Simsek, Endothelial dysfunction, inflammation, and apoptosis in diabetes mellitus, Mediators of Inflammation, 2010(792393) (2010), 15.

[271] W.P.T.M. van Doorn, Y.D. Foreman, N.C. Schaper, H.H.C.M. Savelberg, A. Koster, C.J.H. van der Kallen, et al., Machine learning-based glucose prediction with use of continuous glucose and physical activity monitoring data: The Maastricht Study. PLoS ONE 16(6) (2021), e0253125. https://doi.org/10.1371/journal.pone.0253125

[272] Y. Vengrenyuk, S. Carlier, S. Xanthos, L. Cardoso, P. Ganatos, R. Virmani, and S. Weinbaum, A hypothesis for vulnerable plaque rupture due to stress-induced debonding around cellular microcalcifications in thin fibrous caps. Proceedings of the National Academy of Sciences USA, 103(40) (2016), 14678-14683.

[273] J.B. Walsh, An introduction to stochastic partial differential equations. In *Ecole d'Été de Probabilités de Saint-Flour XIV*. Springer, 1986, pp. 265-439.

[274] H. Wang, J. Li, Y. Kuang, Mathematical Modeling and qualitative analysis of insulin therapies, Math. Biosci. 210 (2007), 17.

[275] H. Wang, J. Li, Y. Kuang, Enhanced Modeling of the glucose-insulin system and its application in insulin therapies, J. Biol. Dynam. 3 (1) (2009), 22.

[276] Z. Wang, and T.S. Deisboeck, Computational modeling of brain tumors: discrete, continuum or hybrid? Scientific Model. Simul 15 (2008), 381-393.

[277] J.P. Ward and J.R. King, Mathematical Modeling of avascular tumour growth. IMA J. Math. Appl. Med. Biol 14 (1997), 36-69.

[278] J.P. Ward and J.R. King, Mathematical Modeling of drug transport in tumour multicell spheroids and monolayer cultures. Math. Biosci 181 (2003), 177-207.

[279] M.P. Wautier, O. Chappey, S. Corda, D.M. Stern, A.M. Schmidt, and J.L. Wautier. Activation of NADPH oxidase by AGE links oxidant stress to altered gene expression via RAGE. Am J Physiol Endocrinol Metab. 280 (2001), 685-694.

[280] C. Weber, and H. Noels, Atherosclerosis: current pathogenesis and therapeutic options. Nat Med 17 (2011), 1410-1422.

[281] S. Wiggins, *Introduction to Applied Nonlinear Dynamical Systems and Chaos*, Springer, 2003.

[282] S.B. Williams, J.A. Cusco, M.A. Rody, et al., Impaired nitric oxide-mediated vasodilation in patients with non-insulin-dependent diabetes mellitus. J. Am Coll Cardiol. 27 (1996), 567-574.

[283] D. Wodarz, Viruses as antitumor weapons: Defining conditions for tumor remission, Cancer Res., 61 (2001), 3501-3507.

[284] D. Wodarz and N. Komarova, Towards predictive computational models of oncolytic virus therapy: Basis for experimental validation and model selection, PloS ONE, 4 (2009), e4271.

[285] J. Wu, Asymptotic stability of a free boundary problem for the growth of multi-layer tumours in the necrotic phase, Nonlinearty 32(8) (2019), 2955-2974.

[286] J. Wu, and S. Cui, Asymptotic behavior of solutions of a free boundary problem modeling the growth of tumors with stokes equations Discrete. Contin. Dyn. Syst 24 (2009), 625-651.

[287] J. Wu, and S. Cui, Bifurcation analysis of a mathematical model for the growth of solid tumors in the presence of external inhibitors Math. Methods Appl. Sci. 38(9) (2015), 1813-1823.

[288] X. Xie, Well-posedness of a mathematical model for diabetic atherosclerosis, J. Math. Anal. Appl. 505(2) (2022), Paper No. 125606, pp. 18.

[289] X. Xie, Well-posedness of a mathematical model for diabetic atherosclerosis with advanced glycation end-products, Applicable Analysis 101(11) (2022), 3989-4013, DOI:10.1080/00036811.2022.2060210

[290] X. Xie, Steady solution and its stability of a mathematical model of diabetic atherosclerosis, Journal of biological dynamics, 17(1) (2023), Article: 2257734.

[291] X. Xie, Mild solution of a stochastic model of diabetic atherosclerosis with free boundary, 2023, submitted.

[292] X. Xie and L. Kadhim, Long time behavior of solutions to free boundary problems modeling tumor evolution, Applicable Analysis 104(1) (2025), 128-141.

[293] Y. Xie, et al., Patient-specific fluid-structure interaction Modeling of coronary plaques from optical coherence tomography and angiography. Computer Methods in Biomechanics and Biomedical Engineering, 26(5) (2023), 457-470.

[294] B. Xu, R. Chibber, D. Ruggiero, E. Kohner, J. Ritter, and A. Ferro. Impairment of vascular endothelial nitric oxide synthase activity by advanced glycation end products. FASEB J. 17 (2003), 1289-1291.

[295] Y. Xu, and R. Gilbert, Some inverse problems raised from a mathematical model of ductal carcinoma in situ 2009. Math. Comput. Model 49 (2009), 814-828.

[296] C. Yang, D. Tang, and C. Yuan, Multiphysics modeling of atherosclerotic plaque progression and rupture. Annals of Biomedical Engineering, 45(6) (2017), 1444-1460.

[297] N. Yang, and K. Vafai, Modeling of low-density lipoprotein (LDL) transport in the artery-effects of hypertension. Int. J. Heat Mass Transf. 49 (2006), 850–867.

[298] N. Yang, and K. Vafai, Low-density lipoprotein (LDL) transport in an artery—a simplified analytical solution. Int. J. Heat Mass Transf. 51 (2008), 497–505.

[299] A. Yin, D.J.A.R. Moes, J.G.C. van Hasselt, J.J. Swen, and H.-J. Guchelaar, A Review of Mathematical Models for Tumor Dynamics and Treatment Resistance Evolution of Solid Tumors, CPT Pharmacometrics Syst. Pharmacol. 8 (2019), 720-737.

[300] K. Yosida. Functional analysis. Classics in Mathematics. Springer-Verlag, Berlin, 1995

[301] Y. Yuan, and L.J.S. Allen, Stochastic Models for Virus and Immune System Dynamics, Math Biosci. 234(2) (2011), 84-94.

[302] X. Zhang, B. Hu, and Z. Zhang, Bifurcation for a free-boundary problem modeling small plaques with reverse cholesterol transport, J. Math. Anal. Appl. 517(1) (2023), Paper No. 126604, 45.

[303] Y. Zhang, T.A. Holt, and N. Khovanova, A data driven nonlinear stochastic model for blood glucose dynamics, Computer method and programs in biomedicine, 125 (2016), 18-25.

[304] X. Zhao, and B. Hu, Bifurcation for a free boundary problem modeling a small arterial plaque, Journal of Differential Equations, 288 (2021), 250-287.

[305] X. Zhao, and B. Hu, On the first bifurcation point for a free boundary problem modeling small arterial plaque, Mathematical Methods in Applied Sciences, 45 (2022), 4974-4988.

[306] J. Zheng, and S. Cui, Analysis of a tumor-model free boundary problem with a nonlinear boundary condition, J. Math. Anal. Appl. 478(2) (2019), 806-824.

[307] J. Zheng, and S. Cui, Analysis of a tumor model free boundary problem with action of an inhibitor and nonlinear boundary conditions, J. Math. Anal. Appl. 496(1) (2021), Paper No. 124793, pp. 35.

[308] J. Zheng, R. Li, and Y. Zhuang, Analysis of the growth of a radial tumor with triple-layered structure Discrete Contin. Dyn. Syst. 44(7) (2024), 1958-1981.

[309] Y. Zhuang, Analysis of a high-dimensional free boundary problem on tumor growth with time-dependent nutrient supply and inhibitor action, J. Differential Equations 416 (2025), 1222-1259.

[310] Y. Zhuang, and S. Cui, Analysis of a free boundary problem modeling the growth of multicell spheroids with angiogenesis J. Differential Equations 265(2) (2018), 620-644.

[311] F. Zhou, and S. Cui, Bifurcation for a free boundary problem modeling the growth of multi-layer tumors. Nonlinear Anal. Theory Methods Appl 68 (2008), 2128-2145.

[312] F. Zhou, J. Escher, and S. Cui, Well-posedness and stability of a free boundary problem modeling the growth of multi-layer tumors. J. Diff. Eqns 244 (2008), 2909-2933.

[313] F. Zhou, and J. Wu, Stability and bifurcation analysis of a free boundary problem Modeling multi-layer tumours with Gibbs-Thomson relation, European J. Appl. Math. 26(4) (2015), 401-425.

Index

For Product Safety Concerns and Information please contact our EU representative GPSR@taylorandfrancis.com Taylor & Francis Verlag GmbH, Kaufingerstraße 24, 80331 München, Germany

Batch number: 10777146

Printed by Printforce, the Netherlands